Anti-Obesity Drug Discovery and Development

(Volume 4)

Edited by

Atta-ur-Rahman, *FRS*

Honorary Life Fellow, Kings College, University of Cambridge, Cambridge, UK

&

M. Iqbal Choudhary

H.E.J. Research Institute of Chemistry, International Center for Chemical and Biological Sciences, University of Karachi, Karachi, Pakistan

Anti-Obesity Drug Discovery and Development

Volume # 4

Editors: Atta-ur-Rahman and M. Iqbal Choudhary

ISSN (Online): 2210-2698

ISSN (Print): 2467-9615

ISBN (Online): 978-1-68108-558-6

ISBN (Print): 978-1-68108-559-3

General:

1. Any dispute or claim arising out of or in connection with this License Agreement or the Work (including non-contractual disputes or claims) will be governed by and construed in accordance with the laws of the U.A.E. as applied in the Emirate of Dubai. Each party agrees that the courts of the Emirate of Dubai shall have exclusive jurisdiction to settle any dispute or claim arising out of or in connection with this License Agreement or the Work (including non-contractual disputes or claims).

2. Your rights under this License Agreement will automatically terminate without notice and without the need for a court order if at any point you breach any terms of this License Agreement. In no event will any delay or failure by Bentham Science Publishers in enforcing your compliance with this License Agreement constitute a waiver of any of its rights.

3. You acknowledge that you have read this License Agreement, and agree to be bound by its terms and conditions. To the extent that any other terms and conditions presented on any website of Bentham Science Publishers conflict with, or are inconsistent with, the terms and conditions set out in this License Agreement, you acknowledge that the terms and conditions set out in this License Agreement shall prevail.

Bentham Science Publishers Ltd.
Executive Suite Y - 2
PO Box 7917, Saif Zone
Sharjah, U.A.E.
Email: subscriptions@benthamscience.org

BENTHAM SCIENCE

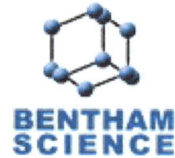

CONTENTS

PREFACE

Obesity disorders are on the rise globally, and have reached to epidemic proportions in certain regions of the world. Obesity is regarded as the mother of many illnesses, as it increase the chances of onset of conditions, such as cardiovascular diseases, diabetes, certain cancers, chronic kidney diseases, gallbladder stones, osteoarthritis, gout, respiratory problems, as well as psychological disorders and social isolation. Therefore, treatment of obesity by life style modifications, chemotherapy, and surgery has *multiple* benefits by causing reduction of many diseases. Unfortunately, the aetiology of obesity is extremely complex, and it is equally difficult to treat. It is not just the consumption of extra calories or lack of physical activities that causes obesity, there are many other complex underlying causes.

The treatment of obesity often requires a personalized approach. Current therapies for obesity and weight reduction are associated with severe after effects, creating the need for extensive research in obesity prevention and treatment. Drugs which are safe and effective are urgently required not only to treat obesity, but also to prevent and treat associated disorders. Extensive work in this field has also created a *niche* for authoritative reviews on the topic. The current book series is an attempt to fulfil this need.

The first three volumes of the ebook series *"Anti-Obesity Drug Discovery and Development"* have been very well received as very useful additions to the global literature in this dynamic area of research. Volume 4 is also a humble effort to continue this scholarly tradition. The 4th volume of this widely recognized book series comprises six invited reviews on various aspects of anti-obesity drug discovery and treatment of obesity related diseases, and they have been contributed by leading experts in this field. Each of these reviews is focused on drug discovery and development against obesity and related disorders, including new knowledge of molecular and cellular basis of obesity diseases, rationale for multi-target approach, outcomes of pre-clinical and clinical studies on new anti-obesity drugs and drug delivery systems, and potential of natural products in obesity treatment. Each chapter addresses a different aspect of the topic, and comprehensively reviews the state of the art, both in terms of understanding of the disease, as well as the therapeutic interventions developed so far.

The first review contributed by Wan and Kwan starts with a commentary on the relationship between diet and obesity, and the onset of various cancers. A comprehensive write-up on the role of dietary modulations in the prevention and treatment of cancer is presented. Diets rich in omega-3 polyunsaturated fatty acids, fiber, anti-oxidants, including polyphenols are known to reduce the chances of obesity and cancer. Some of them are anti-angiogenic which prevent the progression of cancer, especially solid tumors. However, it is often difficult to generalize the dietary recommendations, as individuals may have different life styles, gut microbiota, metabolic rates, as well as genetic make-up. Based on this, the authors have also introduced the interesting concept of "personalized nutrition", *as one size doesn't fit all*. In order to design personalized nutrition, system biology approach, and "omic" techniques can be employed.

Polycystic ovary syndrome (POCS) is among the most common endocrine disorders in women of reproductive age, leading to a whole range of problems, including infertility, metabolic and psychological problems. POCS is highly prevalent in obese females (40% - 60%), and thus obesity is regarded as one of the risk factors for POCS. Weight loss through life style changes is the first-line treatment in overweight PCOS women. Insulin-sensitizing drugs such as metformin, glucagon-like peptide-1, and antiobesity drugs such as Orlistat are used. Turkcuoglu and Melekoglu present a comprehensive review on the role of anti-obesity medications in the prevention of a common health disorder polycystic ovary syndrome (POCS).

Rolo *et al* . review the role of mitochondrial dysfunction in obesity. Mitochondria play a crucial role in energy metabolism. Extreme events during obesity disorders, such as chronic inflammation, oxidative stress, increased nutrient supply, etc. lead to mitochondrial dysfunctions. The authors discuss how restoration of mitochondrial health can contribute to the prevention and treatment of obesity. They highlight emerging interventions which can help in boosting mitochondrial activity and repair mitochondrial damage.

Orlistat is one of the most widely used drugs for the treatment of obesity. It functions by preventing the absorption of fats from the human diet through lipase inhibition, and thus reduces caloric intake. However Orlistat is notorious for its gastrointestinal side effects, including steatorrhea or oily, loose stools. Sunil K. Jain has reviewed recently developed new formulations of Orlistat which can reduce the associated side effects of this useful drug. These include calcium silicate based floating microspheres, and floating granules. Merits and demerits as well as safety profiles of these drug delivery systems have been comprehensively reviewed.

The chapter contributed by Lakshmi and Thiyagarajan is primarily focused on a multi-targeted approach towards the treatment of obesity disorder. Various mechanisms are involved in the on-set and progression of obesity. Based on this approach, multi-target drugs are needed for the successful treatment of obesity. Examples of such agents include glucagon-like peptides-1 mimetics and insulin secretagogues reported for anti-obesity activity. Natural products, mostly obtained from medicinal plants, can exhibit multi-targeted action, due to their diverse and complex structures. Some of these natural products, such as polyphenols, alkaloids, sterols, glycosides, terpenes, saponins, etc can work through diverse mechanisms, such as appetite suppression, metabolic enzyme inhibitions, increased insulin secretion, etc, all relevant to obesity control.

Augustine *et al* . have focussed on plant-based anti-obesity drugs in the next chapter. The authors have presented a comprehensive review on anti-obesity properties of several plant species, along with the known mechanisms of action. The review provides a strong rationale of the need of further research on the use of medicinal plants, particularly those used in traditional systems of medicine, as safe and effective anti-obesity agents.

We would like to express our sincere thanks to all the contributors for their excellent scholarly works. We also appreciate efforts of the efficient team of Bentham Science Publishers for the timely publication of the 4th volume of the book series. The organizational and communication skills of Ms. Faryal Sami (Manager Publications), Mr. Shehzad Naqvi (Editorial Manager Publications) and the excellent management of Mr. Mahmood Alam (Director Publications) are also gratefully acknowledged. We sincerely hope that the volume will provide readers with a better understanding of the subject, and motivate them to conduct good quality research on obesity.

M. Iqbal Choudhary
H.E.J. Research Institute of Chemistry
International Center for Chemical and
Biological Sciences
University of Karachi
Pakistan

Atta-ur-Rahman, *FRS*
Honorary Life Fellow
Kings College
University of Cambridge
UK

List of Contributors

Anabela Pinto Rolo CNC – Center for Neuroscience and Cell Biology, University of Coimbra, Portugal
Department of Life Sciences, University of Coimbra, Portugal

Anu Augustine Department of Biotechnology and Microbiology, Kannur University, Thalassery Campus, India

Arun Subash Koorapally Department of Biotechnology and Microbiology, Kannur University, Thalassery Campus, India

Baddireddi Subhadra Lakshmi Centre for Food Technology, Anna University, Chennai, India
Department of Biotechnology, Anna University, Chennai, India

Carlos Marques Palmeira CNC – Center for Neuroscience and Cell Biology, University of Coimbra, Portugal
Department of Life Sciences, University of Coimbra, Portugal

Gopal Thiyagarajan Department of Biotechnology, Anna University, Chennai, India

Hiu Yee Kwan School of Chinese Medicine, Hong Kong Baptist University, Hong Kong, China

Ilgın Turkcuoglu Department of Obstetrics and Gynecology, Division of Reproductive Endocrinology and Infertility 44280, Faculty of Medicine, University of Inonu, Malatya, Turkey

Jennifer Man Fan Wan Food and Nutrition Division, School of Biological Sciences, The University of Hong Kong, Hong Kong, China

João Alves Amorim CNC – Center for Neuroscience and Cell Biology, University of Coimbra, Portugal

João Soeiro Teodoro CNC – Center for Neuroscience and Cell Biology, University of Coimbra, Portugal
Department of Life Sciences, University of Coimbra, Portugal

Megha Valsaraj Department of Biotechnology and Microbiology, Kannur University, Thalassery Campus, India

Navaneetha Saseendran Department of Biotechnology and Microbiology, Kannur University, Thalassery Campus, India

Rauf Melekoglu Faculty of Medicine, Department of Obstetrics and Gynecology, Division of Perinatology, University of Inonu, Malatya, Turkey

Sunil K. Jain Guru Ghasidas Vishwavidyalaya, Institute of Pharmaceutical Sciences, Bilaspur, Chhattisgarh, India

CHAPTER 1

Dietary Modulation, Obesity and Cancer Prevention

Jennifer Man Fan Wan[1,*] and **Hiu Yee Kwan**[2]

[1] Food and Nutrition Division, School of Biological Sciences, The University of Hong Kong, Hong Kong, China

[2]School of Chinese Medicine, Hong Kong Baptist University, Hong Kong, China

Abstract: Cancer is the leading cause of morbidity and mortality worldwide, and the number of new cases is expected to rise. Among all the risk factors for cancers, lifestyle, eating habit and obesity are considered the most significant determining factors. In this chapter, we review evidence indicating that diet and obesity play significant roles in both the initiation and promotion of the cancer development. Furthermore, we also critically summarize how cancers can be prevented or its growth be inhibited by dietary modulation and reducing obesity. The evidence reviewed here overwhelmingly suggests that nutritional recommendations for cancer prevention should focus on improving host immunity. Specifically, this means consuming diets high in omega-3 polyunsaturated fatty acids (PUFAs) in a low omega-6 to omega-3 ratio, and rich in fiber and anti-angiogenic compounds such as omega-3 PUFAs, antioxidants and polyphenols. Given the causal link between obesity and cancer, reduced obesity, for instance, by dietary modulation may help to reduce cancer risk. Nevertheless, the conventional studies of the anti-cancer and/ or anti-obesity effects of dietary components or compounds may be complicated by the influences from background diet, life style, gut microbiome, age, environmental factors, genetic factors, drug therapy, and an individual's physical and pathological conditions. Therefore, in order to have the most effective dietary modulation for an individual for cancer prevention and treatment, "personalized nutrition" may be an alternative approach. Facing the challenge of how to optimize the individual's nutrition, we believe "omic" technologies and system biology will have great potential for designing "personalized nutrition" that can prevent the onset and slow down, if not reverse, the progression of the cancer.

Keywords: Cancer, Carcinogen, Dietary component, Epidemiology, Genomics, Lipidomics, Metabolomics, Obesity, Oncogenic signaling pathway, Proteomics.

* **Corresponding author Jennifer Man Fan Wan:** Food and Nutrition Division, School of Biological Sciences, The University of Hong Kong, Hong Kong, China; Tel: 852-22990838; E-mail: jmfwan@hku.hk;
Hiu Yee Kwan: School of Chinese Medicine, Hong Kong Baptist University, Hong Kong, China; Tel: 852-34112016; E-mail: hykwan@hkbu.edu.hk

Atta-ur-Rahman & M. Iqbal Choudhary (Eds.)
All rights reserved-© 2018 Bentham Science Publishers

INTRODUCTION

Cancer is the leading cause of death around the world. Approximately, 14 million new cases and 8.2 million cancer-related deaths were reported in 2012; and the number of new cases is expected to rise by about 70% over the next two decades [1]. On 30th May 2017, the 70th World Health Assembly adopted a draft resolution on cancer prevention and control with 18 sponsors and more than 40 Member States and 11 non-governmental organizations speaking in support of the resolution.

The rates of cancer are significantly affected by environmental, biological, economic and social factors. The cancer promoting factors include industrial chemicals, cigarette smoking, air and water pollutants, irradiation, hormones and drugs, genetic factors and oncogenic viruses; while life-style and eating habits are considered the most significant risk factors. The 2007 report of the World Cancer Research Fund (WCRF)/American Institute of Cancer Research (AICR) entitled "Food, Nutrition, Physical Activity, and the Prevention of Cancer: A Global Perspective" stressed that, after smoking, unhealthy diets, physical inactivity and excessive body weight are the next most important preventable causes of cancer. Nutritional factors have been estimated to contribute to 20-60% of cancers worldwide and to approximately one-third of deaths from cancers in Western countries [2]. Obesity is another important factor for cancer cause. Evidences from systemic reviews, meta-analysis and large-scale prospective studies demonstrate that being overweight or obese increases the risk of cancers of the oesophagus (adenocarcinoma), colorectal, breast (postmenopausal), endometrium and kidney [3, 4].

Geographical differences in cancer incidence also exist. These may be associated with different dietary patterns in different regions. For instance, esophageal cancer incidence is relatively high in the Middle East, China and Southern Africa. Evidence suggests that this relatively high incidence correlates with the widespread habit of smoking, extensive consumption of alcohol and low intake of vitamins A and C and riboflavin in the populations [5 - 7]. Stomach cancer incidence is relatively high in Japan and Asia, and is probably related to the high intake of smoked, salted and pickled vegetables [5, 8]. Liver cancer is common in Africa and Southeast Asia where the people may have lipotrope deficiency and have high intake of protein, alcohol and mycotoxin [9]. Breast, prostate and colorectal cancer incidences are found high in Western countries, which are likely due to obesity, high intake of dietary fat and low intake of fiber [5, 10, 11]. The common cancers with known diet-related factors are listed in Table **1**.

Table 1. Diet-related factors associated with specific cancers.

Cancer	Diet-related factor
Breast	Alcohol, Obesity, Central fat
Colorectal	Dietary fat, Meat, Obesity, Alcohol
Esophageal	Alcohol, Pickled vegetable, Obesity
Endometrial	Obesity, Dietary fat
Pancreatic	Meat, Dietary fat, Obesity
Liver	Alcohol, Iron overloaded
Prostate	Dietary fat, Vitamin A supplements and low calcium, High fructose diet

Cancer is a largely preventable disease if healthy lifestyle is adopted, 30-50% of cancers could be prevented. In 2009, the WCRF global network published another report entitled "Policy and Action for Cancer Prevention" which stresses that a healthy lifestyle can help reduce cancer risks. The most important factors are to maintain a healthy body mass index (BMI), limit the consumption of energy-dense food, surgery drinks and red meat, avoid salty foods and processed meat and consume diets high in plant-based foods. Alcohol consumption should be modest and dietary supplements specifically to prevent cancers are not recommended.

HOW DIET RELATES TO CANCERS?

The relationship between diet and cancer is complex. Dietary factors can act at the initiation stage and /or the developmental stage of cancer. Dietary carcinogens can initiate DNA damage and gene mutation which may result in uncontrolled cellular division and abnormal differentiation. Dietary factors may influence the cancer development by affecting the oncogenic signaling pathways related to angiogenesis, cancer cell invasion and metastasis, cancer cell proliferation and the host immunity. Excess calories and fat intake lead to obesity can also promote cancer growth by favoring the inflammatory and oxidative stress environment of the host.

Dietary Factors that Promote the Cancer Initiation

Dietary factors can initiate the formation of cancer in four possible ways. These are *via* (i) ingestion of powerful, direct-acting carcinogens or their precursors; (ii) ingestion of carcinogens that are produced *via* food processing such as cooking; (iii) ingestion of carcinogens that are produced in stored food such as the contaminants; and (iv) formation of carcinogen in the body.

Ingestion of Powerful, Direct-Acting Carcinogens or their Precursors

Carcinogens may be present in natural foods. The crude cycad material is carcinogenic because it contains cycasin that shows distinct resemblance with dimethylnitrosamine. Cycasin can be converted to methylazoxymethanol (MAM) which will be metabolized to human carcinogen formaldehyde. A study showed that miR-17-5p and miR-18d are the formaldehyde-responsive miRNAs which modulate MAM-associated genes involved in tumor suppression, DNA repair, amyloid deposition, and neurotransmission [12]. Besides, the complex taxon embraced in the *Pteridium* genus, popularly known as bracken fern, is one of the few vascular plants known to induce cancers. Epidemiological studies in Japan and Brazil showed a close association between bracken consumption and cancers of the upper alimentary tract [13]. Another well-studied example of direct-acting carcinogen is safrole (4-allyl-1,2-methylenedioxybenzene), the major chemical constituent of the aromatic oil present in sassafras root bark. An electrophilic metabolite of safrole, safrole 2',3'-oxide (SFO), is shown to react with DNA bases to form detectable DNA adducts *in vitro*. In animal models, safrole is a hepatocarcinogen [14] that may convert SFO to N7-guanine DNA adduct [15]. On the contrary, other studies showed that safrole induced G0/G1 phase arrest, induced apoptosis in human leukemia cells [16, 17]; and had cytotoxicity in human prostate cancer cells [18]. Prior to the regulation set up by the Food and Drug Administration in 1960, safrole and safrole-containing sassafras extracts were used as flavoring agents in beverages such as root beer.

Ingestion of Carcinogens that are Produced *via* Food Processing

Cooking of muscle meats such as beef, pork, fish or poultry using high-temperature methods will form heterocyclic amines (HCAs) and polycyclic aromatic hydrocarbons (PAHs) [19]. HCAs are formed when amino acids, sugars and creatine react at high temperature. PAHs are formed when fat and juices from meat drip onto the fire and causes flames. The flames contain PAHs that will adhere to the meat surface. Besides, N-nitrosamines such as dimethylnitrosamine, methylnitrosourea from nitrates are used in meat as preservatives. The N-nitro compounds will bind with DNA bases to form DNA adducts. Repeatedly used deep frying oils will produce free radicals. The heat-induced reaction of amino groups of amino acids, peptides, and proteins with carbonyl groups of reducing sugars such as glucose may result in the concurrent formation of Maillard browning products [20], also known as advanced glycation end-products. For instance, acrylamide, a cancer-causing agent, is released by the thermal treatment of certain amino acids (asparagine, for example), particularly in combination with reducing sugars, and of early Maillard reaction products.

Ingestion of Carcinogens Produced in Stored Food

Carcinogen metabolites of mycotoxins such as ochratoxin and aflatoxins, two types of mycotoxins, are contaminant of a wide range of food commodities. Aflatoxin produces by *Aspergillus* species of fungi, such as *A. flavus* and *A. parasitic*, are found particularly in contaminated peanuts. Aflatoxins are lipid-soluble and cannot be destroyed under common cooking conditions. However, they become unstable when exposed to ultraviolet light. Aflatoxins B1/G1 are the most potent hepato-carcinogens; they bind to guanine residues of DNA to form DNA adducts [21]. Found in wide range of commodities including beverages such as beer and wine, orchratoxin comes in three secondary metabolites forms, A,B and C, produced by *Penicillium* and *Aspergillus* species. Ochtatoxin A has been labeled as a carcinogen and a nephrotoxin, and has been linked to tumors in the human urinary tract [22].

Formation of Carcinogens in the Body

N-nitro compounds (secondary amines or N-substituted amides) naturally occur in many foods such as fish, meat, beer and cheese as well as in preservatives, colorings and flavor enhancers. They are formed in small amounts in the gastrointestinal tract and bladder by a reaction between nitrites and various nitrosable compounds such as dimethylnitrosamine, N-nitrosodimethylamine, dimethylnitrosamine, dibutylnitrosamine. These compounds can bind to the guanine of DNA bases to form DNA adducts.

Carcinogens can be transported, activated or detoxified in our body. The metabolism of carcinogens is catalyzed by enzymes in the endoplasmic reticulum and other parts of the cell [23]. Genetic and environmental factors will affect the activities and the balance of these enzymes [23]. Colon and intestinal cancers are associated with the intake or excretion of cholesterol and bile acids, and the alternation of the microflora of the bowel [24]. Secondary bile acid metabolites formed in the presence of certain gut bacteria such as deoxycholic and lithocholic acids are carcinogenic. In addition, the redox balance system of our body can also control the formation, activation and deactivation of free radicals from both lipid oxidation and oxidative stress [25].

DIETARY FACTORS THAT PROMOTE THE CANCER DEVELOPMENT

Dietary factors can promote cancer growth and metastasis indirectly *via* affecting the host's immune defense system. Depending on the degree of their saturation and their omega-6/omega-3 ratio, dietary fatty acids can alter both structural and functional properties of the phospholipid-cellular membrane. For instance, they can affect membrane fluidity and eicosanoid metabolism (*via* phospholipids turnover). This will in turn affect cell membrane receptor activities and hence the signal transduction and transport pathways. The cancer promoting mechanisms of diets rich in saturated fatty acids (SFAs) and the omega-6 polyunsaturated fatty acids (PUFAs) as compared to omega-3 PUFAs such as docosahexaenoic acid (DHA) and eicosapentaenoic acid (EPA), for instance, are said to be involved in the pathways of signal transduction, hormonal control, oncogene activation, cancer suppressor gene deactivation, immune dysfunction, metastasis, angiogenesis, and disruption of cell cycle progression *via* the checkpoint cyclins [26 - 37].

In addition, fried foods and fatty acids can easily undergo lipid oxidation and produce free radicals that provoke our immune system, extend oxidative stress, and cause inflammation which indirectly favors cancer progression. The excessive intake of high calories in a diet high in fat, red meat and simple carbohydrate-enriched foods may lead to obesity which is a predisposing factor in the initiation and growth of a variety of cancers.

GENERAL MECHANISM OF HOW OBESITY CAN CAUSE AND PROMOTE CANCER

Based on World Health Organization's definition, non-Asian people with body mass index (BMI) $\geq$ 30 are classified as obese, while those with a BMI $\geq$ 25 are classified as overweight (Table **2**). In general, obesity is characterized as excess accumulation of adipose tissues, and is always associated with an increased production of metabolic hormones coupled with a chronic low-grade state of inflammation that links to various diseases such as diabetes as well as certain kinds of cancers.

Table 2. Body mass index (BMI) cutoff values for adults.

BMI (kg/m^2) classification		
	WHO	**Asian**
Underweight	<18.5	<18.5
Normal range	18.5-24.9	18.5-22.9
Overweight (Pre-obese)	≥25.0	23.0-24.9
Obese	≥30.3	≥25.0
Obese class I	30.0-34.9	25.0-29.9
Obese class II	35.0-39.9	≥30.0
Obese class III	≥40.0	

Adipose tissues consist of mature adipocytes, stromal-vascular cells such as fibroblast, smooth muscle cells, pericytes, endothelial cells and adipogenic progenitor cells. In normal physiological conditions, adipose tissues release both protein and non-protein factors (Table **3**) such as adipokines, inflammatory mediators and growth factors, which have their own important physiological functions. However, in obese subjects, the excess accumulated adipose tissues may be dysfunctional [38] which produce high levels of proinflammatory cytokines and hormones, along with altered adipokines profiles. The macrophages may also accumulate in the white adipose tissues and contribute to the production of inflammatory mediators in concert with the adipocytes [39]. Furthermore, hyperlipidemia in obesity leads to insulin resistance which also plays a role in cancer growth. Fatty acids released from white adipocytes may serve as an energy source for cancer cells [40 - 42]. All these pathogenic conditions will promote cancer initiation, progression, growth and recurrence by activating various oncogenic signaling pathways as illustrated in Fig. (**1**). Indeed, the National Cancer Institute in USA suggests that obesity has a profound influence on cancer risk and progression such as cancers of the breast, colon, endometrium, gallbladder, thyroid, adenocarcinoma of the oesophagus, kidney and pancreas. Researchers also estimate that overweight and obesity are found correlated with 17,000 cases of cancer each year in the UK [43].

Table 3. Protein and non-protein factors released by white adipose tissue that may cause cancer or promote cancer growth.

Factor released by white adipose tissue	Example
Adipokine	Leptin
	Adiponectin
	Resistin
	Visfatin
Cytokines and other immune-related proteins	Tumor necrosis factor-α (TNF-α)
	Interleukin-6 (IL-6)
	Prostaglandins
	Monocyte chemotactic protein-1 (MCP-1)
	Macrophage migration inhibitory factor
Growth factor	Fibroblast growth factor-1 (FGF-1)
	Vascular endothelial growth factor (VEGF)
	Insulin-like growth factor-1 (IGF-1)
	Angiotensin
	Transforming growth factor-β (TGF-β)

(Table 3) cont.....

Factor released by white adipose tissue	Example
Fatty acids	Saturated fatty acids such as palmitic acid; other Fatty acids with specific oncogenic Targets/functions yet to be identified

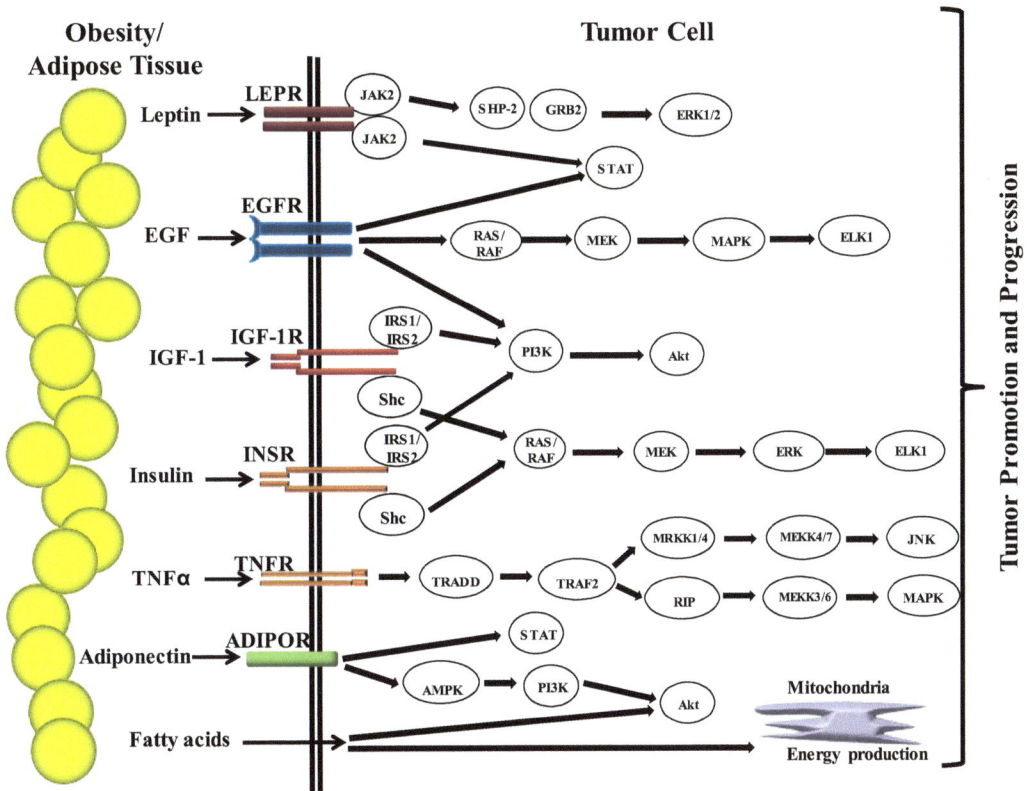

Fig. (1). Oncogenic signaling pathways involved in cancer initiation, progression and growth in obesity. ADIPOR, Adiponectin receptor; Akt, known as protein kinase B; AMPK, 5' AMP-activated protein kinase; ELK, ETS domain-containing protein; ERK, extracellular-signal-regulated kinases; EGF, epidermal growth factor; EGFR, Epidermal growth factor receptor; Grb2, Growth factor receptor-bound protein 2; IGF, insulin-like growth factor; IGF-1R, Insulin-like growth factor-1 receptor; INSR, Insulin receptor; IRS, Insulin receptor substrate; JAK, Janus kinase; MAPK, Mitogen-activated protein kinases; MEK, Mitogen-activated protein kinase; MEKK, Mitogen-activated protein/ERK kinase kinases; PI3K, Phosphoinositide 3-kinase; Shc, Src homology 2 domain containing transforming protein; SHP-2, SH2-containing a ubiquitously expressed tyrosine-specific protein phosphatase; STAT, Signal transducers and activators of transcription; TNF, Tumor necrosis factors; TNFR, Tumor necrosis factors receptor; TRADD, TNFRSF1A-associated *via* death domain; TRAF, TNF receptor-associated factors.

DIETARY COMPONENTS WITH CANCER PREVENTION POTENTIAL

Diets that prevent cancer initiation and growth include diets rich in omega-3 PUFAs such as fish oil, walnut, linseeds, extra-virgin olive oil, fax seed, fruits and vegetables, particularly alliums and cruciferous vegetables (Table **4**). The anticancer bioactive components include selenium, folic acid, vitamin B12, vitamin D, antioxidants such as carotenoids (alpha-carotene, beta-carotene, lycopene, lutein, crytoxanthin), and ascorbic acid [44]. The anticancer mechanisms of these active compounds include inhibiting tumor angiogenesis, maintaining a redox balance in the body, inducing cancer cell cycle arrest, reducing metastasis and enhancing immune function. For instance, lycopene from tomatoes, vitamins A,C and E from vegetables [45, 46], green tea catechins [47], polyphenols from mushrooms and grapes [48] have been shown to possess anti-angiogenesis potential.

Table 4. Epidemiological and experimental studies showing the modulatory effects of dietary components on cancers.

Dietary factor	Cancer	Modulatory effect
ω-3 PUFAs	Breast	• Have beneficial roles for both the prevention and treatment of breast cancer • Inhibit breast cancer cell growth • Induce G1 cell cycle arrest • Down-regulate Wnt/β-catenin signaling and HER2 signaling pathways
	Colon	• Have beneficial roles for both the prevention and treatment of colon cancer • Modulate cyclooxygenase-2 (COX-2) and β-catenin signaling pathways • Reduce VEGF expression by negative regulation of the COX-2/prostaglandin pathway
	Liver	• Have beneficial roles for both the prevention and treatment of liver cancer • Modulate COX2 activity, heat shock, N-myc and oxidative stress-related pathways • Activate JNK-related cell death pathway followed by mitochondrial injury and apoptosis. • Docosahexaenoic acid (DHA) affects cell cycle progression and delays S-phase duration *via* suppression of cell cycle regulatory proteins
Calcium	Colon	• Controversial findings or modestly reduces risk of colorectal cancer • Low intakes of calcium in younger women are associated with an increased risk of multiple and advanced colorectal adenoma.

(Table 4) cont.....

Dietary factor	Cancer	Modulatory effect
Vitamin D	Colon	• Vitamin D3 lowers colon cancer incidence • Reduces polyp recurrence leads to a better overall survival rate • Inhibits the ability of macrophages to activate Wnt signaling in a vitamin D receptor-dependent manner • Induces differentiation • Controls the detoxification metabolism and cell phenotype • Sensitizes cells to apoptosis • Inhibits the colon carcinoma cells proliferation
Folate	Colon	• Lowers risk of colorectal cancer • Maintains genomic stability by regulating DNA biosynthesis, repair and methylation.
	Breast, Prostate, Esophagus,	• Reduces cancer risks
Polyphenols	Colon	• Have antiangiogenic activity by downregulating the hypoxia-inducible factor-1 (HIF-1α)/mPGEs-1/VEGF axis • Decrease arachidonic acid release and arachidonic acid metabolite synthesis • Affect cyclin D1 expression by modulating STAT5B and ATF-2, • Inhibit β-catenin signaling pathway and TNF α-activated NFκB signaling pathways
Carotenoids	Lung	• Modestly reduce risk of lung cancers
	Colorectal	• Reduces cancer risk
Lycopene	Prostate	• Has antioxidant effects • Prevents DNA damage • Mediates cell cycle arrest • Induces apoptosis • Inhibits IGF-1 signaling pathway • Has controversial findings in clinical studies
Lignans	Coloretcal, Breast, Prostate, Oesophageal	• Reduce cancer risks

The anticancer properties of vegetables and fruits as well as most natural food components are attributed to their antioxidants. Antioxidants are capable of deactivating or preventing the formation of short-lived ions, active species which will bind to DNA causing mutation. Some antioxidants are enzymes in our body such as superoxide dismutases (SOD), catalase and glutathione peroxide, but their activities are dependent on the presence of other dietary nutrients such as zinc, iron and selenium. Other antioxidants can come from dietary sources such as vitamin C, vitamin E and vitamin A. In human, vitamin C is the major water-soluble antioxidant and vitamin E is the major lipid-soluble membrane-localized antioxidant. Other plant food constituents such as carotenoids and flavonoids also have antioxidant activities [49], they are rich in certain foods, such as soybeans, green tea, coffee, wine, citrus and fruits and in some herbs, such as rosemary, sage. These antioxidants can reduce the metabolically activated intermediates such as the oxidative free radicals and excited molecular oxygen which are capable of forming DNA adducts and destroy proteins and sugar molecules. Other food components may induce cell cycle arrest such as genisten [50], and a Chinese medicine mushroom cordyceps [51] which are G2/M phase inhibitors. The polysaccharopeptides derived from the Chinese mushroom *Coriolus versicolor* are S phase-specific inhibitors [52]. Omega-3 PUFAs are S-phase suppressors for breast [53] and colon cancer [33]. We are the very first few scientists to demonstrate that omega-3 fatty acid-enriched fish oil protected mammary tumor growth by inhibiting DNA synthesis in the S-phase [54]. Besides, omega-3 PUFAs also possess anti-inflammatory properties. Reports show that omega-3 PUFAs suppress nuclear factor-κB, modulate cyclooxygenase activity and upregulated anti-inflammatory lipid mediators such as protectins, maresins, and resolvins [55]. Omega-3 PUFAs have also been shown to lower estrogen and prolactin production, and to suppress matrix metalloproteinase-9 induction and tumor angiogenesis [27, 55 - 58].

It has been long recognized that the ratio of omega-6 to omega-3 PUFAs or (ω6/ω3) is a key factor in the promotion or suppression of cancer pathogenesis. Very high ω6/ω3 ratio promotes cancer growth, while increasing levels of omega-3 PUFA in a low ω6/ω3 ratio exerts suppressive effects on cancers. For instance, the lower ω6/ω3 ratio in women with breast cancer was associated with decreased risk; and diets high in omega-6 PUFA have a clear stimulating influence [59, 60]. Different ratios of ω6/ω3 PUFAs affect the estrogen receptor expression of human breast cancer cells [61].

Olive oil, the integral ingredient of the Mediterranean diet, has a potential chemopreventive effect in reducing incidence and mortality rates of breast, colon, prostate and liver cancers [62 - 65]. Olive oil is high in oleic acid, squalene, terpenoids, polyphenols, hydroxytyrosol, tyrosol, phenyl propionic acids and antioxidants. Squalene inhibits the catalytic activity of beta-hydroxy-be-a-methyglytaryl-CoA reductase and reduces farnesyl for prenylation of the ras oncogene [66]. Olive oil also suppresses Her-2/neu overexpression, which interacts synergistically with anti-Her-2/neu immunotherapy by promoting apoptotic cell death of breast cancer cells with Her-2/neu oncogene amplification [67].

In addition, dietary fiber and probiotics can reduce the amount and duration of carcinogens in contact with the epithelial cells of the intestinal lining and thereby reduce colon cancer risk. The short chain fatty acids (such as butyrate and propionate) derived from dietary fiber can inhibit activity of the gut bacterial enzyme, 7-dehydroxylase, that produces the carcinogenic secondary bile acids lithocholic acid and deoxycholic acids from the primarily bile acids and it decreases opportunity for their contact with the proliferative crypt cells of the colon. Foods such as, pectin, bran, oatmeal, barely and lignin are cancer preventive as they can bind with bile and decrease its absorption. A large European study involving 10 countries found a 25% lower risk of colon cancer associated with higher fiber intake compared to low intake [68].

DIETARY COMPONENTS THAT AFFECT BODY WEIGHT

Obesity mainly arises from prolonged imbalance between energy intake and expenditure. Macronutrients such as lipids, carbohydrate and protein are energy-providing chemical substances. The excess consumed high calories will be stored as triglyceride in the adipose tissues. Dietary fatty acids can regulate gene expressions in a hormone-independent manner, which is mediated either directly by specific bindings to nuclear receptors that change the trans-activating activity of these transcription factors, or indirectly by changing the expression levels of the regulatory transcriptional factors. For instance, in colorectal cancer cells, butyrate changes the expressions of genes involved in the regulation of cell proliferation and apoptosis [69, 70]. PUFAs decrease the activities of hepatic lipogenic enzymes [71, 72].

Over-consumption of carbohydrate also leads to obesity. Interestingly, overfeeding carbohydrate accounts for around 40% of the increase of fat mass coming from *de novo* fatty acid synthesis [73]. In addition, over-consumption of carbohydrate induces hypertriacyglycerolaemia (HPTG) [74, 75] that is characterized by elevated levels of plasma triglyceride. Studies suggest that the sugar components of the diet may be responsible for the HPTG rather than the total carbohydrate [75]. Indeed, studies of the dose-dependent effect of substituting sucrose or fructose for starch have indicated that the greater the amount of sugars in the diet, the greater the increase in plasma triglyceride level [76]. Increase in sugar-sweetened soft drink consumption is strongly associated with weight gain; that is presumably because sugar-sweetened beverages do not induce satiety to the same extent as solid forms of carbohydrate. Interestingly, although dietary fiber is associated with less weight gain in some observational studies [77], a cross-sectional study showed that higher carbohydrate and fibre intake was positively associated with obesity in women [78]. Recently, the Committee on Nutrition of the European Society for Paediatric Gastroenterology, Hepatology and Nutrition has summarized the role of the nutrition-related factors on obesity prevention [79] and the study suggests that no single nutrient is unequivocally associated with the development of obesity.

Many dietary factors are reported to have regulatory roles on body weight (Table 5). Among these, the anti-obesity properties of dietary polyphenols have received great attention. Polyphenols are a class of naturally-occurring phytochemicals, of which some such as catechins, anthocynines, resveratrol and curcumin modulate pathways involved in energy metabolism and adiposity [80]. For instance, green tea contains five major catechins, namely catechin, epicatechin, gallate, epigallocatechin and epigallocatechin gallate. These catechins exhibit anti-obesity effects by suppressing adipocyte differentiation and proliferation *via* reducing levels of phosphorylated extracellular signal-regulated kinases-1/2, cyclin-dependent kinase-2 and cyclin D1 proteins [81] and also by inducing apoptosis in mature adipocytes [82]. Furthermore, catechines inhibit fat absorption from the gut, and suppress catecholo-methyl transferase which inhibits fatty acid oxidation in brown adipose tissue [83]. Resveratrol is another well-studied polyphenol, present in red grapes, red wine and peanuts; while curcumin is a bioactive polyphenol present in the spice turmeric. Mounting evidence suggests that both resveratrol and curcumin possess potent anti-obesity properties.

Table 5. Epidemiological and experimental studies showing the regulatory roles of dietary components on body weight.

Dietary factor	Impacts on body weight	Mechanism
Fiber	Reduces body weight	● Has low energy value ● Fermentation of soluble fiber produces glucagon-like peptide and peptide YY, which induces satiety and reduces food intake
Trans fat	Increases body weight	● Increases intra-abdominal deposition of fat in the absence of caloric excess
SFAs	Increase body weight	● Obesigenic
ω-3-PUFAs	Controversial finding	● Do not have an important role in regulation of body weight ● Only the α-linolenic acid is inversely associated with body fat measures.
Polyphenols	Reduce body weight	● Increase sympathetic activity and stimulate thermogenesis ● Modulate fat metabolism gene expressions ● Suppress adipogenesis by targeting insulin receptor ● Inhibit intestinal absorption of lipids ● Induce lipolytic activity ● Reduce glucose uptake in adipocytes
Polyphenol - Resveratrol	Reduces body weight	● Increases mitochondrial activity in brown adipose tissue and muscle by activating peroxisome proliferator-activated receptor-γ coactivator1-α (PGC1-α) ● Inhibits pre-adipocyte differentiation and proliferation in a Sirt1-dependent manner, ● Increases expression of uncoupling protein-1 in white adipocytes

(Table 5) cont.....

Dietary factor	Impacts on body weight	Mechanism
Polyphenol - Curcumin	Reduces body weight	• Anti-angiogenesis by downregulating VEGF, bFGF, epidermal growth factor (EGF) and HIF-1α • Reduces liver cholesterol • Reduces weight gain, blood triglyceride and free fatty acid levels • Downregulates the conversion of acetyl-CoA to malonyl-CoA that leads to upregulation of carnitine palmitoyltransferase-1 • Inhibits glycerol-3-phosphate acyl transferase-1 activity which esterifies fatty acids to glycerol to form triglycerides for storage • Reduces expressions of peroxisome proliferator-activated receptor-γ (PPARγ) and CCAAT/enhancer-binding protein-α (C/EBP-α) which are the key transcription factors in adipogenesis and lipogenesis
Caffeine	Reduces body weight	• Increases sympathetic nervous system activity and hence increase oxygen consumption and fat oxidation

PROSPECTIVE FOR THE ANTI-CANCER STUDY

Cancer is a complex disease that involves of gene-environment interactions. In the studies of the anti-cancer and/ or anti-obesity effects of dietary components or compounds, the results may be complicated by influences from background diet, life style, gut microbiome, age, environmental factors, genetic factors, drug therapy, and an individual's physical and pathological conditions. Improvement in nutritional intervention for cancer treatment and prevention requires a new paradigm that focuses on revising systemic dysfunction and tailoring treatment to specific stages in the process. It requires the move from a reductionist framework of seeking for multidisciplinary system biology approach aimed to reversing multiple levels of dysfunction. Indeed, the effectiveness of drug treatment encounters the same problems; clinical intervention can be strongly influenced by the individual's biochemical state at the time of treatment [84]. Recently, a new field, pharmacometabonomics has been emerged, which uses the pre-dose metabolite profiling in the bio-fluids or fecal extracts to predict the responses of an individual to a chemical intervention and to identify surrogate markers for subsequent drug administration [85 - 88]. It seems reasonable to postulate that a similar concept can be applied to studying the effects of (i) dietary components/compounds consumption or (ii) body weight control in the cancer progression. The metabolite profiling of an individual before dietary intervention can be used as a reference to predict the individual's responses to the dietary intervention, and biomarkers can be identified to evaluate the efficacy of the dietary treatment. In addition, high-dimensional data analysis and mathematical modeling can provide further understanding of the mechanisms and pathways modeling can provide further understanding of the mechanisms and pathways involved in these dietary effects. Indeed, metabolomics is particularly well-suited for personalized medicine since it reflects the metabolic phenotype downstream of genetics together with environmental effects at a given time in the individual. Thanks to advanced technology, choices of methodologies have evolved for the study of metabolomes with tissue, urine or serum samples, for instance, (i) magic angle spinning-nuclear magnetic resonance (MAS-NMR); (ii) proton nuclear magnetic resonance (^{1}H-NMR); (iii) gas chromatography-mass spectrometry (GC-MS); (iv) ultra-performance liquid chromatography-quadrupole time-of-flight mass spectrometry (UPLC-QTOF-MS); (v) capillary electrophoresis-MS (CE-MS); (vi) fourier transform ion-cyclotron-MS (FTICR-MS); (vii) ion mobility-mass spectrometry (IMMS) and (viii) direct infusion traveling wave ion mobility mass spectrometry. This new "omic" generation provides an exciting new dimension to the study of cancer prevention/ treatment with focus on identifying and developing new biomarkers, and it provides novel and contemporary paradigm for dietary intervention.

It is newly accepted that the nutrients can alter molecular processes such as DNA structure, gene expression, and metabolism, and those in turn may alter disease initiation, development or progression. Scientists are working hard to uncover gene-nutrient association for all types of cancers. Once these associations are better understood with the aim of the "omic technology and system biology", nutrition recommendation can be then "personalized" for cancer prevention and management (Fig. **2**).

SUMMARY

Dietary factors and obesity are having significant effects on the cancer risk, with different dietary elements either increase or reduce the risk of cancer. Specific foods are linked to specific cancers. To reduce cancer risk, the most important factors are to maintain a healthy BMI; limit the consumption of energy-dense food, sugary drinks and red meat; avoid salty foods and processed meat, and consume diets high in plant-based foods or rich in omega-3 PUFAs, dietary fiber, antioxidants and polyphenols which can enhance the host immunity.

More sophisticated research methodologies are certainly needed to understand the cause and appropriate control of cancer advancement. The biggest challenge for the scientists, nutritionists and physicians at present and future is how to optimize an individual's nutrition in the form of "personalized nutrition" through dietary interventions that can prevent the onset and modulate the progression of the cancer disease.

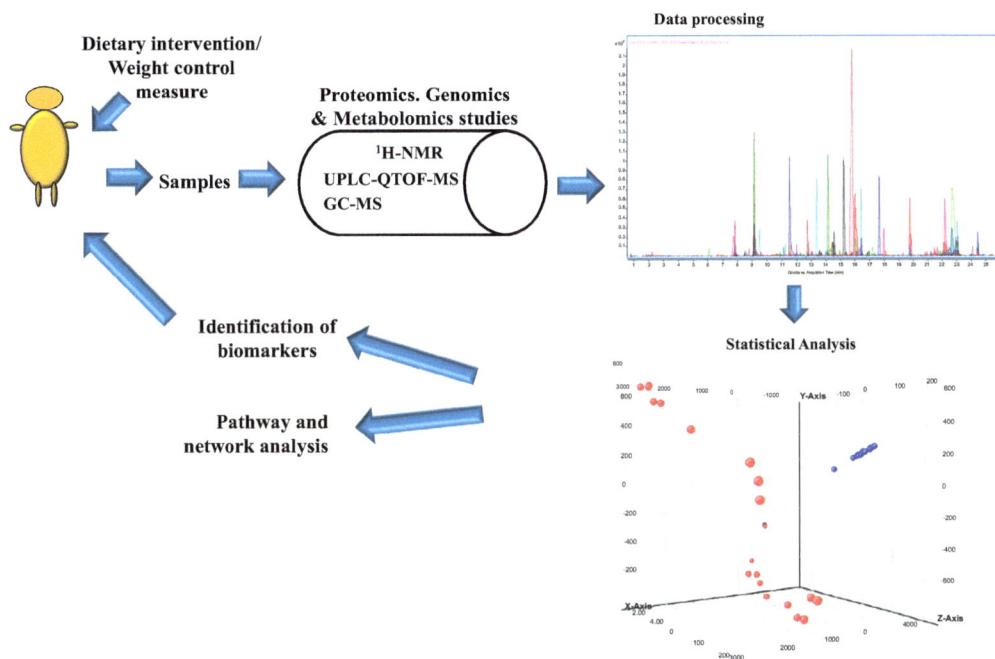

Fig. (2). The application of omic technology and system biology in the anti-cancer study. GC-MS, Gas chromatography-mass spectrometry; NMR, Nuclear magnetic resonance; UPLC-QTOF-MS, ultra-performance liquid chromatography-quadrupole time-of-flight mass spectrometry.

ABBREVIATIONS

ADIPOR	Adiponectin receptor
Akt	known as protein kinase B
AMPK 5'	AMP-activated protein kinase
BMI	Body mass index
C/EBP-α	CCAAT/enhancer-binding protein-α
CE-MS	Capillary electrophoresis-MS
COX-2	Cyclooxygenase-2
DHA	Docosahexaenoic acid
EGF	Epidermal growth factor
EGFR	Epidermal growth factor receptor
ELK	ETS domain-containing protein
ERK	Extracellular-signal-regulated kinases
FGF-1	Fibroblast growth factor-1
FTICR-MS	Fourier transform ion-cyclotron-MS
GC-MS	Gas chromatography-mass spectrometry

Grb2	Growth factor receptor-bound protein 2
HCAs	Heterocyclic amines
HIF-1α	Hypoxia-inducible factor-1α
HPTG	Hypertriacyglycerolaemia
IFN-γ	Interferon-γ
IGF	Insulin-like growth factor
IGF-1	Insulin-like growth factor-1
IGF-1R	Insulin-like growth factor-1 receptor
IL-6	Interleukin-6
IMMS	Ion mobility-mass spectrometry
INSR	Insulin receptor
IRS	Insulin receptor substrate
JAK	Janus kinase
MAM	Methylazoxymethanol
MAPK	Mitogen-activated protein kinases
MAS-NMR	Magic angle spinning-nuclear magnetic resonance
MCP-1	Monocyte chemotactic protein-1
MEK	Mitogen-activated protein kinase
MEKK	Mitogen-activated protein/ERK kinase kinases
NMR	Nuclear magnetic resonance
PAHs	Polycyclic aromatic hydrocarbons
PGC1-α	Peroxisome proliferator-activated receptor-γ coactivator1-α
PI3K	Phosphoinositide 3-kinase
PPARγ	Peroxisome proliferator-activated receptor-γ
PUFAs	Polyunsaturated fatty acids
ROS	Reactive oxygen species
SFO	Safrole 2'3'-oxide
Shc	Src homology 2 domain containing transforming protein
SHP-2	SH2-containing a ubiquitously expressed tyrosine-specific protein phosphatase
STAT	Signal transducers and activators of transcription
TGF-β	Transforming growth factor-β
TNF	Tumor necrosis factors
TNFR	Tumor necrosis factors receptor
TNF-α	Tumor necrosis factor-α
TRADD	TNFRSF1A-associated *via* death domain

TRAF	TNF receptor-associated factors
UPLC-QTOF-MS	Ultra-performance liquid chromatography-quadrupole time-of-flight mass spectrometry
VEGF	Vascular endothelial growth factor

CONSENT FOR PUBLICATION

Not applicable.

CONFLICT OF INTEREST

The author (editor) declares no conflict of interest, financial or otherwise.

ACKNOWLEDGEMENTS

We gratefully acknowledge Martha Annette Dahlen for her invaluable help with the final editing. This work was the Early Career Scheme (#22103017), partially supported by Health and Medical Research Fund (HMRF/14-15/03), the Hong Kong Baptist University grants FRG2/16-17/076 and FRG2/16-17/010.

REFERENCES

[1]   Report WC. World Health Organization Edited by Bernard Stewart and Christopher P Wild 2014.

[2]   McCullough ML, Giovannucci EL. Diet and cancer prevention. Oncogene 2004; 23(38): 6349-64.
       [http://dx.doi.org/10.1038/sj.onc.1207716] [PMID: 15322510]

[3]   Pischon T, Nöthlings U, Boeing H. Obesity and cancer. Proc Nutr Soc 2008; 67(2): 128-45.
       [http://dx.doi.org/10.1017/S0029665108006976] [PMID: 18412987]

[4]   Wolin KY, Carson K, Colditz GA. Obesity and cancer. Oncologist 2010; 15(6): 556-65.
       [http://dx.doi.org/10.1634/theoncologist.2009-0285] [PMID: 20507889]

[5]   Key TJ, Schatzkin A, Willett WC, Allen NE, Spencer EA, Travis RC. Diet, nutrition and the prevention of cancer. Public Health Nutr 2004; 7(1A): 187-200.
       [http://dx.doi.org/10.1079/PHN2003588] [PMID: 14972060]

[6]   Holmes RS, Vaughan TL. Epidemiology and pathogenesis of esophageal cancer. Semin Radiat Oncol 2007; 17(1): 2-9.
       [http://dx.doi.org/10.1016/j.semradonc.2006.09.003] [PMID: 17185192]

[7]   Lee CH, Lee JM, Wu DC, *et al.* Independent and combined effects of alcohol intake, tobacco smoking and betel quid chewing on the risk of esophageal cancer in Taiwan. Int J Cancer 2005; 113(3): 475-82.
       [http://dx.doi.org/10.1002/ijc.20619] [PMID: 15455377]

[8]   Wang XQ, Terry PD, Yan H. Review of salt consumption and stomach cancer risk: epidemiological and biological evidence. World J Gastroenterol 2009; 15(18): 2204-13.
       [http://dx.doi.org/10.3748/wjg.15.2204] [PMID: 19437559]

[9]   Leong TY, Leong AS. Epidemiology and carcinogenesis of hepatocellular carcinoma. HPB 2005; 7(1): 5-15.
       [http://dx.doi.org/10.1080/13651820410024021] [PMID: 18333156]

[10]   Rasool S, Kadla SA, Rasool V, Ganai BA. A comparative overview of general risk factors associated with the incidence of colorectal cancer. Tumour Biol 2013; 34(5): 2469-76.

[http://dx.doi.org/10.1007/s13277-013-0876-y] [PMID: 23832537]

[11]   Usmani K. The human environment today and its impact on society. J Environ Pathol Toxicol Oncol 1992; 11(5-6): 283-5.
[PMID: 1464808]

[12]   Spencer P, Fry RC, Kisby GE. Unraveling 50-Year-Old Clues Linking Neurodegeneration and Cancer to Cycad Toxins: Are microRNAs Common Mediators? Front Genet 2012; 3: 192.
[http://dx.doi.org/10.3389/fgene.2012.00192] [PMID: 23060898]

[13]   Alonso-Amelot ME, Avendaño M. Human carcinogenesis and bracken fern: a review of the evidence. Curr Med Chem 2002; 9(6): 675-86.
[http://dx.doi.org/10.2174/0929867023370743] [PMID: 11945131]

[14]   Daimon H, Sawada S, Asakura S, Sagami F. *In vivo* genotoxicity and DNA adduct levels in the liver of rats treated with safrole. Carcinogenesis 1998; 19(1): 141-6.
[http://dx.doi.org/10.1093/carcin/19.1.141] [PMID: 9472705]

[15]   Shen LC, Chiang SY, Lin MH, Chung WS, Wu KY. *In vivo* formation of N7-guanine DNA adduct by safrole 2′,3′-oxide in mice. Toxicol Lett 2012; 213(3): 309-15.
[http://dx.doi.org/10.1016/j.toxlet.2012.07.006] [PMID: 22820429]

[16]   Yu CS, Huang AC, Yang JS, *et al.* Safrole induces G0/G1 phase arrest *via* inhibition of cyclin E and provokes apoptosis through endoplasmic reticulum stress and mitochondrion-dependent pathways in human leukemia HL-60 cells. Anticancer Res 2012; 32(5): 1671-9.
[PMID: 22593445]

[17]   Yu FS, Yang JS, Yu CS, *et al.* Safrole suppresses murine myelomonocytic leukemia WEHI-3 cells *in vivo*, and stimulates macrophage phagocytosis and natural killer cell cytotoxicity in leukemic mice. Environ Toxicol 2013; 28(11): 601-8.
[http://dx.doi.org/10.1002/tox.20756] [PMID: 24150866]

[18]   Chang HC, Cheng HH, Huang CJ, *et al.* Safrole-induced Ca2+ mobilization and cytotoxicity in human PC3 prostate cancer cells. J Recept Signal Transduct Res 2006; 26(3): 199-212.
[http://dx.doi.org/10.1080/10799890600662595] [PMID: 16777715]

[19]   Chiang VS, Quek SY. The relationship of red meat with cancer: Effects of thermal processing and related physiological mechanisms. Crit Rev Food Sci Nutr 2017; 57(6): 1153-73.
[http://dx.doi.org/10.1080/10408398.2014.967833] [PMID: 26075652]

[20]   Friedman M. Biological effects of Maillard browning products that may affect acrylamide safety in food: biological effects of Maillard products. Adv Exp Med Biol 2005; 561: 135-56.
[http://dx.doi.org/10.1007/0-387-24980-X_12] [PMID: 16438296]

[21]   Abnet CC. Carcinogenic food contaminants. Cancer Invest 2007; 25(3): 189-96.
[http://dx.doi.org/10.1080/07357900701208733] [PMID: 17530489]

[22]   Bayman P, Baker JL. Ochratoxins: a global perspective. Mycopathologia 2006; 162(3): 215-23.
[http://dx.doi.org/10.1007/s11046-006-0055-4] [PMID: 16944288]

[23]   Pelkonen O, Vähäkangas K. Metabolic activation and inactivation of chemical carcinogens. J Toxicol Environ Health 1980; 6(5-6): 989-99.
[http://dx.doi.org/10.1080/15287398009529921] [PMID: 7463530]

[24]   Louis P, Hold GL, Flint HJ. The gut microbiota, bacterial metabolites and colorectal cancer. Nat Rev Microbiol 2014; 12(10): 661-72.
[http://dx.doi.org/10.1038/nrmicro3344] [PMID: 25198138]

[25]   Sarsour EH, Kumar MG, Chaudhuri L, Kalen AL, Goswami PC. Redox control of the cell cycle in health and disease. Antioxid Redox Signal 2009; 11(12): 2985-3011.
[http://dx.doi.org/10.1089/ars.2009.2513] [PMID: 19505186]

[26]   Chiu LC, Ooi V, Wan JM. Eicosapentaenoic acid modulates cyclin depression and arrests cell cycle

progression in human leek K-562 cells. Int J Oncol 2001; 19: 846-9.

[27]   Lee CY, Sit WH, Fan ST, *et al.* The cell cycle effects of docosahexaenoic acid on human metastatic hepatocellular carcinoma proliferation. Int J Oncol 2010; 36(4): 991-8.
[PMID: 20198345]

[28]   Istfan NW, Wan J, Chen ZY. Fish oil and cell proliferation kinetics in a mammary carcinoma tumor model. Adv Exp Med Biol 1995; 375: 149-56.
[http://dx.doi.org/10.1007/978-1-4899-0949-7_13] [PMID: 7645425]

[29]   Wan JM, Teo TC, Babayan VK, Blackburn GL. Invited comment: lipids and the development of immune dysfunction and infection. JPEN J Parenter Enteral Nutr 1988; 12(6) (Suppl.): 43S-52S.
[http://dx.doi.org/10.1177/014860718801200603] [PMID: 3063838]

[30]   Chiu LC, Wan JM. Induction of apoptosis in HL-60 cells by eicosapentaenoic acid (EPA) is associated with downregulation of bcl-2 expression. Cancer Lett 1999; 145(1-2): 17-27.
[http://dx.doi.org/10.1016/S0304-3835(99)00224-4] [PMID: 10530765]

[31]   Man-Fan Wan J, Kanders BS, Kowalchuk M, *et al.* Omega 3 fatty acids and cancer metastasis in humans. World Rev Nutr Diet 1991; 66: 477-87.
[http://dx.doi.org/10.1159/000419315] [PMID: 2053364]

[32]   Larsson SC, Kumlin M, Ingelman-Sundberg M, Wolk A. Dietary long-chain n-3 fatty acids for the prevention of cancer: a review of potential mechanisms. Am J Clin Nutr 2004; 79(6): 935-45.
[PMID: 15159222]

[33]   Calviello G, Serini S, Piccioni E. n-3 polyunsaturated fatty acids and the prevention of colorectal cancer: molecular mechanisms involved. Curr Med Chem 2007; 14(29): 3059-69.
[http://dx.doi.org/10.2174/092986707782793934] [PMID: 18220742]

[34]   Calviello G, Di Nicuolo F, Gragnoli S, *et al.* n-3 PUFAs reduce VEGF expression in human colon cancer cells modulating the COX-2/PGE2 induced ERK-1 and -2 and HIF-1alpha induction pathway. Carcinogenesis 2004; 25(12): 2303-10.
[http://dx.doi.org/10.1093/carcin/bgh265] [PMID: 15358633]

[35]   Johnson IT, Lund EK. Review article: nutrition, obesity and colorectal cancer. Aliment Pharmacol Ther 2007; 26(2): 161-81.
[http://dx.doi.org/10.1111/j.1365-2036.2007.03371.x] [PMID: 17593063]

[36]   Maillard V, Bougnoux P, Ferrari P, *et al.* N-3 and N-6 fatty acids in breast adipose tissue and relative risk of breast cancer in a case-control study in Tours, France. Int J Cancer 2002; 98(1): 78-83.
[http://dx.doi.org/10.1002/ijc.10130] [PMID: 11857389]

[37]   Calviello G, Palozza P, Piccioni E, *et al.* Dietary supplementation with eicosapentaenoic and docosahexaenoic acid inhibits growth of Morris hepatocarcinoma 3924A in rats: effects on proliferation and apoptosis. Int J Cancer 1998; 75(5): 699-705.
[http://dx.doi.org/10.1002/(SICI)1097-0215(19980302)75:5<699::AID-IJC7>3.0.CO;2-U]   [PMID: 9495237]

[38]   Matafome P, Santos-Silva D, Sena CM, Seiça R. Common mechanisms of dysfunctional adipose tissue and obesity-related cancers. Diabetes Metab Res Rev 2013; 29(4): 285-95.
[http://dx.doi.org/10.1002/dmrr.2395] [PMID: 23390053]

[39]   Weisberg SP, McCann D, Desai M, Rosenbaum M, Leibel RL, Ferrante AW Jr. Obesity is associated with macrophage accumulation in adipose tissue. J Clin Invest 2003; 112(12): 1796-808.
[http://dx.doi.org/10.1172/JCI200319246] [PMID: 14679176]

[40]   Nieman KM, Kenny HA, Penicka CV, *et al.* Adipocytes promote ovarian cancer metastasis and provide energy for rapid tumor growth. Nat Med 2011; 17(11): 1498-503.
[http://dx.doi.org/10.1038/nm.2492] [PMID: 22037646]

[41]   Kwan HY, Fu X, Liu B, *et al.* Subcutaneous adipocytes promote melanoma cell growth by activating the Akt signaling pathway: role of palmitic acid. J Biol Chem 2014; 289(44): 30525-37.

[http://dx.doi.org/10.1074/jbc.M114.593210] [PMID: 25228694]

[42]   Straka S, Lester JL, Cole RM, *et al.* Incorporation of eicosapentaenioic and docosahexaenoic acids into breast adipose tissue of women at high risk of breast cancer: a randomized clinical trial of dietary fish and n-3 fatty acid capsules. Mol Nutr Food Res 2015; 59(9): 1780-90.
[http://dx.doi.org/10.1002/mnfr.201500161] [PMID: 26081224]

[43]   Parkin DM, L . Cancers attributable to overweight and obesity in the UK in 2010. Br J Cancer 2011; 105 (Suppl. 2): S34-7.
[http://dx.doi.org/10.1038/bjc.2011.481] [PMID: 22158318]

[44]   Donaldson MS. Nutrition and cancer: a review of the evidence for an anti-cancer diet. Nutr J 2004; 3: 19.
[http://dx.doi.org/10.1186/1475-2891-3-19] [PMID: 15496224]

[45]   Tang FY, Meydani M. Green tea catechins and vitamin E inhibit angiogenesis of human microvascular endothelial cells through suppression of IL-8 production. Nutr Cancer 2001; 41(1-2): 119-25.
[http://dx.doi.org/10.1080/01635581.2001.9680622] [PMID: 12094614]

[46]   Telang S, Clem AL, Eaton JW, Chesney J. Depletion of ascorbic acid restricts angiogenesis and retards tumor growth in a mouse model. Neoplasia 2007; 9(1): 47-56.
[http://dx.doi.org/10.1593/neo.06664] [PMID: 17325743]

[47]   Gu JW, Makey KL, Tucker KB, *et al.* EGCG, a major green tea catechin suppresses breast tumor angiogenesis and growth *via* inhibiting the activation of HIF-1α and NFκB, and VEGF expression. Vasc Cell 2013; 5(1): 9.
[http://dx.doi.org/10.1186/2045-824X-5-9] [PMID: 23638734]

[48]   Daleprane JB, Freitas VdaS, Pacheco A, *et al.* Anti-atherogenic and anti-angiogenic activities of polyphenols from propolis. J Nutr Biochem 2012; 23(6): 557-66.
[http://dx.doi.org/10.1016/j.jnutbio.2011.02.012] [PMID: 21764281]

[49]   Yang CS, Landau JM, Huang MT, Newmark HL. Inhibition of carcinogenesis by dietary polyphenolic compounds. Annu Rev Nutr 2001; 21: 381-406.
[http://dx.doi.org/10.1146/annurev.nutr.21.1.381] [PMID: 11375442]

[50]   Han H, Zhong C, Zhang X, *et al.* Genistein induces growth inhibition and G2/M arrest in nasopharyngeal carcinoma cells. Nutr Cancer 2010; 62(5): 641-7.
[http://dx.doi.org/10.1080/01635581003605490] [PMID: 20574925]

[51]   Wang H, Zhang J, Sit WH, Lee CY, Wan JM. Cordyceps cicadae induces G2/M cell cycle arrest in MHCC97H human hepatocellular carcinoma cells: a proteomic study. Chin Med 2014; 9: 15.
[http://dx.doi.org/10.1186/1749-8546-9-15] [PMID: 24872842]

[52]   Wan JM, Sit WH, Yang X, Jiang P, Wong LL. Polysaccharopeptides derived from Coriolus versicolor potentiate the S-phase specific cytotoxicity of camptothecin (CPT) on human leukaemia HL-60 cells. Chin Med 2010; 27(5): 16-26.
[http://dx.doi.org/10.1186/1749-8546-5-16] [PMID: 20423495]

[53]   Bagga D, Anders KH, Wang HJ, Glaspy JA. Long-chain n-3-to-n-6 polyunsaturated fatty acid ratios in breast adipose tissue from women with and without breast cancer. Nutr Cancer 2002; 42(2): 180-5.
[http://dx.doi.org/10.1207/S15327914NC422_5] [PMID: 12416257]

[54]   Istfan NW, Wan JM, Bistrian BR, Chen ZY. DNA replication time accounts for tumor growth variation induced by dietary fat in a breast carcinoma model. Cancer Lett 1994; 86(2): 177-86.
[http://dx.doi.org/10.1016/0304-3835(94)90076-0] [PMID: 7982205]

[55]   Nabavi SF, Bilotto S, Russo GL, *et al.* Omega-3 polyunsaturated fatty acids and cancer: lessons learned from clinical trials. Cancer Metastasis Rev 2015; 34(3): 359-80.
[http://dx.doi.org/10.1007/s10555-015-9572-2] [PMID: 26227583]

[56]   Szymczak M, Murray M, Petrovic N. Modulation of angiogenesis by omega-3 polyunsaturated fatty acids is mediated by cyclooxygenases. Blood 2008; 111(7): 3514-21.

[http://dx.doi.org/10.1182/blood-2007-08-109934] [PMID: 18216296]

[57] Taguchi A, Kawana K, Tomio K, *et al.* Matrix metalloproteinase (MMP)-9 in cancer-associated fibroblasts (CAFs) is suppressed by omega-3 polyunsaturated fatty acids *in vitro* and *in vivo.* PLoS One 2014; 9(2): e89605.
[http://dx.doi.org/10.1371/journal.pone.0089605] [PMID: 24586907]

[58] Jing K, Wu T, Lim K. Omega-3 polyunsaturated fatty acids and cancer. Anticancer Agents Med Chem 2013; 13(8): 1162-77.
[http://dx.doi.org/10.2174/18715206113139990319] [PMID: 23919748]

[59] Simopoulos AP. The importance of the ratio of omega-6/omega-3 essential fatty acids. Biomed Pharmacother 2002; 56(8): 365-79.
[http://dx.doi.org/10.1016/S0753-3322(02)00253-6] [PMID: 12442909]

[60] Escrich E, Solanas M, Moral R. Olive oil and other dietary lipids in breast cancer. Cancer Treat Res 2014; 159: 289-309.
[http://dx.doi.org/10.1007/978-3-642-38007-5_17] [PMID: 24114487]

[61] Zhang F, Chen Y, Long J, Dong L, Wang Y, Chen Y. Effect of n-3 and n-6 polyunsaturated fatty acids on lipid metabolic genes and estrogen receptor expression in MCF-7 breast cancer cells. Clin Lab 2015; 61(3-4): 397-403.
[PMID: 25975008]

[62] Stark AH, Madar Z. Olive oil as a functional food: epidemiology and nutritional approaches. Nutr Rev 2002; 60(6): 170-6.
[http://dx.doi.org/10.1301/002966402320243250] [PMID: 12078915]

[63] Stoneham M, Goldacre M, Seagroatt V, Gill L. Olive oil, diet and colorectal cancer: an ecological study and a hypothesis. J Epidemiol Community Health 2000; 54(10): 756-60.
[http://dx.doi.org/10.1136/jech.54.10.756] [PMID: 10990479]

[64] Hodge AM, English DR, McCredie MR, *et al.* Foods, nutrients and prostate cancer. Cancer Causes Control 2004; 15(1): 11-20.
[http://dx.doi.org/10.1023/B:CACO.0000016568.25127.10] [PMID: 14970730]

[65] Kwan HY, Chao X, Su T, *et al.* The anticancer and antiobesity effects of Mediterranean diet. Crit Rev Food Sci Nutr 2017; 57(1): 82-94.
[PMID: 25831235]

[66] Newmark HL. Squalene, olive oil, and cancer risk. Review and hypothesis. Ann N Y Acad Sci 1999; 889: 193-203.
[http://dx.doi.org/10.1111/j.1749-6632.1999.tb08735.x] [PMID: 10668494]

[67] Menendez JA, Vellon L, Colomer R, Lupu R. Oleic acid, the main monounsaturated fatty acid of olive oil, suppresses Her-2/neu (erbB-2) expression and synergistically enhances the growth inhibitory effects of trastuzumab (Herceptin) in breast cancer cells with Her-2/neu oncogene amplification. Ann Oncol 2005; 16(3): 359-71.
[http://dx.doi.org/10.1093/annonc/mdi090] [PMID: 15642702]

[68] Bingham SA, Day NE, Luben R, *et al.* European Prospective Investigation into Cancer and Nutrition. Dietary fibre in food and protection against colorectal cancer in the European Prospective Investigation into Cancer and Nutrition (EPIC): an observational study. Lancet 2003; 361(9368): 1496-501.
[http://dx.doi.org/10.1016/S0140-6736(03)13174-1] [PMID: 12737858]

[69] Iacomino G, Tecce MF, Grimaldi C, Tosto M, Russo GL. Transcriptional response of a human colon adenocarcinoma cell line to sodium butyrate. Biochem Biophys Res Commun 2001; 285(5): 1280-9.
[http://dx.doi.org/10.1006/bbrc.2001.5323] [PMID: 11478796]

[70] Tabuchi Y, Arai Y, Kondo T, Takeguchi N, Asano S. Identification of genes responsive to sodium butyrate in colonic epithelial cells. Biochem Biophys Res Commun 2002; 293(4): 1287-94.

[http://dx.doi.org/10.1016/S0006-291X(02)00365-0] [PMID: 12054516]

[71]   Jump DB, Clarke SD. Regulation of gene expression by dietary fat. Annu Rev Nutr 1999; 19: 63-90.
        [http://dx.doi.org/10.1146/annurev.nutr.19.1.63] [PMID: 10448517]

[72]   Jump DB. Dietary polyunsaturated fatty acids and regulation of gene transcription. Curr Opin Lipidol
        2002; 13(2): 155-64.
        [http://dx.doi.org/10.1097/00041433-200204000-00007] [PMID: 11891418]

[73]   Jeffcoat R. Obesity - a perspective based on the biochemical interrelationship of lipids and
        carbohydrates. Med Hypotheses 2007; 68(5): 1159-71.
        [http://dx.doi.org/10.1016/j.mehy.2006.06.009] [PMID: 17257774]

[74]   Parks EJ. Dietary carbohydrate's effects on lipogenesis and the relationship of lipogenesis to blood
        insulin and glucose concentrations. Br J Nutr 2002; 87 (Suppl. 2): S247-53.
        [http://dx.doi.org/10.1079/BJN/2002544] [PMID: 12088525]

[75]   Chong MF, Fielding BA, Frayn KN. Metabolic interaction of dietary sugars and plasma lipids with a
        focus on mechanisms and de novo lipogenesis. Proc Nutr Soc 2007; 66(1): 52-9.
        [http://dx.doi.org/10.1017/S0029665107005290] [PMID: 17343772]

[76]   Hallfrisch J, Reiser S, Prather ES. Blood lipid distribution of hyperinsulinemic men consuming three
        levels of fructose. Am J Clin Nutr 1983; 37(5): 740-8.
        [PMID: 6846212]

[77]   van Dam RM, Seidell JC. Carbohydrate intake and obesity. Eur J Clin Nutr 2007; 61 (Suppl. 1): S75-
        99.
        [http://dx.doi.org/10.1038/sj.ejcn.1602939] [PMID: 17992188]

[78]   Duvigneaud N, Wijndaele K, Matton L, *et al.* Dietary factors associated with obesity indicators and
        level of sports participation in Flemish adults: a cross-sectional study. Nutr J 2007; 6: 26.
        [http://dx.doi.org/10.1186/1475-2891-6-26] [PMID: 17883880]

[79]   Agostoni C, Braegger C, Decsi T, *et al.* ESPGHAN Committee on Nutrition. Role of dietary factors
        and food habits in the development of childhood obesity: A commentary. J Pediatr Gastroenterol Nutr
        2011; 52: 662-9.

[80]   Meydani M, Hasan ST. Dietary polyphenols and obesity. Nutrients 2010; 2(7): 737-51.
        [http://dx.doi.org/10.3390/nu2070737] [PMID: 22254051]

[81]   Lin JK, Lin-Shiau SY. Mechanisms of hypolipidemic and anti-obesity effects of tea and tea
        polyphenols. Mol Nutr Food Res 2006; 50(2): 211-7.
        [http://dx.doi.org/10.1002/mnfr.200500138] [PMID: 16404708]

[82]   Lin J, Della-Fera MA, Baile CA. Green tea polyphenol epigallocatechin gallate inhibits adipogenesis
        and induces apoptosis in 3T3-L1 adipocytes. Obes Res 2005; 13(6): 982-90.
        [http://dx.doi.org/10.1038/oby.2005.115] [PMID: 15976140]

[83]   Hursel R, Westerterp-Plantenga MS. Thermogenic ingredients and body weight regulation. Int J Obes
        2010; 34(4): 659-69.
        [http://dx.doi.org/10.1038/ijo.2009.299] [PMID: 20142827]

[84]   Wilson ID. Drugs, bugs, and personalized medicine: pharmacometabonomics enters the ring. Proc Natl
        Acad Sci USA 2009; 106(34): 14187-8.
        [http://dx.doi.org/10.1073/pnas.0907721106] [PMID: 19706501]

[85]   Clayton TA, Lindon JC, Cloarec O, *et al.* Pharmaco-metabonomic phenotyping and personalized drug
        treatment. Nature 2006; 440(7087): 1073-7.
        [http://dx.doi.org/10.1038/nature04648] [PMID: 16625200]

[86]   Everett JR, Loo RL, Pullen FS. Pharmacometabonomics and personalized medicine. Ann Clin
        Biochem 2013; 50(Pt 6): 523-45.
        [http://dx.doi.org/10.1177/0004563213497929] [PMID: 23888060]

[87]   Nicholson JK, Wilson ID, Lindon JC. Pharmacometabonomics as an effector for personalized medicine. Pharmacogenomics 2011; 12(1): 103-11.
[http://dx.doi.org/10.2217/pgs.10.157] [PMID: 21174625]

[88]   Nicholson JK, Everett JR, Lindon JC. Longitudinal pharmacometabonomics for predicting patient responses to therapy: drug metabolism, toxicity and efficacy. Expert Opin Drug Metab Toxicol 2012; 8(2): 135-9.
[http://dx.doi.org/10.1517/17425255.2012.646987] [PMID: 22248264]

CHAPTER 2

The Role of Anti-Obesity Medications in Polycystic Ovary Syndrome

Ilgın Turkcuoglu[1],* and **Rauf Melekoglu[2]**

[1] *Department of Obstetrics and Gynecology, Division of Reproductive Endocrinology and Infertility 44280, Faculty of Medicine, University of Inonu, Malatya, Turkey*

[2] *Faculty of Medicine, Department of Obstetrics and Gynecology, Division of Perinatology, University of Inonu, 44280, Malatya, Turkey*

Abstract: The polycystic ovary syndrome (PCOS) is the most common endocrinopathy and the most frequent cause of anovulatory infertility in women of reproductive age. PCOS can lead to various clinical consequences including reproductive, metabolic and psychological problems. Obesity has been defined as having excess body fat that is closely related to insulin resistance, and the estimated incidence of obesity in PCOS has been reported to be 40% to 60%. The initial management option includes lifestyle interventions in patients with PCOS complicated by obesity and insulin resistance. For the dietary management, it is important to have reduced body weight and maintain a lower long-term body weight by preventing further weight gain. Although these lifestyle interventions can provide modest weight loss, in some cases it is necessary to use pharmacologic agents to gain optimal weight loss and maintain optimal weight in the long term. Studies including the use of pharmacologic agents for the treatment of obesity and insulin resistance have increased over the last decade. Pharmacologic agents including orlistat, metformin, glucagon-like peptide-1 receptors (exenatide and liraglutide), phentermine, topiramate, lorcaserin are available for the treatment of obesity and studies have also focused on the effectiveness of these anti-obesity medications in patients with PCOS in the recent years. It has been demonstrated that anti-obesity drugs have beneficial effects on metabolic parameters and weight loss in the obese patients with PCOS used in conjunction with diet and lifestyle modification. However, the administration of these drugs for the PCOS treatment should be under constant medical supervision due to the requirement of monitorization of possible side effects and dose adjustment.

Keywords: Adipokines, Diet, Infertility, Insulin resistance, Metformin, Obesity, Orlistat, Overweight, Polycystic ovary syndrome, Topiramate.

---

* Corresponding author Ilgın Turkcuoglu: Faculty of Medicine, Department of Obstetrics and Gynecology, Division of Reproductive Endocrinology and Infertility, The University of Inonu, 44 280, Malatya, Turkey; Tel: +90533 3347528; Fax: +90342 3600290; E-mail: dr.ilgin@yahoo.com

Atta-ur-Rahman & M. Iqbal Choudhary (Eds.)
All rights reserved-© 2018 Bentham Science Publishers

INTRODUCTION

The polycystic ovary syndrome (PCOS) is the most common endocrinopathy and the most frequent cause of anovulatory infertility in women of reproductive age [1, 2] which has serious effects on short and long-term women's health [3, 4]. PCOS is a heterogeneous disorder with the wide spectrum of clinical symptoms and associated morbidities [5]. It is characterized by hyperandrogenism, ovulatory dysfunction and polycystic ovarian morphologic features. The major health problems related to PCOS are reproductive abnormalities [6, 7], increased insulin resistance [8], increased risk of type 2 diabetes mellitus [9], coronary heart disease [10], dyslipidemia [11], cerebrovascular morbidity [12], anxiety, poor self-esteem and depression [13]. In pregnant women, there is considerably increased risk for the development of gestational diabetes mellitus, preeclampsia, fetal macrosomia, small-for-gestational-age infants, and perinatal mortality [14 - 17].

Although there have been several efforts to establish diagnostic criteria, there is no global consensus regarding PCOS diagnosis. Three organizations have been proposed over the past three decades to establish diagnostic criteria (Table **1**). The first effort to determine the PCOS criteria was carried out by National Institute of Child Health and Human Development of the United States National Institutes of Health (NIH) conference in April 1990 [18]. They reported that clinical or biochemical hyperandrogenism and chronic oligo-anovulation, after the exclusion of related disorders were accepted as diagnostic PCOS features. The second definition was based on the Rotterdam consensus that was sponsored by the European Society of Human Reproduction and Embryology (ESHRE) and the American Society for Reproductive Medicine (ASRM) in May 2003. As a result of this meeting, ultrasound characteristics for polycystic ovarian morphology were added to the NIH 1990 criteria. The Rotterdam PCOS criteria were defined as the presence of two of the following three findings: (1) signs of clinical or biochemical hyperandrogenism; (2) chronic ovulatory dysfunction; and (3) polycystic ovaries on ultrasonography, after exclusion of secondary diseases [19]. The Rotterdam criteria led to a substantial increment in the number of cases diagnosed with PCOS and expanded the heterogeneity of PCOS compared with the NIH criteria [20]. Subsequently, in 2006, a task force by the Androgen Excess & PCOS Society (AE- PCOS) implemented that the diagnosis of PCOS should be based on the presence of clinical or biochemical hyperandrogenism and ovarian dysfunction (ovarian dysfunction or polycystic ovarian morphology), excluding other causes [21, 22].

Due to the global use of varying PCOS diagnostic criteria, the NIH in 2012 conducted an Evidence-Based Methodology PCOS Workshop that evaluated the "benefits and drawbacks" of available diagnostic criteria. The panel concluded the application of the broader ESHRE/ ASRM 2003 criteria with comprehensive definition of the PCOS phenotype including the following phenotype classification: phenotype A: Hyperandrogenism (clinical or biochemical), ovulatory dysfunction and polycystic ovarian morphology; phenotype B: hyperandrogenism and ovulatory dysfunction; phenotype C: hyperandrogenism and polycystic ovarian morphology; and phenotype D: ovulatory dysfunction and polycystic ovarian morphology. The different diagnostic criteria of PCOS are summarized in Table **1**.

Table 1. Different diagnostic criteria for polycystic ovary syndrome.

Diagnostic criteria	NIH 1990	ESHRE/ASRM 2003	AE-PCOS 2006	NIH 2012 extension of ESHRE/ASRM 2003
Criteria	• Hyperandrogenism • Oligo-anovulation	• Hyperandrogenism • Ovulatory dysfunction • Polycystic ovarian morphology.	• Hyperandrogenism • Ovarian dysfunction (Ovulatory dysfunction and/or polycystic ovarian morphology)	• Hyperandrogenism • Ovulatory dysfunction • Polycystic ovarian morphology.
Diagnosis of PCOS	Both of the criteria required	Two of three criteria required	Both of the criteria required	Two of three criteria required and identification of specific phenotypes included: A: Hyperandrogenism + Ovulatory Dysfunction + Polycystic ovarian morphology. B: Hyperandrogenism + Ovulatory Dysfunction C: Hyperandrogenism + Polycystic ovarian morphology. D: Ovulatory Dysfunction + Polycystic ovarian morphology.
Exclusion of mimicking disorder (congenital adrenal hyperplasia, non-classical adrenal hyperplasia, idiopathic hyperandrogenism, idiopathic hirsutism, hyperprolactinemia, thyroid diseases, tumors that secrete androgen, Cushing disease)				

* PCOS: Polycystic ovarian syndrome, NIH: National Institute of Health. AE-PCOS: Androgen Excess & PCOS Society; ASRM: American Society for Reproductive Medicine; ESHRE: European Society of Human Reproduction and Embryology.

Different phenotypes of PCOS emerged due to ESHRE/ ASRM 2003 diagnostic criteria led to cases with different metabolic and health risks [23]. Nevertheless, this phenotypic approach provided some advantages including determination of the women with PCOS having metabolic dysfunction risk (phenotypes A and B) and implementation of homogenous definition in epidemiologic research and clinical trials related with PCOS.

Although the precise frequency of this disorder is not known, the worldwide prevalence of PCOS varies from 4% to 21% [24, 25], based on the diagnostic criteria used. The prevalence was reported between 5% and 10% according to the National Institutes of Health (NIH) 1990 criteria and up to 21% based on the Rotterdam consensus workshop. This wide variation in the prevalence of PCOS can be attributed to the differences in the definition of the PCOS, the geographic and ethnic heterogeneity in the study populations, the use of insensitive circulating androgen measures, inter-observer variation for the evaluation of hirsutism and the absence of standardization in the assessment of the exclusion of mimicking disorder.

PCOS is closely associated with obesity. The incidence of obesity in PCOS has been reported to be 40% to 60%. The prevalence of obesity is increasing all over the world in all age groups, including women of reproductive age, independent of PCOS. Therefore, one can predict a rise in the incidence of obesity in PCOS as well. Obesity is defined as having excess body fat that is closely related to insulin resistance. However, independent of obesity, in PCOS, the incidence of insulin resistance is 40% to 70% and is higher compared to general population [26]. Obesity in PCOS patient may be attributed to the higher incidence of eating disorders, decreased postprandial cholecystokinin and reduced postprandial thermogenesis.

The most commonly proposed pathophysiologic factors in PCOS are hyperandrogenism and insulin resistance. Insulin stimulates the ovarian androgen production and decreases the hepatic sex hormone– binding globulin (SHBG) production which lead to increased free androgens, causing clinical or biochemical hyperandrogenemia, one of the diagnostic criteria of PCOS. Obesity worsens the metabolic profile and aggravates the pathophysiological pathway through insulin resistance in PCOS [27].

Obesity has major effects on women's health especially on the reproductive function that leads fertility problems in reproductive period. Adipose tissue is closely related to the gonads by the secretion of adipokines, such as adiponectin, leptin, and resistin. Particularly, leptin has a significant role in the regulation of early embryo cleavage and development, stimulation of hypothalamic-pituitary axis and inhibition of ovarian follicular development [28]. Elevated serum and follicular leptin levels in obese women affect on specific follicular cell receptors and cause a reduction in insulin-induced steroidogenesis in granulosa and theca cells [29]. Leptin also has an inhibitory effect on luteinizing hormone-stimulated estradiol production in the granulosa cells. These effects may partially be responsible for the poor reproductive performance in obese women. In contrast to leptin, there is a reduction in adiponectin levels in obesity and adiponectin levels are negatively correlated with plasma insulin [30]. Therefore, adiponectin may contribute a significant link between obesity, insulin resistance, and hyperandrogenism. The serum levels and the effects of adipokines on the reproductive system in obese patients are summarized in Table **2**.

Table 2. The serum levels and effects of adipokines on the reproductive system in obese patients.

Adipokines secreted from adipose tissue	Serum concentrations in obese patients	Effects
Leptin	↑	• stimulation of hypothalamic-pituitary axis and inhibition of ovarian follicular development • cause a reduction in insulin-induced steroidogenesis in granulosa and theca cells by binding specific follicular cell receptors • the inhibitory effect on LH-stimulated oestradiol production in the granulosa cells • regulation of early embryo cleavage and development
Resistin	↑	• decreases the ability of insulin to suppress hepatic glucose output or increase glucose uptake by muscle • induces insulin resistance
Ghrelin	↓	• disturbs the ability to regulate hunger and satiation process
Adiponectin	↓	• reduces the ability of insulin to suppress hepatic glucose production • diminishes insulin sensitivity and the development of insulin resistance

The additional effect of obesity on steroid hormones is hyperandrogenism as a result of hyperinsulinemia. Hyperinsulinemia in obese patients may be attributed to the impacts of decreased levels of adiponectin and increased levels of resistin [31] or probably a polymorphism characterized by glycine-to-arginine substitution at codon 972 (Gly972Arg) of the insulin receptor substrate [32]. Besides, inhibition of the hepatic production of sex hormone-binding globulin and insulin-like growth factor binding protein-I and stimulation of ovarian P450c17a activity have been considered the leading causes of hyperandrogenemia [33]. Hyperandrogenemia has been shown to be related to increased risk of anovulatory infertility in obese women. The hyperandrogenism causes anovulation due to the stimulation of granulosa cell apoptosis [34]. Also, it creates a negative feedback on gonadotropin secretion as a result of the peripheral conversion of androgens to estrogen and has possible adverse effects on the endometrium and developing oocyte. The relationship between obesity, insulin resistance, hyperandrogenism, and PCOS is shown in Fig. (**1**).

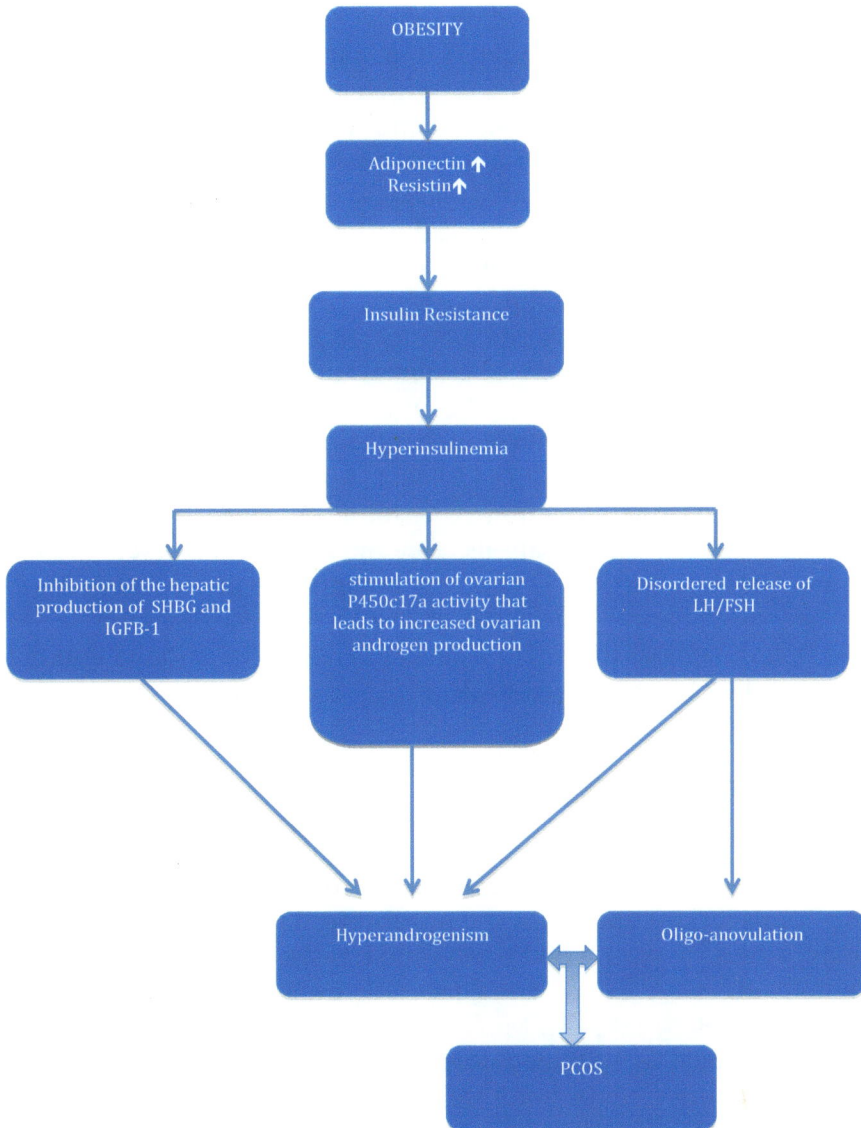

Fig. (1). The relationship between obesity, insulin resistance, hyperandrogenism and PCOS.

PCOS is commonly associated with anovulatory infertility that is also closely related to obesity. Hyperandrogenemia and insulin resistance are the most commonly proposed pathophysiological characteristics in PCOS [35 - 38]. Also, obesity in PCOS patient may be attributed to the higher incidence of eating disorders, decreased postprandial cholecystokinin and reduced postprandial thermogenesis [39 - 41]. The incidence of obesity in PCOS has been reported to be 40% to 60%. Besides, insulin resistance exists in most of the women with PCOS (40% to 70%) independent of obesity. The major factor in the etiology of PCOS is the insulin which stimulates the ovarian androgen production and decreases the hepatic SHBG production, which leads to increased free androgens. In PCOS, it is important to identify and correct the risk factors for the reproductive failure before the initiation of treatment. Recognizing the presence and distribution of obesity is important because obesity is linked to the failure or delayed response to the medical or surgical treatment as well as to the clomiphene citrate, gonadotropins, and laparoscopic ovarian drilling treatments. Weight loss is considered as the first-line therapy in obese women with PCOS due to the presence of an association between obesity and poor reproductive outcomes. Several studies reported that there is a significant increase in live birth rates in obese women with or without PCOS. Furthermore, numerous studies demonstrated that weight loss contributes to the improvement of the spontaneous ovulation rates in women with PCOS [30, 37]. An increase in pregnancy rates has been reported even at 5% reduction in baseline weight [38]. The treatment of obesity involves lifestyle modifications (diet and regular exercise), pharmacologic treatment and bariatric surgery [39]. Even though bariatric surgery provides the best weight maintenance after weight loss, a combination of lifestyle modifications and medical treatment is usually enough to gain the optimal weight loss [41]. The following pharmacologic agents are available for the treatment of obesity and insulin resistance in PCOS.

Orlistat, Sibutramine, and Rimonabant

Orlistat is approved by the Food and Drug Administration (FDA) in 1999 as the first gastrointestinal lipase inhibitor drug for the medical treatment of obesity [42, 43]. Dietary triglycerides and lipids are metabolized to absorbable free fatty acids and monoglycerides by gastric and pancreatic lipases for the intestinal absorption. Orlistat inhibits digestive gastric and pancreatic carboxyl ester lipase and reduces the absorption of dietary fat [44]. McNeely *et al.* demonstrated that incorporation of orlistat (360 mg/day, in 3 divided doses) in a hypocaloric diet for 12 weeks had a significant contribution to the body weight loss compared with placebo in obese patients (5% *vs.* 3.5%) [42]. Besides, several randomized controlled trials showed beneficial effects of orlistat on long-term (2-4 years) body weight reduction [45 - 47]. Also, orlistat was found to be associated with improvement in blood pressure, serum lipid levels and insulin resistance [47, 48]. Jayagopal *et al.* conducted the first randomized controlled trial about the benefit of orlistat in PCOS, and they demonstrated a significant reduction in weight and total testosterone levels in patients treated by orlistat. They concluded that orlistat might prove to be a useful adjunct in the treatment of PCOS [49]. The effects of orlistat (120 mg, three times a day for three months) added to a reduced-energy diet were investigated in obese women with or without PCOS. Although changes in weight, waist-to-hip ratio, and insulin resistance were similar in both groups, only androgen levels were found to be decreased in women with PCOS [50]. Also, it was shown that orlistat combined with lifestyle changes leads to substantial weight loss in women with PCOS, resulting in an improvement in insulin resistance and hyperandrogenemia and has beneficial effects on cardiovascular risk factors, including blood pressure and dyslipidemia [51]. Gastrointestinal side effects including abdominal pain, dyspepsia, flatulence, bloating and diarrhea are observed as the most common side effects related to orlistat treatment. Supplementation of daily multivitamins is found helpful to prevent fat-soluble vitamin deficiencies [52]. Excretion of orlistat occurs almost entirely by feces within 3-5 days with minimal systemic absorption and no accumulation [53, 54]. In 2012, a safety label warning about the risk of increased urinary oxalate levels was approved, thus monitoring of renal function is critical in patients at risk for renal insufficiency. Also, 32 cases complicated with serious liver injury have been reported in patients using orlistat from 1999 to 2008 [55].

Sibutramine, a centrally acting agent that inhibits noradrenaline/serotonin reuptake selectively, has been used widely after approval by the FDA in 1997. It has been demonstrated that sibutramine treatment of at least 12 months provided a mean weight loss of 4.2 kg compared with placebo [56]. Park *et al.* showed that 68.2% of obese patients present 5% or more of weight reduction with the sibutramine therapy for 12 weeks [57]. Nisoli *et al.* showed the improvement of plasma triglyceride, total cholesterol, low-density lipoprotein (LDL) cholesterol, high-density lipoprotein (HDL) cholesterol, glucose, and insulin levels with sibutramine treatment [58]. However, a meta-analysis that evaluated ten trials with 1213 participants who were treated with sibutramine or placebo showed no significant decrease in total cholesterol levels after adjustment for weight loss [59]. Lindholm *et al.* examined the effectiveness of sibutramine treatment with lifestyle intervention for weight loss in obese women with PCOS in a randomized, double-blind, placebo-controlled trial. They demonstrated that 15 mg once daily sibutramine treatment for six months period provided significant weight loss compared with placebo (7.8±5.1 kg *vs.* 2.8±6.2 kg). Also, they found that sibutramine treatment resulted in a significant reduction in apolipoprotein B, triglycerides, and cystatin C levels. They concluded that sibutramine treatment in combination with lifestyle modifications is beneficial for weight loss in obese patients with PCOS, particularly among young obese patients with PCOS with low SHBG levels [60]. Wadden *et al.* assigned 224 obese women to four groups (sibutramine alone, lifestyle modification alone, sibutramine plus group lifestyle modification and sibutramine plus brief therapy) for examining the efficiency of sibutramine treatment combined with brief lifestyle modification. They found that the combination of sibutramine and group lifestyle modification resulted in more weight reduction than either medication or lifestyle modification alone [61]. Also, sibutramine added to a reduced-energy diet led to more spontaneous pregnancies and greater decreases in body weight, triglycerides, lipoprotein ApoA and androgens compared with placebo and diet, diet alone, or ethinylestradiol plus cyproterone acetate [62]. Sibutramine is a well tolerated anti-obesity drug due to mild common side effect including headache, constipation, insomnia and dry mouth. However, due to the presence of concerns over its safety (especially cardiovascular side effects including increased heart rate and blood pressure), it was temporarily withdrawn from the Italian market, because 47 adverse events (arrhythmias, primarily tachycardia, and hypertension) and two deaths were reported from cardiovascular disease in the country [63]. After that, a randomized, double-blind, placebo-controlled study titled as Sibutramine Cardiovascular Outcomes trial was conducted [64, 65]. It was demonstrated that patients who were administered sibutramine treatment had an average of 2.2 kg weight loss and 2.0 cm reduction in waist circumference with a decrease in blood pressure and pulse rate after a six week period. In the preliminary report of this study, sibutramine was found related to nonfatal cardiovascular effects such as myocardial infarction or stroke as compared with placebo. FDA suggested healthcare professionals to be informed about not to prescribe sibutramine in patients with known heart disease. Initially, this drug is allowed to be available because of potential benefits outweigh their possible risks with a strong warning about should not be used by people with a history of stroke or myocardial infarct and uncontrolled high blood pressure [66]. Harrison-Woolrych *et al.* performed a prospective observational study in 15686 patients who were prescribed sibutramine for obesity treatment in New Zealand, and they failed to show any higher risk of death from a cardiovascular disease [67]. However, the FDA finally decided to withdraw sibutramine on October 8, 2010, due to the drug's unnecessary cardiovascular risks in the obese patients.

The endocannabinoid system has been known as a critical role in the control of appetite such as glucose metabolism. Rimonabant is the first new class of drug that blocks cannabinoid receptor-1 in the endocannabinoid system selectively and works as an anorectic agent by modulating lipid and glucose metabolism as well as adipose tissue function [68]. The efficiency of Rimonabant on obesity has been extensively tested in the Rimonabant in Obesity program. In this program, four randomized, double-blinded, placebo- controlled phase 3 clinical study were evaluated, and it was demonstrated that rimonabant treatment was associated with significant reduction in body weight and waist circumference over a 1 to 2 year period [69 - 72]. Also, the improvement was shown in cardiometabolic risk factors, including blood pressure, insulin resistance and serum triglycerides, C-reactive protein, HDL cholesterol levels in overweight and obese patients. Sathyapalan *et al.* conducted a randomized open-label parallel study to compare the effectiveness of metformin and rimonabant on weight reduction, biochemical hyperandrogenemia, and insulin resistance in patients with PCOS. They found a significant decrease in body weight, waist circumference, hip circumference, waist-hip ratio, free androgen index, testosterone and insulin resistance after 12 weeks of rimonabant treatment. They also noted that there was no remarkable change in all of these parameters in the metformin-treated group [73].

Adverse effects related to rimonabant treatment were identified as psychiatric side effects, including depression, anxiety, and suicidal ideation. The psychiatric adverse events showed 26% of patients treated with rimonabant [74], and the risk of depressive symptoms was increased approximately 2.5 fold higher than the patients treated with placebo. Despite the several favorable clinical data, FDA did not approve marketing authorization for rimonabant as a result of the risks.

Insulin-sensitizing Drugs (Metformin, Rosiglitazone, Pioglitazone, and D-chiro-inositol)

The major insulin-sensitizing agents are metformin and thiazolidinediones including troglitazone, rosiglitazone, pioglitazone, and D-chiro-inositol. Insulin sensitizing drugs are not considered as anti-obesity drugs until some studies indicated the contribution of metformin therapy on weight loss [75].

Metformin is a biguanide antihyperglycemic drug used widely in the treatment of type 2 diabetes mellitus. Also, it is the most studied insulin-lowering drug in the PCOS treatment. The mechanism of action of glycemic control in diabetic individuals is attributed to the decreased hepatic glycogenolysis and increased peripheral glucose uptake. Unlike insulin and sulfonylureas, metformin does not increase the serum insulin levels. Several studies demonstrated the beneficial effect of metformin on ovarian androgen production [76, 77].

The first study about the use of metformin treatment in patients with PCOS was conducted by Velazquez *et al.* [78]. They demonstrated that metformin therapy was associated with increased insulin sensitivity, decreased serum LH, total and free testosterone levels and elevated serum FSH and SHBG levels.

Since that time, several studies evaluated the effect of metformin treatment on obese women with PCOS and demonstrated the improvement in ovulation and the reduction in androgen levels [79, 80]. Moghetti *et al.* examined the effect of long-term (6 months) metformin treatment in obese patients with PCOS, and they demonstrated a significant improvement in hyperinsulinemia and hyper-androgenemia independent of alterations in body weight. Besides, higher plasma insulin, lower serum androstenedione, and less severe menstrual irregularities were identified as predictors of better clinical response to metformin [81].

Despite the high association with the obesity and PCOS, lean women are comprised of 20% to 50% of PCOS patients. Nestler and Jakubowicz [82] demonstrated that similarly with the obese PCOS patients; metformin treatment showed a beneficial effect on fasting and glucose-stimulated insulin levels, gonadotropin-releasing hormone- stimulated LH release, free and total testosterone concentrations in lean patients with PCOS. Lord *et al.* performed a systematic review confirming the efficiency of metformin therapy for ovulation induction in women with PCOS, and they could not demonstrate the contribution of metformin on weight loss [83]. However, another systematic review on the same topic confirmed the contribution of metformin to weight loss [84]. Also, Legro *et al.* compared the three ovulation induction modalities (metformin and placebo, metformin and clomiphene, clomiphene and placebo) in patients with PCOS and they showed that women treated with metformin had better weight loss [85]. Nieuwenhuis-Ruifrok *et al.* assessed the contribution of insulin sensitizing drugs on weight loss, compared with diet or a lifestyle intervention in overweight or obese patients with PCOS in a systematic review. They indicated that metformin treatment of reproductive-aged overweight or obese women with PCOS leads to a significant reduction in body mass index when compared with placebo. They showed that higher dose (1500 mg/day) and longer duration (8 weeks) of metformin treatment showed greater effects on weight reduction. However, they concluded that a structured lifestyle modification program should be considered to obtain optimal weight loss as the first line treatment in obese women with or without PCOS [86]. Tang *et al.* conducted a Cochrane review regarding the use of insulin-sensitizing agents in patients with PCOS, and they confirmed the beneficial effect of metformin on the improvement of clinical pregnancy and ovulation rates. Also, they suggested that metformin has limited effect on the weight loss and metabolic parameters including insulin and lipid profiles in obese patients with PCOS [87].

The most common side effect of metformin is gastrointestinal irritation including nausea, vomiting, diarrhea, cramps, and flatulence [88]. The most severe potential adverse effect of metformin use is lactic acidosis; this complication is uncommon, and the majority of this complication was seen in patients having comorbid conditions, such as hepatic dysfunction or impaired kidney function [89]. Reduction in serum thyroid-stimulating hormone levels in patients treated with metformin [90] has also been reported. However, the clinical significance of this complication is still unknown.

Thiazolidinediones or "glitazones" compose a novel type of potent oral antidiabetic drugs for the treatment of non-insulin dependent diabetes mellitus, and they have potentially beneficial effects in the treatment of obese women with PCOS. The primary mechanism of their action is attributed to the activation of the selective ligand of the nuclear transcription factor gamma isoform of the peroxisome proliferator-activated receptor (PPAR-γ). Activation of PPAR-γ modulates the transcription of several genes associated with glucose metabolism, lipid metabolism and energy balance, including code for lipoprotein lipase and fatty acyl-CoA synthase. This modulation results in reduction in insulin resistance of adipose tissue, liver, and muscle [91]. Despite this common mechanism of action; troglitazone, rosiglitazone, pioglitazone, and D-chiro-inositol differ in their chemical compositions and binding affinities for PPAR-γ. These differences may account for the difference in their safety profiles observed in clinical studies [92].

Troglitazone was the first thiazolidinedione approved in the United States for the treatment of diabetes mellitus. It has been shown that troglitazone has a beneficial effect on the improvement of peripheral insulin sensitivity and reducing the serum insulin levels in patients with type 2 diabetes mellitus. Dunaif *et al.* [93] conducted the first study demonstrating an increment in insulin sensitivity and a reduction in serum LH and androgen levels with troglitazone treatment in obese patients with PCOS. Also, improvements in ovulatory function were shown due to the hormonal and metabolic changes associated with troglitazone treatment [94, 95].

Although Aziz *et al.* demonstrated improvement in insulin resistance, hyperandrogenemia, hirsutism, and ovulatory dysfunction treated with troglitazone in a randomized prospective trial, this treatment was found associated with severe hepatic dysfunction [96]. The liver damage was usually reversible; however, a few cases with hepatic failure leading to mortality or liver transplant were reported [97]. The injury had occurred with both short- and long- term troglitazone therapy. For this reason, troglitazone was withdrawn from the market in March 2000 by FDA.

Rosiglitazone maleate was another thiazolidinedione to be investigated in women with PCOS. Shobokshi and Shaarawy examined the effects of combined rosiglitazone and clomiphene citrate therapy *versus* clomiphene citrate monotherapy on serum insulin-like growth factor 1 (IGF-1) and insulin-like growth factor binding protein 3 (IGFBP-3) levels in patients with PCOS [98]. In this study, combined rosiglitazone and clomiphene treatment provided a better reduction in area under the insulin curve, serum LH, free testosterone, LH: FSH and IGBP1: IGBP-3 ratio compared with clomiphene monotherapy. Consistently, Ghazeeri *et al.* [99] conducted a double-blinded, randomized, prospective trial that examined the effect of rosiglitazone maleate on ovulation induction in obese women with PCOS. They randomized 25 clomiphene citrate-resistant obese women with PCOS to treat with rosiglitazone (4 mg twice a day) plus clomiphene citrate or placebo for two months. They concluded that short-term rosiglitazone treatment improved both spontaneous and clomiphene-induced ovulation, insulin sensitivity and serum androgen levels by increasing SHBG levels. In literature, a limited number of studies exist about the use of rosiglitazone in women with PCOS. Tang *et al.* showed an improvement in ovulation rate with rosiglitazone treatment [87]. On the other hand, these drugs are classified as category C. More recently, there is also a concern about the increased risk of myocardial infarction in rosiglitazone treatment [100]. In contrast to the troglitazone treatment, its use was not found related to increased hepatotoxicity risk [101]. Rosiglitazone was classified as pregnancy category C drug according to FDA for the potential risk of fetal growth restriction that was shown in animal experiments [102].

Pioglitazone is the other thiazolidinedione; that was investigated in women with PCOS. Romualdi *et al.* [103] demonstrated the beneficial effects of pioglitazone on maintaining body weight, body fat distribution and blood pressure on normo-insulinemic and hyperinsulinemic obese women with PCOS. Glueck *et al.* [104] examined the effectiveness of supplementing pioglitazone (45 mg/d) to the treatment of women with PCOS which were not optimally responsive to a 1-year treatment with metformin (2.55 g/d) combined with diet (1500 to 2000 calorie depending on initial BMI). They observed a reduction in serum glucose, insulin, and DHEAS levels, and insulin resistance with the pioglitazone treatment after ten months of treatment. Glintborg *et al.* evaluated the effects of pioglitazone therapy on insulin resistance, beta-cell function, glucose metabolism and LH secretion. They found that pioglitazone treatment was associated with significantly lower levels of fasting insulin and higher insulin sensitivity with increased insulin-stimulated glucose oxidation and insulin-stimulated inhibition of lipid oxidation. In respect to the use of pioglitazone in women with PCOS, with a limited number of studies [105], Tag *et al.* showed the increased ovulation rate with pioglitazone. However, they concluded that thiazolidinediones should not be considered as a primary therapy in the treatment of women with PCOS [87].

Adverse effects related with pioglitazone are similar with rosiglitazone and mild to moderate edema was reported in about 5% of patients. A few case reports about pioglitazone-related hepatotoxicity [106, 107], clinical experience with pioglitazone have not shown significant hepatotoxicity in the majority of the cases

[92]. Pioglitazone is a category C drug for the pregnant women due to the observation of fetal death and growth retardation in animal models.

As a result of binding of insulin to its receptor, inositol phospho-glycan mediators are produced by the hydrolysis of glycosylphosphatidylinositol lipids that are located in the outer cell membrane. Subsequently, these mediators pass the membrane and enter the intracellular metabolic process. It has shown that the inositol-phospho-glycan molecule containing D-chiro-inositol and galactosamine has a critical role in the activation of essential enzymes that control the nonoxidative and oxidative glucose metabolism [108]. It is shown that a defect in D-chiro-inositol–containing phospho-glycan mediator was associated with insulin resistance in nonhuman primates and humans [109, 110].

Nestler *et al.* [111] performed a randomized, prospective, placebo-controlled study which evaluated the effect of D-chiro- inositol in obese women with PCOS. Participants were treated with 1200 mg/d of D-chiro- inositol or placebo for 6 to 8 weeks. It was shown that the administration of D-chiro-inositol had a beneficial effect on the reduction of serum testosterone concentration and improvement in SHBG concentration and ovulation rates. Also, Gerli *et al.* confirmed these findings in a randomized, double-blind placebo-controlled trial that examined the effects of myoinositol on ovarian function and metabolic factors in women with PCOS. They found that myoinositol combined with folic acid is associated with better ovulation frequency, shorter time to first ovulation and rapid follicular maturation [112].

GLP-1 Agonists (Exenatide, Liraglutide), Phentermine and Topiramate

Glucagon and glucagon-like-peptid-1 (GLP-1) are pancreatic and intestinal hormones, respectively, derived from the same proglucagon peptide that is secreted in response to ingestion of carbohydrates, lipids, and mixed meals from the L-cells located in the distal jejunum, ileum, and colon/rectum [113]. Glucagon is a 29 amino acid peptide hormone that is derived from pancreatic islet α cells as well as brainstem [114]. Glucagon leads to elevation of blood glucose by promoting glycogenolysis and gluconeogenesis, as well as β-oxidation of hepatic fatty acid and ketogenesis under conditions of hypoglycemia [115]. GLP-1 is an incretin hormone which is released in postprandial period and associated with an increment in β-cell insulin response, inhibition of gastric emptying, and suppression of appetite [116]. It is proposed that presence of optimal ratios of GLP-1 and glucagon agonism has synergistic and additive effects on weight loss. Activation of glucagon receptors increases the hyperglycemia risk due to the glucose production whereas simultaneous activation of GLP-1 receptors inhibits this effect [117]. There are currently two GLP-1R agonists available (exenatide and liraglutide), with several more are currently being developed. Liraglutide is a GLP-1R analog that reduces blood glucose levels, glucagon secretion, gastric emptying, appetite, and energy intake. At the same time, it increases pancreatic beta cell growth, insulin secretion, and improves insulin sensitivity through mechanisms that are not completely understood. The GLP-1R agonists have been used for the treatment of patients with type-2 diabetes mellitus for the past five years. Liraglutide reduces plasma glucose levels in both fasting and postprandial states. As injected once daily, it has been shown to improve glycemic control in individuals with type-2 diabetes (up to a 1.5% decrease in glycated hemoglobin). It has been demonstrated that GLP-1 receptor agonists have potentially beneficial effects for the treatment of obesity. As much as 5–10% weight loss improves clinical (reproductive and metabolic) outcomes in PCOS women [118].

Phentermine is an approved drug by the FDA in 1959 for short-term (≤12 week) monotherapy of obesity as an adjunct to caloric restriction and lifestyle interventions for overweight individuals with weight-related comorbidities [119]. It is the most commonly prescribed anti-obesity drug in the United States [120]. The recommended dosage is 15–30 mg orally daily to minimize sleep disturbances from central nervous system stimulation. Thus, phentermine can be taken in the early morning. The efficacy and safety of phentermine (30 mg for 12 weeks) in overweight patients with controlled diabetes, hypertension and dyslipidemia have been demonstrated in several studies. Phentermine provides significant body weight reduction in participants compared to placebo (8 kg *vs.* 2 kg). Also, an improvement was shown in total cholesterol and low-density lipoprotein cholesterol with phentermine. Bates *et al.* stated that obesity might be the best predictor of both reproductive and metabolic dysfunction and it negatively affects the response to treatment in women with PCOS. They suggested that pharmaceuticals including metformin, lipid lowering agents and oral contraceptives should be considered by the individual's risk profile and treatment goals [121]. The phase 3 SEQUEL trial about the evaluation of the weight loss and metabolic benefits of controlled-release phentermine/topiramate in obese and overweight adults has demonstrated weight reduction with decreased cardiovascular risk factors and enhanced metabolic function following the use of phentermine/topiramate in conjunction with lifestyle interventions [122].

There is limited evidence about the long-term effectiveness of phentermine monotherapy in the literature. The longest (36 weeks) placebo-controlled trial evaluating the efficacy of continuous or intermittent phentermine monotherapy (30 mg per day) reported a mean weight loss of 12.2 and 13.0 kg, respectively, compared with placebo (4.8 kg) [123]. The most common adverse effects are dry mouth, constipation, tachycardia, hypertension, and palpitations. After prolonged use, abrupt cessation of phentermine may cause extreme fatigue and depression

[124, 125]. The use of phentermine is restricted in individuals with cardiovascular disease, uncontrolled hypertension, hyperthyroidism, glaucoma. Phentermine is a pregnancy category C drug and should not be used by pregnant women.

Topiramate is an anticonvulsant agent with weight loss properties that modulates sodium and gamma-aminobutyric acid (GABA)-activated chloride channels and inhibits carbonic anhydrase. Patients treated with topiramate were found to be associated with reduced calorie intake and weight loss [126]. The appetite suppression mechanism of topiramate is attributed to the modulation of voltage-gated ion channels, improved activity at GABA-A receptors, and inhibition of AMPA/kainite glutamate receptors [127]. It has also been demonstrated that topiramate has an inhibitory effect on compulsive food cravings and addictive behavior. Patients who were treated by topiramate by a starting dose of 25 mg/day that is titrated over eight weeks to 400 mg/day had a significant reduction in binge eating duration and frequency, body weight and compulsive characteristics of binge eating disorders, compared to placebo [128]. Phentermine, which is the potent inhibitor of the norepinephrine transporter, has a suppressive effect on appetite due to activation of pro-opiomelanocortin (POMC) arcuate nucleus neurons. Combination of phentermine and topiramate was approved as a combination therapy by the FDA in 2012 for achieving effective weight loss in obesity with a reduced-calorie diet and regular exercise. In three randomized, placebo- controlled, phase 3 trials, the average expected weight loss over one year was 5%–11% with Phen/TPM *versus* 1%–2% with placebo [129]. Gadde *et al*. conducted a phase 3 trial which examined the efficiency and safety of two different doses of phentermine plus topiramate controlled-release combination (7.5 mg of phentermine/46 mg of topiramate and 15 mg of phentermine/92 mg of topiramate) as a supplement to diet and lifestyle interventions for weight loss. They demonstrated that both doses of phentermine/topiramate combination were associated with a significant weight reduction of 7.8% and 9.8%, respectively, compared to 1.2% with placebo. Also, it has been observed that phentermine/ topiramate combination has a beneficial effect on blood pressure, total cholesterol, high-density lipoprotein, and hemoglobin A1c levels in obese patients with type 2 diabetes [130]. Adverse reactions related to phentermine/topiramate combination were reported as paresthesia, dizziness, insomnia, dysgeusia, altered taste, glaucoma, metabolic acidosis, constipation and dry mouth that occur at a rate of ≥5%. This combination was also found to be associated with heart rate increment; thus, routine monitorization is required before the treatment and if the dose augmentation is considered. Depression and suicide ideation assessment should be performed before the treatment due to topiramate's enhancement effect on suicidal thoughts [131]. The phentermine/topiramate combination is a contraindicated during pregnancy period especially in the first trimester for the possible teratogen effects on fetus including cleft lip with or without cleft palate.

Therefore, it is classified as category X drug for pregnant women due to teratogenic risk. Therefore, effective contraception use should be considered for the women of reproductive age during the treatment period [132]. Although phentermine/topiramate combination has not been investigated especially in the obese, infertile, PCOS patients, it is suggested that antiobesity pharmacologic agents and bariatric surgery are potential future options for the management of obese women with PCOS but require further research [133, 134].

Lorcaserin and Bupropion/ Naltrexone

It is shown that serotonin (5-hydroxytryptophan) has an important function in the short-term regulation of food intake and satiation [135]. Previously, a 5-HT transporter inhibitor, Dexfenfluramine was approved as an appetite suppressant for obese individuals, but it was withdrawn due to severe adverse effects including hallucinations caused by 5-HT2A receptor activation, pulmonary artery hypertension, and cardiac valvulopathy caused by 5-HT2B receptor activation [136]. In 2012, a selective 5-HT2C agonist, lorcaserin was approved by the FDA for the treatment of obesity. It was the second anti-obesity drug that has been approved by the FDA. It is highly selective for 5-HT2C receptors and has no side effects associated with 5-HT2A and 5-HT2B receptor activation [137]. The main effect of lorcaserin is increased satiety that occurs by the regulatory effects of 5-HT2C receptors which are expressed in POMC neurons of the arcuate nucleus [138]. Specifically, lorcaserin stimulates POMC neurons in the arcuate nucleus to release alpha-melanocortin- stimulating hormone (a-MSH), which acts in the paraventricular nucleus to suppress appetite. It was shown that mice lacking melanocortin 4 receptors (MC4R) are not sensitive to 5-HT2C agonist-induced hypophagia, implying that 5-HT2C receptor agonists, such as lorcaserin, increase hypophagia by downstream stimulation of the melanocortin pathway. The recommended dose of lorcaserin is 10 mg twice daily, and it is approved as supplementation therapy to lifestyle intervention (reduced-calorie diet and increased physical activity) in obese patients with a body mass index of ≥ 30, or ≥ 27 kg/m2, with a weight-related comorbidity, like hypertension, type 2 diabetes or dyslipidemia. Besides, it is recommended that the treatment should be discontinued if 5% weight reduction of initial weight is not achieved [139].

O' Neil *et al.* demonstrated the safety and effectiveness of lorcaserin treatment in conjunction with lifestyle interventions in obese patients with type 2 diabetes in a randomized, double-blind, placebo-controlled trial. They showed that lorcaserin (10 mg, twice daily) provided 5% weight reduction in body weight and this decrease was significantly higher than the placebo group. They observed that the weight reduction started at the second week of the treatment and at the end of the treatment period (one year) lorcaserin was administered and found to be associated with higher body weight reduction compared with placebo (4.5% *vs.* 1.5%) [140]. In diabetic patients, in addition to proper anti-diabetic regimen modifications, it is crucial to monitoring glucose levels during the treatment period due to significant hypoglycemia risk (7.4%). The most common side-effects were reported as headache, dry mouth, dizziness, fatigue, nausea, constipation in non-diabetic patients, and hypoglycemia, headache, back pain, cough, and fatigue in diabetic patients. There was no increase in the rate of cardiac valvulopathy in contrast to fenfluramine [141]. Shram *et al.* evaluated the abuse liability of lorcaserin, and they concluded that lorcaserin was well tolerated, and it was associated with lack of abuse liability compared with zolpidem and ketamine in therapeutic doses [142]. Although lorcaserin has not been studied primarily in the obese, infertile, PCOS patients, it is suggested that anti-obesity pharmacologic agents and bariatric surgery are potential future options for the management of obese women with PCOS but require further research [133, 134].

Naltrexone is an opioid receptor antagonist used in opioid and alcohol dependence treatment. Buproprion is a dopamine (DA) and NE transporter inhibitor and is approved for the treatment of depression and nicotine addiction [143]. In 2014, the combination of naltrexone and bupropion was approved by the FDA for adults with a body mass index of 30 and higher or with a body mass index of at least 27 with concomitant obesity-related comorbidities. Apovian *et al.* conducted a double-blind, placebo-controlled study to test the effects of naltrexone/bupropion (NB) combination therapy on weight and weight-related risk factors in overweight and obese individuals. They showed that obese or overweight patients with dyslipidemia or hypertension that received 32 mg/day naltrexone and 360 mg/day bupropion for 56 weeks provided significant body loss compared with placebo (6.4% *vs.* 1.2%). Also, participants that were treated with bupropion/naltrexone combination presented better improvement in cardiometabolic risk markers and weight-related quality of life compared to placebo [144]. Adverse effects associated with bupropion/naltrexone combination therapy include nausea, vomiting, headache, dizziness, insomnia, constipation, dry mouth and diarrhea. This treatment also carries increased risk of suicidal behavior and thoughts, and neuropsychiatric symptoms. Mechanism and adverse effects of all anti-obesity medications including bupropion/naltrexone are summarized in Table **3**.

Table 3. Mechanism and adverse effects of anti-obesity drugs.

Drug	Standard dose	Mechanism of action	Side effects
Orlistat	120 mg three times daily	• inhibits digestive gastric and pancreatic carboxyl ester lipase and reduces the absorption of dietary fat	• gastrointestinal side effects including abdominal pain, dyspepsia, flatulence, bloating, diarrhea • increased urinary oxalate levels • serious liver injury
Sibutramine	10-15 mg once daily	• centrally acting agent that inhibits noradrenaline/serotonin reuptake selectively	• headache, constipation, insomnia, dry mouth • cardiovascular side effects(arrhythmias, primarily tachycardia, hypertension)
Rimonabant	20 mg once daily	• blocks cannabinoid receptor-1 (CB1) in the endocannabinoid system selectively and works as an anorectic agent by modulating lipid and glucose metabolism as well as adipose tissue function	• psychiatric side effects, including depression, anxiety, and suicidal ideation
Metformin	1000-1500 mg once daily	• decreases hepatic glycogenolysis and increases peripheral glucose uptake	• gastrointestinal irritation, including nausea, vomiting, diarrhea, cramps, and flatulence • lactic acidosis • hypothyroidism
Troglitazone	400-800 mg once daily.	• activates the selective ligand of the nuclear transcription factor gamma isoform of the PPAR-γ • improves peripheral insulin sensitivity and reduces the serum insulin levels	• severe hepatic dysfunction
Rosiglitazone	4 mg twice a day	• activates the selective ligand of the nuclear transcription factor gamma isoform of the PPAR-γ • improves peripheral insulin sensitivity and reduces the serum insulin levels	• increased risk of myocardial infarction • peripheral edema and a dilutional reduction in hematocrit level • increased hepatotoxicity risk
Pioglitazone	45 mg once daily	• activates the selective ligand of the nuclear transcription factor gamma isoform of the PPAR-γ • improves peripheral insulin sensitivity and reduces the serum insulin levels	• mild to moderate edema • a small reduction in hemoglobin due to fluid-retaining effect • myalgia • hepatotoxicity

(Table 3) cont.....

Drug	Standard dose	Mechanism of action	Side effects
D-chiro-inositol	1200 mg once daily	• activates essential enzymes that control the nonoxidative and oxidative glucose metabolism	• nausea, tiredness, headache, and dizziness.
GLP-1 agonists (exenatide, liraglutide)	Exenatide 5-10 mcg twice a day Liraglutide 0.6-1.8 mg once daily	• reduces blood glucose levels, • increases insulin secretion • inhibits glucagon secretion • increases pancreatic beta cell growth • suppresses appetite and energy intake • delays gastric emptying, and improves insulin sensitivity	• diarrhea, nausea, vomiting, injection-site reactions and acute pancreatitis
Phentermine	15–30 mg once daily	• central sympathomimetic amine	• dry mouth, constipation, tachycardia, hypertension, palpitations • fatigue, depression
Topiramate	25 mg once daily	• modulates sodium and GABA-activated chloride channels, and inhibits carbonic anhydrase.	• paresthesia, dizziness, insomnia, dysgeusia, altered taste, glaucoma, metabolic acidosis, constipation and dry mouth • tachycardia • suicidal thoughts
Lorcaserin	10 mg, twice daily	• 5-HT2C agonist • stimulates POMC neurons in the arcuate nucleus to release a-MSH, which acts in the paraventricular nucleus to suppress appetite	• headache, dry mouth, dizziness, fatigue, nausea, and constipation in non-diabetic patients • hypoglycemia, headache, back pain, cough, and fatigue in diabetic patients
Bupropion/ naltrexone	32 mg/day naltrexone and 360 mg/day bupropion	• Naltrexone: opioid receptor antagonist; prevents β-endorphi--mediated negative feedback on α-MSH release • Bupropion: DA and NE transporter inhibitor; stimulates hypothalamic POMC neurons that release α-MSH resulting in decreased food intake and increased energy expenditure	• nausea, vomiting, headache, dizziness, insomnia, constipation, dry mouth, diarrhea, increased risk of suicidal behavior and neuropsychiatric symptoms

The exact mechanism of action of bupropion/naltrexone combination therapy as an anti-obesity drug is poorly understood. It is suggested that modulatory effect of bupropion/naltrexone combination on homeostatic (hypothalamic melanocortin system) and nonhomeostatic systems (mesolimbic dopaminergic system) provides activation of POMC neurons in the arcuate nucleus and results in releasing a-

MSH which acts as a potent anorectic neuropeptide by binding to MC4Rs [145]. β-endorphin is a μ-opioid receptor agonist that is released simultaneously with α-MSH secretion and inhibits α-MSH releasing by a negative feedback mechanism under physiological conditions [146]. Naltrexone prevents the β-endorphi--mediated negative feedback by blocking μ-opioid receptors and inhibiting the subsequent increase in POMC activity [147]. There is no study about the use of bupropion/naltrexone combination, especially in the obese, infertile, PCOS patients. However, this approved that anti-obesity drugs could be potential future options for the management of obese women with PCOS but require further research [133, 134].

Other Drugs

Several weight-loss medications are no longer available due to concerns regarding their adverse effects. Aminorex, an amphetamine-like agent, was found to be associated with pulmonary hypertension. Fenfluramine and dexfenfluramine, serotonin 2B receptor agonists, were observed to be linked with cardiac valvulopathy. Phenylpropanolamine, a norepinephrine-releasing agent, was found to be linked to stroke. Besides, there are also new drugs developed for the treatment of obesity. Tesofensine, which is a sympathomimetic drug in the family of Sibutramine, inhibits the reuptake of noradrenaline, dopamine and serotonin. It was developed for the Parkinson and Alzheimer disease previously, but afterward, significant weight reduction effect was observed. Cetilistat is another drug that inhibits pancreatic lipase and breaks down the triglycerides in the intestine. Also, Beloranib is another candidate drug for the obesity treatment that inhibits methionine aminopeptidase 2. Long-term phase 3 trials for new drugs continue for the treatment of obesity [148].

In summary, it is concluded that anti-obesity drugs have beneficial effects on metabolic parameters and weight loss in the obese patient with PCOS used in conjunction with diet and lifestyle modification. The administration of these drugs to the PCOS treatment should be under constant medical supervision due to the requirement of monitorization of possible side effects and dose adjustment.

CONSENT FOR PUBLICATION

Not applicable.

CONFLICT OF INTEREST

The author (editor) declares no conflict of interest, financial or otherwise.

ACKNOWLEDGEMENTS

None declared.

REFERENCES

[1]   Azziz R, Woods KS, Reyna R, Key TJ, Knochenhauer ES, Yildiz BO. The prevalence and features of the polycystic ovary syndrome in an unselected population. J Clin Endocrinol Metab 2004; 89(6): 2745-9.
[http://dx.doi.org/10.1210/jc.2003-032046] [PMID: 15181052]

[2]   Yildiz BO, Bozdag G, Yapici Z, Esinler I, Yarali H. Prevalence, phenotype and cardiometabolic risk of polycystic ovary syndrome under different diagnostic criteria. Hum Reprod 2012; 27(10): 3067-73.
[http://dx.doi.org/10.1093/humrep/des232] [PMID: 22777527]

[3]   Puurunen J, Piltonen T, Morin-Papunen L, *et al.* Unfavorable hormonal, metabolic, and inflammatory alterations persist after menopause in women with PCOS. J Clin Endocrinol Metab 2011; 96(6): 1827-34.
[http://dx.doi.org/10.1210/jc.2011-0039] [PMID: 21450988]

[4]   Shaw LJ, Bairey Merz CN, Azziz R, *et al.* Postmenopausal women with a history of irregular menses and elevated androgen measurements at high risk for worsening cardiovascular event-free survival: results from the National Institutes of Health--National Heart, Lung, and Blood Institute sponsored Women's Ischemia Syndrome Evaluation. J Clin Endocrinol Metab 2008; 93(4): 1276-84.
[http://dx.doi.org/10.1210/jc.2007-0425] [PMID: 18182456]

[5]   Diamanti-Kandarakis E, Dunaif A. Insulin resistance and the polycystic ovary syndrome revisited: an update on mechanisms and implications. Endocr Rev 2012; 33(6): 981-1030.
[http://dx.doi.org/10.1210/er.2011-1034] [PMID: 23065822]

[6]   Ferriman D, Purdie AW. The aetiology of oligomenorrhoea and/or hirsuties: a study of 467 patients. Postgrad Med J 1983; 59(687): 17-20.
[http://dx.doi.org/10.1136/pgmj.59.687.17] [PMID: 6866869]

[7]   Balen AH, Conway GS, Kaltsas G, *et al.* Polycystic ovary syndrome: the spectrum of the disorder in 1741 patients. Hum Reprod 1995; 10(8): 2107-11.
[http://dx.doi.org/10.1093/oxfordjournals.humrep.a136243] [PMID: 8567849]

[8]   DeUgarte CM, Bartolucci AA, Azziz R. Prevalence of insulin resistance in the polycystic ovary syndrome using the homeostasis model assessment. Fertil Steril 2005; 83(5): 1454-60.
[http://dx.doi.org/10.1016/j.fertnstert.2004.11.070] [PMID: 15866584]

[9]   Norman RJ, Masters L, Milner CR, Wang JX, Davies MJ. Relative risk of conversion from normoglycaemia to impaired glucose tolerance or non-insulin dependent diabetes mellitus in polycystic ovarian syndrome. Hum Reprod 2001; 16(9): 1995-8.
[http://dx.doi.org/10.1093/humrep/16.9.1995] [PMID: 11527911]

[10]   Krentz AJ, von Mühlen D, Barrett-Connor E. Searching for polycystic ovary syndrome in postmenopausal women: evidence of a dose-effect association with prevalent cardiovascular disease. Menopause 2007; 14(2): 284-92.
[http://dx.doi.org/10.1097/GME.0b013e31802cc7ab] [PMID: 17245231]

[11]   Legro RS, Kunselman AR, Dunaif A. Prevalence and predictors of dyslipidemia in women with polycystic ovary syndrome. Am J Med 2001; 111(8): 607-13.
[http://dx.doi.org/10.1016/S0002-9343(01)00948-2] [PMID: 11755503]

[12]   Wild S, Pierpoint T, McKeigue P, Jacobs H. Cardiovascular disease in women with polycystic ovary syndrome at long-term follow-up: a retrospective cohort study. Clin Endocrinol (Oxf) 2000; 52(5): 595-600.
[http://dx.doi.org/10.1046/j.1365-2265.2000.01000.x] [PMID: 10792339]

[13]   Jedel E, Waern M, Gustafson D, *et al.* Anxiety and depression symptoms in women with polycystic ovary syndrome compared with controls matched for body mass index. Hum Reprod 2010; 25(2): 450-6.
[http://dx.doi.org/10.1093/humrep/dep384] [PMID: 19933236]

[14]   Boomsma CM, Eijkemans MJ, Hughes EG, Visser GH, Fauser BC, Macklon NS. A meta-analysis of pregnancy outcomes in women with polycystic ovary syndrome. Hum Reprod Update 2006; 12(6): 673-83.
[http://dx.doi.org/10.1093/humupd/dml036] [PMID: 16891296]

[15]   Qin JZ, Pang LH, Li MJ, Fan XJ, Huang RD, Chen HY. Obstetric complications in women with polycystic ovary syndrome: a systematic review and meta-analysis. Reprod Biol Endocrinol 2013; 11: 56.
[http://dx.doi.org/10.1186/1477-7827-11-56] [PMID: 23800002]

[16]   Kjerulff LE, Sanchez-Ramos L, Duffy D. Pregnancy outcomes in women with polycystic ovary syndrome: a metaanalysis. Am J Obstet Gynecol 2011; 204(6): 558.e1-6.
[http://dx.doi.org/10.1016/j.ajog.2011.03.021] [PMID: 21752757]

[17]   Hart R, Doherty DA. The potential implications of a PCOS diagnosis on a woman's long-term health using data linkage. J Clin Endocrinol Metab 2015; 100(3): 911-9.
[http://dx.doi.org/10.1210/jc.2014-3886] [PMID: 25532045]

[18]   Zawadzki JK, Dunaif A. Diagnostic criteria for polycystic ovary syndrome; towards a rational approach.Polycystic ovary syndrome. Boston: Blackwell Scientific 1992; pp. 377-84.

[19]   Rotterdam ESHRE/ASRM-Sponsored PCOS Consensus Workshop Group. Revised 2003 consensus on diagnostic criteria and long-term health risks related to polycystic ovary syndrome. Fertil Steril 2004; 81(1): 19-25.
[http://dx.doi.org/10.1016/j.fertnstert.2003.10.004] [PMID: 14711538]

[20]   National Institutes of Health. Evidence-based methodology workshop on polycystic ovary syndrome 2012.https://prevention.nih.gov/docs/programs/pcos/FinalReport.pdf

[21]   Azziz R, Carmina E, Dewailly D, *et al.* Androgen Excess Society. Positions statement: criteria for defining polycystic ovary syndrome as a predominantly hyperandrogenic syndrome: an Androgen Excess Society guideline. J Clin Endocrinol Metab 2006; 91(11): 4237-45.
[http://dx.doi.org/10.1210/jc.2006-0178] [PMID: 16940456]

[22]   Azziz R, Carmina E, Dewailly D, *et al.* Task Force on the Phenotype of the Polycystic Ovary Syndrome of The Androgen Excess and PCOS Society. The Androgen Excess and PCOS Society criteria for the polycystic ovary syndrome: the complete task force report. Fertil Steril 2009; 91(2): 456-88.
[http://dx.doi.org/10.1016/j.fertnstert.2008.06.035] [PMID: 18950759]

[23]   Çelik E, Türkçüoğlu I, Ata B, *et al.* Metabolic and carbohydrate characteristics of different phenotypes of polycystic ovary syndrome. J Turk Ger Gynecol Assoc 2016; 17(4): 201-8.
[http://dx.doi.org/10.5152/jtgga.2016.16133] [PMID: 27990089]

[24]   Boyle JA, Cunningham J, O'Dea K, Dunbar T, Norman RJ. Prevalence of polycystic ovary syndrome in a sample of Indigenous women in Darwin, Australia. Med J Aust 2012; 196(1): 62-6.
[http://dx.doi.org/10.5694/mja11.10553] [PMID: 22256938]

[25]   Ma YM, Li R, Qiao J, *et al.* Characteristics of abnormal menstrual cycle and polycystic ovary syndrome in community and hospital populations. Chin Med J (Engl) 2010; 123(16): 2185-9.
[PMID: 20819662]

[26]   Linné Y. Effects of obesity on women's reproduction and complications during pregnancy. Obes Rev 2004; 5(3): 137-43.
[http://dx.doi.org/10.1111/j.1467-789X.2004.00147.x] [PMID: 15245382]

[27]   Türkçüoğlu I, Kafkasli A, Meydanli MM, Ozyalin F, Taşkapan C. Independent predictors of

cardiovascular risk in polycystic ovarian syndrome. Gynecol Endocrinol 2011; 27(11): 915-9.
[http://dx.doi.org/10.3109/09513590.2010.551566] [PMID: 21294689]

[28]   Moschos S, Chan JL, Mantzoros CS. Leptin and reproduction: a review. Fertil Steril 2002; 77(3): 433-44.
[http://dx.doi.org/10.1016/S0015-0282(01)03010-2] [PMID: 11872190]

[29]   Spicer LJ. Leptin: a possible metabolic signal affecting reproduction. Domest Anim Endocrinol 2001; 21(4): 251-70.
[http://dx.doi.org/10.1016/S0739-7240(01)00120-5] [PMID: 11872320]

[30]   Gil-Campos M, Cañete RR, Gil A. Adiponectin, the missing link in insulin resistance and obesity. Clin Nutr 2004; 23(5): 963-74.
[http://dx.doi.org/10.1016/j.clnu.2004.04.010] [PMID: 15380884]

[31]   Gosman GG, Katcher HI, Legro RS. Obesity and the role of gut and adipose hormones in female reproduction. Hum Reprod Update 2006; 12(5): 585-601.
[http://dx.doi.org/10.1093/humupd/dml024] [PMID: 16775192]

[32]   Sir-Petermann T, Angel B, Maliqueo M, et al. Insulin secretion in women who have polycystic ovary syndrome and carry the Gly972Arg variant of insulin receptor substrate-1 in response to a high-glycemic or low-glycemic carbohydrate load. Nutrition 2004; 20(10): 905-10.
[http://dx.doi.org/10.1016/j.nut.2004.08.017] [PMID: 15474880]

[33]   Douglas CC, Gower BA, Darnell BE, Ovalle F, Oster RA, Azziz R. Role of diet in the treatment of polycystic ovary syndrome. Fertil Steril 2006; 85(3): 679-88.
[http://dx.doi.org/10.1016/j.fertnstert.2005.08.045] [PMID: 16500338]

[34]   Billig H, Chun SY, Eisenhauer K, Hsueh AJ. Gonadal cell apoptosis: hormone-regulated cell demise. Hum Reprod Update 1996; 2(2): 103-17.
[http://dx.doi.org/10.1093/humupd/2.2.103] [PMID: 9079407]

[35]   McCartney CR, Prendergast KA, Chhabra S, et al. The association of obesity and hyperandrogenemia during the pubertal transition in girls: obesity as a potential factor in the genesis of postpubertal hyperandrogenism. J Clin Endocrinol Metab 2006; 91(5): 1714-22.
[http://dx.doi.org/10.1210/jc.2005-1852] [PMID: 16492701]

[36]   Diamanti-Kandarakis E, Papailiou J, Palimeri S. Hyperandrogenemia: pathophysiology and its role in ovulatory dysfunction in PCOS. Pediatr Endocrinol Rev 2006; 3 (Suppl. 1): 198-204.
[PMID: 16641860]

[37]   Franks S, McCarthy MI, Hardy K. Development of polycystic ovary syndrome: involvement of genetic and environmental factors. Int J Androl 2006; 29(1): 278-85.
[http://dx.doi.org/10.1111/j.1365-2605.2005.00623.x] [PMID: 16390494]

[38]   Ibáñez L, Ferrer A, Ong K, Amin R, Dunger D, de Zegher F. Insulin sensitization early after menarche prevents progression from precocious pubarche to polycystic ovary syndrome. J Pediatr 2004; 144(1): 23-9.
[http://dx.doi.org/10.1016/j.jpeds.2003.08.015] [PMID: 14722514]

[39]   Legro RS. Detection of insulin resistance and its treatment in adolescents with polycystic ovary syndrome. J Pediatr Endocrinol Metab 2002; 15 (Suppl. 5): 1367-78.
[PMID: 12510993]

[40]   Robinson S, Chan SP, Spacey S, Anyaoku V, Johnston DG, Franks S. Postprandial thermogenesis is reduced in polycystic ovary syndrome and is associated with increased insulin resistance. Clin Endocrinol (Oxf) 1992; 36(6): 537-43.
[http://dx.doi.org/10.1111/j.1365-2265.1992.tb02262.x] [PMID: 1424179]

[41]   Hirschberg AL, Naessén S, Stridsberg M, Byström B, Holtet J. Impaired cholecystokinin secretion and disturbed appetite regulation in women with polycystic ovary syndrome. Gynecol Endocrinol 2004; 19(2): 79-87.

[http://dx.doi.org/10.1080/09513590400002300] [PMID: 15624269]

[42]   McNeely W, Benfield P. Orlistat. Drugs 1998; 56(2): 241-9.
       [http://dx.doi.org/10.2165/00003495-199856020-00007] [PMID: 9711448]

[43]   Heal DJ, Gosden J, Smith SL. What is the prognosis for new centrally-acting anti-obesity drugs?
       Neuropharmacology 2012; 63(1): 132-46.
       [http://dx.doi.org/10.1016/j.neuropharm.2012.01.017] [PMID: 22313529]

[44]   Hogan S, Fleury A, Hadvary P, *et al.* Studies on the antiobesity activity of tetrahydrolipstatin, a potent
       and selective inhibitor of pancreatic lipase. Int J Obes 1987; 11 (Suppl. 3): 35-42.
       [PMID: 3440690]

[45]   Hauptman J, Lucas C, Boldrin MN, Collins H, Segal KR. Orlistat in the long-term treatment of obesity
       in primary care settings. Arch Fam Med 2000; 9(2): 160-7.
       [http://dx.doi.org/10.1001/archfami.9.2.160] [PMID: 10693734]

[46]   Heymsfield SB, Segal KR, Hauptman J, *et al.* Effects of weight loss with orlistat on glucose tolerance
       and progression to type 2 diabetes in obese adults. Arch Intern Med 2000; 160(9): 1321-6.
       [http://dx.doi.org/10.1001/archinte.160.9.1321] [PMID: 10809036]

[47]   Torgerson JS, Hauptman J, Boldrin MN, Sjöström L. XENical in the prevention of diabetes in obese
       subjects (XENDOS) study: a randomized study of orlistat as an adjunct to lifestyle changes for the
       prevention of type 2 diabetes in obese patients. Diabetes Care 2004; 27(1): 155-61.
       [http://dx.doi.org/10.2337/diacare.27.1.155] [PMID: 14693982]

[48]   Siebenhofer A, Horvath K, Jeitler K, *et al.* Long-term effects of weight-reducing drugs in hypertensive
       patients. Cochrane Database Syst Rev 2009; (3): CD007654.
       [PMID: 19588440]

[49]   Jayagopal V, Kilpatrick ES, Holding S, Jennings PE, Atkin SL. Orlistat is as beneficial as metformin
       in the treatment of polycystic ovarian syndrome. J Clin Endocrinol Metab 2005; 90(2): 729-33.
       [http://dx.doi.org/10.1210/jc.2004-0176] [PMID: 15536162]

[50]   Panidis D, Farmakiotis D, Rousso D, Kourtis A, Katsikis I, Krassas G. Obesity, weight loss, and the
       polycystic ovary syndrome: effect of treatment with diet and orlistat for 24 weeks on insulin resistance
       and androgen levels. Fertil Steril 2008; 89(4): 899-906.
       [http://dx.doi.org/10.1016/j.fertnstert.2007.04.043] [PMID: 17980364]

[51]   Panidis D, Tziomalos K, Papadakis E, *et al.* The role of orlistat combined with lifestyle changes in the
       management of overweight and obese patients with polycystic ovary syndrome. Clin Endocrinol (Oxf)
       2014; 80(3): 432-8.
       [http://dx.doi.org/10.1111/cen.12305] [PMID: 23909452]

[52]   Padwal RS, Majumdar SR. Drug treatments for obesity: orlistat, sibutramine, and rimonabant. Lancet
       2007; 369(9555): 71-7.
       [http://dx.doi.org/10.1016/S0140-6736(07)60033-6] [PMID: 17208644]

[53]   Zhi J, Melia AT, Funk C, *et al.* Metabolic profiles of minimally absorbed orlistat in obese/overweight
       volunteers. J Clin Pharmacol 1996; 36(11): 1006-11.
       [http://dx.doi.org/10.1177/009127009603601104] [PMID: 8973989]

[54]   Sjöström L, Rissanen A, Andersen T, *et al.* European Multicentre Orlistat Study Group. Randomised
       placebo-controlled trial of orlistat for weight loss and prevention of weight regain in obese patients.
       Lancet 1998; 352(9123): 167-72.
       [http://dx.doi.org/10.1016/S0140-6736(97)11509-4] [PMID: 9683204]

[55]   FDA drug safety communication. Completed safety review of Xenical/Alli (orlistat) and severe liver
       injury 2010. Available at: http://www.fda.gov/Drugs/DrugSafety/PostmarketDrugSafetyInformation
       forPatientsandProviders/ucm213038.htm

[56]   Rucker D, Padwal R, Li SK, Curioni C, Lau DC. Long term pharmacotherapy for obesity and
       overweight: updated meta-analysis. BMJ 2007; 335(7631): 1194-9.

[http://dx.doi.org/10.1136/bmj.39385.413113.25] [PMID: 18006966]

[57]   Park CY, Kim YS, Ryu MS, Nam SY, Park HS, Kim SM. A phase 3 double-blind, parallel-group, placebo-controlled trial of the efficacy and safety of sibutramine (Reductil) in the treatment of obese patients. J Korean Soc Study Obes 2001; 10: 336-47.

[58]   Nisoli E, Carruba MO. An assessment of the safety and efficacy of sibutramine, an anti-obesity drug with a novel mechanism of action. Obes Rev 2000; 1(2): 127-39.
[http://dx.doi.org/10.1046/j.1467-789x.2000.00020.x] [PMID: 12119986]

[59]   Mannucci E, Dicembrini I, Rotella F, Rotella CM. Orlistat and sibutramine beyond weight loss. Nutr Metab Cardiovasc Dis 2008; 18(5): 342-8.
[http://dx.doi.org/10.1016/j.numecd.2007.03.010] [PMID: 17928208]

[60]   Lindholm A, Bixo M, Björn I, *et al.* Effect of sibutramine on weight reduction in women with polycystic ovary syndrome: a randomized, double-blind, placebo-controlled trial. Fertil Steril 2008; 89(5): 1221-8.
[http://dx.doi.org/10.1016/j.fertnstert.2007.05.002] [PMID: 17603048]

[61]   Wadden TA, Berkowitz RI, Womble LG, *et al.* Randomized trial of lifestyle modification and pharmacotherapy for obesity. N Engl J Med 2005; 353(20): 2111-20.
[http://dx.doi.org/10.1056/NEJMoa050156] [PMID: 16291981]

[62]   Sabuncu T, Harma M, Harma M, Nazligul Y, Kilic F. Sibutramine has a positive effect on clinical and metabolic parameters in obese patients with polycystic ovary syndrome. Fertil Steril 2003; 80(5): 1199-204.
[http://dx.doi.org/10.1016/S0015-0282(03)02162-9] [PMID: 14607575]

[63]   Bosello O, Carruba MO, Ferrannini E, Rotella CM. Sibutramine lost and found. Eat Weight Disord 2002; 7(3): 161-7.
[http://dx.doi.org/10.1007/BF03327453] [PMID: 12452247]

[64]   James WP, Caterson ID, Coutinho W, *et al.* SCOUT Investigators. Effect of sibutramine on cardiovascular outcomes in overweight and obese subjects. N Engl J Med 2010; 363(10): 905-17.
[http://dx.doi.org/10.1056/NEJMoa1003114] [PMID: 20818901]

[65]   Torp-Pedersen C, Caterson I, Coutinho W, *et al.* SCOUT Investigators. Cardiovascular responses to weight management and sibutramine in high-risk subjects: an analysis from the SCOUT trial. Eur Heart J 2007; 28(23): 2915-23.
[http://dx.doi.org/10.1093/eurheartj/ehm217] [PMID: 17595194]

[66]   Astrup A. Drug management of obesity--efficacy *versus* safety. N Engl J Med 2010; 363(3): 288-90.
[http://dx.doi.org/10.1056/NEJMe1004076] [PMID: 20647205]

[67]   Harrison-Woolrych M, Ashton J, Herbison P. Fatal and non-fatal cardiovascular events in a general population prescribed sibutramine in New Zealand: a prospective cohort study. Drug Saf 2010; 33(7): 605-13.
[http://dx.doi.org/10.2165/11532440-000000000-00000] [PMID: 20553061]

[68]   Di Marzo V, Bifulco M, De Petrocellis L. The endocannabinoid system and its therapeutic exploitation. Nat Rev Drug Discov 2004; 3(9): 771-84.
[http://dx.doi.org/10.1038/nrd1495] [PMID: 15340387]

[69]   Van Gaal LF, Rissanen AM, Scheen AJ, Ziegler O, Rössner S. RIO-Europe Study Group. Effects of the cannabinoid-1 receptor blocker rimonabant on weight reduction and cardiovascular risk factors in overweight patients: 1-year experience from the RIO-Europe study. Lancet 2005; 365(9468): 1389-97.
[http://dx.doi.org/10.1016/S0140-6736(05)66374-X] [PMID: 15836887]

[70]   Pi-Sunyer FX, Aronne LJ, Heshmati HM, Devin J, Rosenstock J. RIO-North America Study Group. Effect of rimonabant, a cannabinoid-1 receptor blocker, on weight and cardiometabolic risk factors in overweight or obese patients: RIO-North America: a randomized controlled trial. JAMA 2006; 295(7): 761-75.

[http://dx.doi.org/10.1001/jama.295.7.761] [PMID: 16478899]

[71] Després JP, Golay A, Sjöström L. Rimonabant in Obesity-Lipids Study Group. Effects of rimonabant on metabolic risk factors in overweight patients with dyslipidemia. N Engl J Med 2005; 353(20): 2121-34.
[http://dx.doi.org/10.1056/NEJMoa044537] [PMID: 16291982]

[72] Scheen AJ, Finer N, Hollander P, Jensen MD, Van Gaal LF. RIO-Diabetes Study Group. Efficacy and tolerability of rimonabant in overweight or obese patients with type 2 diabetes: a randomised controlled study. Lancet 2006; 368(9548): 1660-72.
[http://dx.doi.org/10.1016/S0140-6736(06)69571-8] [PMID: 17098084]

[73] Sathyapalan T, Cho LW, Kilpatrick ES, Coady AM, Atkin SL. A comparison between rimonabant and metformin in reducing biochemical hyperandrogenaemia and insulin resistance in patients with polycystic ovary syndrome (PCOS): a randomized open-label parallel study. Clin Endocrinol (Oxf) 2008; 69(6): 931-5.
[http://dx.doi.org/10.1111/j.1365-2265.2008.03260.x] [PMID: 18410553]

[74] Samat A, Tomlinson B, Taheri S, Thomas GN. Rimonabant for the treatment of obesity. Recent Patents Cardiovasc Drug Discov 2008; 3(3): 187-93.
[http://dx.doi.org/10.2174/157489008786264014] [PMID: 18991793]

[75] Knowler WC, Barrett-Connor E, Fowler SE, *et al.* Diabetes Prevention Program Research Group. Reduction in the incidence of type 2 diabetes with lifestyle intervention or metformin. N Engl J Med 2002; 346(6): 393-403.
[http://dx.doi.org/10.1056/NEJMoa012512] [PMID: 11832527]

[76] Attia GR, Rainey WE, Carr BR. Metformin directly inhibits androgen production in human thecal cells. Fertil Steril 2001; 76(3): 517-24.
[http://dx.doi.org/10.1016/S0015-0282(01)01975-6] [PMID: 11532475]

[77] Duleba AJ, Pawelczyk LA, Yuen BH, Moon YS. Insulin actions on ovarian steroidogenesis are not modulated by metformin. Hum Reprod 1993; 8(8): 1194-8.
[http://dx.doi.org/10.1093/oxfordjournals.humrep.a138227] [PMID: 8408516]

[78] Velazquez EM, Mendoza S, Hamer T, Sosa F, Glueck CJ. Metformin therapy in polycystic ovary syndrome reduces hyperinsulinemia, insulin resistance, hyperandrogenemia, and systolic blood pressure, while facilitating normal menses and pregnancy. Metabolism 1994; 43(5): 647-54.
[http://dx.doi.org/10.1016/0026-0495(94)90209-7] [PMID: 8177055]

[79] Pirwany IR, Yates RW, Cameron IT, Fleming R. Effects of the insulin sensitizing drug metformin on ovarian function, follicular growth and ovulation rate in obese women with oligomenorrhoea. Hum Reprod 1999; 14(12): 2963-8.
[http://dx.doi.org/10.1093/humrep/14.12.2963] [PMID: 10601079]

[80] Kolodziejczyk B, Duleba AJ, Spaczynski RZ, Pawelczyk L. Metformin therapy decreases hyperandrogenism and hyperinsulinemia in women with polycystic ovary syndrome. Fertil Steril 2000; 73(6): 1149-54.
[http://dx.doi.org/10.1016/S0015-0282(00)00501-X] [PMID: 10856473]

[81] Moghetti P, Castello R, Negri C, *et al.* Metformin effects on clinical features, endocrine and metabolic profiles, and insulin sensitivity in polycystic ovary syndrome: a randomized, double-blind, placebo-controlled 6-month trial, followed by open, long-term clinical evaluation. J Clin Endocrinol Metab 2000; 85(1): 139-46.
[PMID: 10634377]

[82] Nestler JE, Jakubowicz DJ. Lean women with polycystic ovary syndrome respond to insulin reduction with decreases in ovarian P450c17 alpha activity and serum androgens. J Clin Endocrinol Metab 1997; 82(12): 4075-9.
[PMID: 9398716]

[83] Lord JM, Flight IH, Norman RJ. Insulin-sensitising drugs (metformin, troglitazone, rosiglitazone,

pioglitazone, D-chiro-inositol) for polycystic ovary syndrome. Cochrane Database Syst Rev 2003; (3): CD003053.
[PMID: 12917943]

[84]   Harborne L, Fleming R, Lyall H, Sattar N, Norman J. Metformin or antiandrogen in the treatment of hirsutism in polycystic ovary syndrome. J Clin Endocrinol Metab 2003; 88(9): 4116-23.
[http://dx.doi.org/10.1210/jc.2003-030424] [PMID: 12970273]

[85]   Legro RS, Barnhart HX, Schlaff WD, *et al.* Cooperative Multicenter Reproductive Medicine Network. Clomiphene, metformin, or both for infertility in the polycystic ovary syndrome. N Engl J Med 2007; 356(6): 551-66.
[http://dx.doi.org/10.1056/NEJMoa063971] [PMID: 17287476]

[86]   Nieuwenhuis-Ruifrok AE, Kuchenbecker WK, Hoek A, Middleton P, Norman RJ. Insulin sensitizing drugs for weight loss in women of reproductive age who are overweight or obese: systematic review and meta-analysis. Hum Reprod Update 2009; 15(1): 57-68.
[http://dx.doi.org/10.1093/humupd/dmn043] [PMID: 18927072]

[87]   Tang T, Lord JM, Norman RJ, Yasmin E, Balen AH. Insulin-sensitising drugs (metformin, rosiglitazone, pioglitazone, D-chiro-inositol) for women with polycystic ovary syndrome, oligo amenorrhoea and subfertility. Cochrane Database Syst Rev 2012; (5): CD003053.
[PMID: 22592687]

[88]   Bolen S, Feldman L, Vassy J, *et al.* Systematic review: comparative effectiveness and safety of oral medications for type 2 diabetes mellitus. Ann Intern Med 2007; 147(6): 386-99.
[http://dx.doi.org/10.7326/0003-4819-147-6-200709180-00178] [PMID: 17638715]

[89]   Khurana R, Malik IS. Metformin: safety in cardiac patients. Heart 2010; 96(2): 99-102.
[PMID: 19564648]

[90]   Vigersky RA, Filmore-Nassar A, Glass AR. Thyrotropin suppression by metformin. J Clin Endocrinol Metab 2006; 91(1): 225-7.
[http://dx.doi.org/10.1210/jc.2005-1210] [PMID: 16219720]

[91]   Seli E, Duleba AJ. Treatment of PCOS with metformin and other insulin-sensitizing agents. Curr Diab Rep 2004; 4(1): 69-75.
[http://dx.doi.org/10.1007/s11892-004-0014-8] [PMID: 14764283]

[92]   Lebovitz HE. Differentiating members of the thiazolidinedione class: a focus on safety. Diabetes Metab Res Rev 2002; 18 (Suppl. 2): S23-9.
[http://dx.doi.org/10.1002/dmrr.252] [PMID: 11921435]

[93]   Dunaif A, Scott D, Finegood D, Quintana B, Whitcomb R. The insulin-sensitizing agent troglitazone improves metabolic and reproductive abnormalities in the polycystic ovary syndrome. J Clin Endocrinol Metab 1996; 81(9): 3299-306.
[PMID: 8784087]

[94]   Hasegawa I, Murakawa H, Suzuki M, Yamamoto Y, Kurabayashi T, Tanaka K. Effect of troglitazone on endocrine and ovulatory performance in women with insulin resistance-related polycystic ovary syndrome. Fertil Steril 1999; 71(2): 323-7.
[http://dx.doi.org/10.1016/S0015-0282(98)00454-3] [PMID: 9988406]

[95]   Mitwally MF, Kuscu NK, Yalcinkaya TM. High ovulatory rates with use of troglitazone in clomiphene-resistant women with polycystic ovary syndrome. Hum Reprod 1999; 14(11): 2700-3.
[http://dx.doi.org/10.1093/humrep/14.11.2700] [PMID: 10548604]

[96]   Azziz R, Ehrmann D, Legro RS, *et al.* PCOS/Troglitazone Study Group. Troglitazone improves ovulation and hirsutism in the polycystic ovary syndrome: a multicenter, double blind, placebo-controlled trial. J Clin Endocrinol Metab 2001; 86(4): 1626-32.
[PMID: 11297595]

[97]   Graham DJ, Green L, Senior JR, Nourjah P. Troglitazone-induced liver failure: a case study. Am J

Med 2003; 114(4): 299-306.
[http://dx.doi.org/10.1016/S0002-9343(02)01529-2] [PMID: 12681458]

[98]   Shobokshi A, Shaarawy M. Correction of insulin resistance and hyperandrogenism in polycystic ovary syndrome by combined rosiglitazone and clomiphene citrate therapy. J Soc Gynecol Investig 2003; 10(2): 99-104.
[http://dx.doi.org/10.1016/S1071-5576(02)00260-5] [PMID: 12593999]

[99]   Ghazeeri G, Kutteh WH, Bryer-Ash M, Haas D, Ke RW. Effect of rosiglitazone on spontaneous and clomiphene citrate-induced ovulation in women with polycystic ovary syndrome. Fertil Steril 2003; 79(3): 562-6.
[http://dx.doi.org/10.1016/S0015-0282(02)04843-4] [PMID: 12620440]

[100] Lago RM, Singh PP, Nesto RW. Congestive heart failure and cardiovascular death in patients with prediabetes and type 2 diabetes given thiazolidinediones: a meta-analysis of randomised clinical trials. Lancet 2007; 370(9593): 1129-36.
[http://dx.doi.org/10.1016/S0140-6736(07)61514-1] [PMID: 17905165]

[101] Salzman A, Patel J. Rosiglitazone therapy is not associated with hepatotoxicity. Diabetologia 1999; 42 (Suppl. 1): A98.

[102] Yki-Järvinen H. Thiazolidinediones. N Engl J Med 2004; 351(11): 1106-18.
[http://dx.doi.org/10.1056/NEJMra041001] [PMID: 15356308]

[103] Romualdi D, Guido M, Ciampelli M, *et al.* Selective effects of pioglitazone on insulin and androgen abnormalities in normo- and hyperinsulinaemic obese patients with polycystic ovary syndrome. Hum Reprod 2003; 18(6): 1210-8.
[http://dx.doi.org/10.1093/humrep/deg264] [PMID: 12773448]

[104] Glueck CJ, Moreira A, Goldenberg N, Sieve L, Wang P. Pioglitazone and metformin in obese women with polycystic ovary syndrome not optimally responsive to metformin. Hum Reprod 2003; 18(8): 1618-25.
[http://dx.doi.org/10.1093/humrep/deg343] [PMID: 12871871]

[105] Glintborg D, Hermann AP, Andersen M, *et al.* Effect of pioglitazone on glucose metabolism and luteinizing hormone secretion in women with polycystic ovary syndrome. Fertil Steril 2006; 86(2): 385-97.
[http://dx.doi.org/10.1016/j.fertnstert.2005.12.067] [PMID: 16782094]

[106] May LD, Lefkowitch JH, Kram MT, Rubin DE. Mixed hepatocellular-cholestatic liver injury after pioglitazone therapy. Ann Intern Med 2002; 136(6): 449-52.
[http://dx.doi.org/10.7326/0003-4819-136-6-200203190-00008] [PMID: 11900497]

[107] Maeda K. Hepatocellular injury in a patient receiving pioglitazone. Ann Intern Med 2001; 135(4): 306.
[http://dx.doi.org/10.7326/0003-4819-135-4-200108210-00029] [PMID: 11511159]

[108] Larner J. Multiple pathways in insulin signaling: fitting the covalent and allosteric puzzle pieces together. Endocr J 1994; 2(3): 167-71.

[109] Ortmeyer HK, Bodkin NL, Lilley K, Larner J, Hansen BC. Chiroinositol deficiency and insulin resistance. I. Urinary excretion rate of chiroinositol is directly associated with insulin resistance in spontaneously diabetic rhesus monkeys. Endocrinology 1993; 132(2): 640-5.
[http://dx.doi.org/10.1210/endo.132.2.8425483] [PMID: 8425483]

[110] Asplin I, Galasko G, Larner J. chiro-inositol deficiency and insulin resistance: a comparison of the chiro-inositol- and the myo-inositol-containing insulin mediators isolated from urine, hemodialysate, and muscle of control and type II diabetic subjects. Proc Natl Acad Sci USA 1993; 90(13): 5924-8.
[http://dx.doi.org/10.1073/pnas.90.13.5924] [PMID: 8392181]

[111] Nestler JE, Jakubowicz DJ, Reamer P, Gunn RD, Allan G. Ovulatory and metabolic effects of D-chiro-inositol in the polycystic ovary syndrome. N Engl J Med 1999; 340(17): 1314-20.
[http://dx.doi.org/10.1056/NEJM199904293401703] [PMID: 10219066]

[112] Gerli S, Papaleo E, Ferrari A, Di Renzo GC. Randomized, double blind placebo-controlled trial: effects of myo-inositol on ovarian function and metabolic factors in women with PCOS. Eur Rev Med Pharmacol Sci 2007; 11(5): 347-54.
[PMID: 18074942]

[113] Tan T, Bloom S. Gut hormones as therapeutic agents in treatment of diabetes and obesity. Curr Opin Pharmacol 2013; 13(6): 996-1001.
[http://dx.doi.org/10.1016/j.coph.2013.09.005] [PMID: 24060699]

[114] Sadry SA, Drucker DJ. Emerging combinatorial hormone therapies for the treatment of obesity and T2DM. Nat Rev Endocrinol 2013; 9(7): 425-33.
[http://dx.doi.org/10.1038/nrendo.2013.47] [PMID: 23478327]

[115] Cryer PE. Minireview: Glucagon in the pathogenesis of hypoglycemia and hyperglycemia in diabetes. Endocrinology 2012; 153(3): 1039-48.
[http://dx.doi.org/10.1210/en.2011-1499] [PMID: 22166985]

[116] Baggio LL, Drucker DJ. Biology of incretins: GLP-1 and GIP. Gastroenterology 2007; 132(6): 2131-57.
[http://dx.doi.org/10.1053/j.gastro.2007.03.054] [PMID: 17498508]

[117] Pocai A. Glucagon signaling in the heart: Activation or inhibition? Mol Metab 2014; 4(2): 81-2.
[http://dx.doi.org/10.1016/j.molmet.2014.12.004] [PMID: 25685695]

[118] Clements JN, Shealy KM. Liraglutide: an injectable option for the management of obesity. Ann Pharmacother 2015; 49(8): 938-44.
[http://dx.doi.org/10.1177/1060028015586806] [PMID: 25986009]

[119] Sweeting AN, Tabet E, Caterson ID, Markovic TP. Management of obesity and cardiometabolic risk - role of phentermine/extended release topiramate. Diabetes Metab Syndr Obes 2014; 7: 35-44.
[PMID: 24550678]

[120] Hampp C, Kang EM, Borders-Hemphill V. Use of prescription antiobesity drugs in the United States. Pharmacotherapy 2013; 33(12): 1299-307.
[http://dx.doi.org/10.1002/phar.1342] [PMID: 24019195]

[121] Bates GW, Legro RS. Longterm management of Polycystic Ovarian Syndrome (PCOS). Mol Cell Endocrinol 2013; 373(1-2): 91-7.
[http://dx.doi.org/10.1016/j.mce.2012.10.029] [PMID: 23261983]

[122] Garvey WT, Ryan DH, Look M, *et al.* Two-year sustained weight loss and metabolic benefits with controlled-release phentermine/topiramate in obese and overweight adults (SEQUEL): a randomized, placebo-controlled, phase 3 extension study. Am J Clin Nutr 2012; 95(2): 297-308.
[http://dx.doi.org/10.3945/ajcn.111.024927] [PMID: 22158731]

[123] Munro JF, MacCuish AC, Wilson EM, Duncan LJ. Comparison of continuous and intermittent anorectic therapy in obesity. BMJ 1968; 1(5588): 352-4.
[http://dx.doi.org/10.1136/bmj.1.5588.352] [PMID: 15508204]

[124] Yanovski SZ, Yanovski JA. Long-term drug treatment for obesity: a systematic and clinical review. JAMA 2014; 311(1): 74-86.
[http://dx.doi.org/10.1001/jama.2013.281361] [PMID: 24231879]

[125] Fleming JW, McClendon KS, Riche DM. New obesity agents: lorcaserin and phentermine/topiramate. Ann Pharmacother 2013; 47(7-8): 1007-16.
[http://dx.doi.org/10.1345/aph.1R779] [PMID: 23800750]

[126] Ben-Menachem E, Axelsen M, Johanson EH, Stagge A, Smith U. Predictors of weight loss in adults with topiramate-treated epilepsy. Obes Res 2003; 11(4): 556-62.
[http://dx.doi.org/10.1038/oby.2003.78] [PMID: 12690085]

[127] Bray GA, Hollander P, Klein S, *et al.* A 6-month randomized, placebo-controlled, dose-ranging trial of

topiramate for weight loss in obesity. Obes Res 2003; 11(6): 722-33.
[http://dx.doi.org/10.1038/oby.2003.102] [PMID: 12805393]

[128] McElroy SL, Hudson JI, Capece JA, Beyers K, Fisher AC, Rosenthal NR. Topiramate Binge Eating Disorder Research Group. Topiramate for the treatment of binge eating disorder associated with obesity: a placebo-controlled study. Biol Psychiatry 2007; 61(9): 1039-48.
[http://dx.doi.org/10.1016/j.biopsych.2006.08.008] [PMID: 17258690]

[129] Allison DB, Gadde KM, Garvey WT, *et al*. Controlled-release phentermine/topiramate in severely obese adults: a randomized controlled trial (EQUIP). Obesity (Silver Spring) 2012; 20(2): 330-42.
[http://dx.doi.org/10.1038/oby.2011.330] [PMID: 22051941]

[130] Gadde KM, Allison DB, Ryan DH, *et al*. Effects of low-dose, controlled-release, phentermine plus topiramate combination on weight and associated comorbidities in overweight and obese adults (CONQUER): a randomised, placebo-controlled, phase 3 trial. Lancet 2011; 377(9774): 1341-52.
[http://dx.doi.org/10.1016/S0140-6736(11)60205-5] [PMID: 21481449]

[131] Colman E, Golden J, Roberts M, Egan A, Weaver J, Rosebraugh C. The FDA's assessment of two drugs for chronic weight management. N Engl J Med 2012; 367(17): 1577-9.
[http://dx.doi.org/10.1056/NEJMp1211277] [PMID: 23050510]

[132] Margulis AV, Mitchell AA, Gilboa SM, *et al*. National Birth Defects Prevention Study. Use of topiramate in pregnancy and risk of oral clefts. Am J Obstet Gynecol 2012; 207(5): 405.e1-7.
[http://dx.doi.org/10.1016/j.ajog.2012.07.008] [PMID: 22917484]

[133] Berger JJ, Bates GW Jr. Optimal management of subfertility in polycystic ovary syndrome. Int J Womens Health 2014; 6: 613-21.
[PMID: 24966697]

[134] Moran LJ, Pasquali R, Teede HJ, Hoeger KM, Norman RJ. Treatment of obesity in polycystic ovary syndrome: a position statement of the Androgen Excess and Polycystic Ovary Syndrome Society. Fertil Steril 2009; 92(6): 1966-82.
[http://dx.doi.org/10.1016/j.fertnstert.2008.09.018] [PMID: 19062007]

[135] Blundell JE. Is there a role for serotonin (5-hydroxytryptamine) in feeding? Int J Obes 1977; 1(1): 15-42.
[PMID: 361584]

[136] Launay JM, Hervé P, Peoc'h K, *et al*. Function of the serotonin 5-hydroxytryptamine 2B receptor in pulmonary hypertension. Nat Med 2002; 8(10): 1129-35.
[http://dx.doi.org/10.1038/nm764] [PMID: 12244304]

[137] Martin CK, Redman LM, Zhang J, *et al*. Lorcaserin, a 5-HT(2C) receptor agonist, reduces body weight by decreasing energy intake without influencing energy expenditure. J Clin Endocrinol Metab 2011; 96(3): 837-45.
[http://dx.doi.org/10.1210/jc.2010-1848] [PMID: 21190985]

[138] Lam DD, Przydzial MJ, Ridley SH, *et al*. Serotonin 5-HT2C receptor agonist promotes hypophagia *via* downstream activation of melanocortin 4 receptors. Endocrinology 2008; 149(3): 1323-8.
[http://dx.doi.org/10.1210/en.2007-1321] [PMID: 18039773]

[139] Taylor JR, Dietrich E, Powell J. Lorcaserin for weight management. Diabetes Metab Syndr Obes 2013; 6: 209-16.
[http://dx.doi.org/10.2147/DMSO.S36276] [PMID: 23788837]

[140] O'Neil PM, Smith SR, Weissman NJ, *et al*. Randomized placebo-controlled clinical trial of lorcaserin for weight loss in type 2 diabetes mellitus: the BLOOM-DM study. Obesity (Silver Spring) 2012; 20(7): 1426-36.
[http://dx.doi.org/10.1038/oby.2012.66] [PMID: 22421927]

[141] Smith SR, Weissman NJ, Anderson CM, *et al*. Behavioral Modification and Lorcaserin for Overweight and Obesity Management (BLOOM) Study Group. Multicenter, placebo-controlled trial of

lorcaserin for weight management. N Engl J Med 2010; 363(3): 245-56.
[http://dx.doi.org/10.1056/NEJMoa0909809] [PMID: 20647200]

[142] Shram MJ, Schoedel KA, Bartlett C, Shazer RL, Anderson CM, Sellers EM. Evaluation of the abuse potential of lorcaserin, a serotonin 2C (5-HT2C) receptor agonist, in recreational polydrug users. Clin Pharmacol Ther 2011; 89(5): 683-92.
[http://dx.doi.org/10.1038/clpt.2011.20] [PMID: 21412231]

[143] Dwoskin LP, Rauhut AS, King-Pospisil KA, Bardo MT. Review of the pharmacology and clinical profile of bupropion, an antidepressant and tobacco use cessation agent. CNS Drug Rev 2006; 12(3-4): 178-207.
[http://dx.doi.org/10.1111/j.1527-3458.2006.00178.x] [PMID: 17227286]

[144] Apovian CM, Aronne L, Rubino D, *et al.* COR-II Study Group. A randomized, phase 3 trial of naltrexone SR/bupropion SR on weight and obesity-related risk factors (COR-II). Obesity (Silver Spring) 2013; 21(5): 935-43.
[http://dx.doi.org/10.1002/oby.20309] [PMID: 23408728]

[145] Greenway FL, Whitehouse MJ, Guttadauria M, *et al.* Rational design of a combination medication for the treatment of obesity. Obesity (Silver Spring) 2009; 17(1): 30-9.
[http://dx.doi.org/10.1038/oby.2008.461] [PMID: 18997675]

[146] Ibrahim N, Bosch MA, Smart JL, *et al.* Hypothalamic proopiomelanocortin neurons are glucose responsive and express K(ATP) channels. Endocrinology 2003; 144(4): 1331-40.
[http://dx.doi.org/10.1210/en.2002-221033] [PMID: 12639916]

[147] Billes SK, Sinnayah P, Cowley MA. Naltrexone/bupropion for obesity: an investigational combination pharmacotherapy for weight loss. Pharmacol Res 2014; 84: 1-11.
[http://dx.doi.org/10.1016/j.phrs.2014.04.004] [PMID: 24754973]

[148] Narayanaswami V, Dwoskin LP. Obesity: Current and potential pharmacotherapeutics and targets. Pharmacol Ther 2016. pii: S0163-7258(16)30194-2

CHAPTER 3

Sirtuins and Bile Acids: Potential Anti-obesity Strategies Targeting Mitochondria

João Alves Amorim[1,#], João Soeiro Teodoro[1,2,#], Carlos Marques Palmeira[1,2] and Anabela Pinto Rolo[1,2,*]

[1] *CNC – Center for Neuroscience and Cell Biology, University of Coimbra, Portugal*

[2] *Department of Life Sciences, University of Coimbra, Portugal*

Abstract: Obesity is the most prevalent, costly and harmful epidemic of the 21st century. Considered a disease of excess, it is now known that it doesn't take just to have increased food intake with reduced expenditure, but a number of other factors have increasingly been reported to have similar influence. At the center of all metabolic pathways lie mitochondria. The powerhouses of the cell is the cornerstone of cutting-edge research on metabolic alterations in obesity and related conditions. Boosting mitochondrial activity, removing damaged units and producing new, energy-consuming mitochondria are some of the strategies currently used in the development to combat obesity. In this chapter, we will focus on the near-future applicability of therapeutic strategies that achieve this goal. Specifically, we will address how sirtuin-activating compounds and bile acids promote mitochondrial homeostasis in spite of constant fat and carbohydrate insult, resulting in the unclogging of metabolic pathways and promoting the restoration of a normal energetic, redox and functional cellular environment. Activation of sirtuins 1 and 3 stimulates mitochondrial oxidative metabolism and prevents the accumulation of reduced substrates, a major factor driving cellular dysfunction in the setting of obesity. By acting on adipose tissue and stimulating energy expenditure, which may be associated with an increase in fatty acid oxidation, bile acids improve metabolic status.

Keywords: Adipose tissue, Bile acids, Biogenesis, Caloric restriction, Chenodeoxycholic acid, Energy expenditure, Metabolism, Mitochondria, Mitochondrial dysfunction, Mitophagy, Obesity, Sirtuins, Therapeutic strategies, FXR, OXPHOS, PGC-1α, SIRT1, SIRT3, TGR5.

* **Corresponding author Anabela Pinto Rolo:** Department of Life Sciences of the Faculty of Science and Technology of the University of Coimbra, Calçada Martim de Freitas, 3000-456 Coimbra, Portugal; Tel: 239 240 700; Fax: 239 240 701; E-mail: anpiro@ci.uc.pt
# Both authors contributed equally to this work

Atta-ur-Rahman & M. Iqbal Choudhary (Eds.)

INTRODUCTION

Obesity, which is considered a chronic medical disease state, has been rapidly increasing due to an unbalanced diet and reduced physical exercise. The World Health Organization defines obesity as the epidemic of the 21st century with an estimation of more than half a billion adults worldwide being obese, as the prevalence of obesity has nearly doubled between 1980 and 2008 [1]. Comorbidities linked to several metabolic alterations such as metabolic syndrome, steatosis, type 2 diabetes and cardiovascular diseases are triggered by excessive fat deposition [2]. In the past several decades, extensive research has been directed to the development of a safe pharmacological approach to a sustainable weight loss. The close relationship between mitochondrial homeostasis and modulation of energy balance [3] has brought to light pathways which can be targeted by specific molecules acting as anti-obesity drugs [4]. In fact, mitochondrial dysfunction (abnormal dynamics and reduced content, decreased oxidative capacity) has long been described in various key metabolic tissues such as liver, skeletal muscle and adipose tissue, from obese models [5 - 9].

Mitochondria are the powerhouses of the eukaryotic cell. Besides generation of ATP by oxidative phosphorylation (OXPHOS), mitochondria play a key role in the maintenance of cellular homeostasis by regulation of several aspects of cell biology such as metabolism, redox status, calcium signaling and programmed cell death [10, 11]. Mitochondria are the major sites of reactive oxygen species (ROS) generation in the cell, as a result of imperfectly coupled electron transport associated with OXPHOS [12]. Oxidative reactions in mitochondria (β-oxidation, tricarboxylic acid cycle) are associated with the conversion of oxidized cofactors (NAD^+ and FAD) into reduced cofactors (NADH and $FADH_2$). Electrons deriving from oxidation of these reduced cofactors are funneled through the redox carriers of the respiratory chain (complexes I, III, and IV) to the final electron acceptor, molecular oxygen [13]. Electrons released from the ETC incompletely reduce O_2 to form $O2^{.-}$, which is converted into H_2O_2 by manganese superoxide dismutase in the mitochondrial matrix. The primary factor governing mitochondrial ROS generation is the redox state of the respiratory chain [14]. When caloric intake is excessive, the electrochemical potential difference generated by the proton gradient is high, or in conditions of inhibition of the ETC complexes, the life of superoxide generating electron transport intermediates, such as ubisemiquinone, is prolonged resulting in increased ROS generation. Such phenomenon has been shown in mitochondria isolated from skeletal muscle, kidney, liver and adipose tissue from high-fat-fed or obese animals [15 - 17].

Mitochondria's dynamic nature, based on alterations in mitochondrial mass, mitophagy, fusion and fission, allows adjustment of mitochondrial mass and function to different environmental cues [18]. This adaptation is crucial to maintain metabolic homeostasis in fat accumulating tissues including adipose tissue, muscle and liver. In fact, defects in cellular function have already been extensively associated with alterations in mitochondrial dynamics [19]. Mitochondrial biogenesis is triggered in response to stimuli such as nutrient availability, hormones and temperature, all of which are typically involved in the cellular requirement for more ATP. Adaptations in mitochondrial copy number or mitochondrial mass, and the induction of genes implicated in OXPHOS or in intermediary metabolism as well, depend on the balanced contribution of both the nuclear and mitochondrial genomes. This forms a biogenesis program, controlled by several nuclear factors that act coordinately and in a categorized manner. Normally recruited is the Peroxisome Proliferator-Activated Receptor Gamma Coactivator-1 Alpha (PGC-1α). This transcription co-activator is widely regarded as the master regulator of mitochondrial biogenesis, binding to and promoting the activity of various transcription factors that ultimately lead to increased mitochondrial numbers [20]. PGC-1α can also exert a more discrete role, modulating the expression in ways that lead to specific protein transcription as, for example, antioxidant-related proteins or elevating oxidative phosphorylation proteins' levels, without direct elevation of mitochondrial numbers [21]. Other proteins are involved in the biogenesis of mitochondria, but PGC-1α appears to be the key element in driving up the numbers of this organelle inside the cells. Dynamic changes in mitochondrial regulators are associated with post-translational modifications mediated by metabolic sensors, such as sirtuin 1 and AMPK, which are activated by caloric restriction and exercise. Mitochondrial quality control in cells is dependent on the removal of depolarized or dysfunctional mitochondria through mitophagy, a selective form of general autophagy that prevents the accumulation of damaged mitochondria and consequent increased ROS generation [18].

SIRTUIN ACTIVATORS AS A NOVEL ANTI-OBESITY STRATEGY

Sirtuins

More than twenty years ago, a gene involved in extended life span was described for the first time. The *Silent Information Regulator 2* (SIR2) gene, responsible for the sirtuins name, was shown to repress genome instability of budding yeast *Saccharomyces cerevisiae* [22, 23], making sirtuins one of the first families of longevity genes to be revealed [24 - 27]. Meanwhile, several lines of evidence have shown that *SIR2*-like genes can be found in most organisms, mediating organism's health benefits and survival [28]. Over the years, sirtuins have attracted significant attention in order to clarify their activity at the molecular mechanism, and how it promotes survival in a stressful environment. Since nicotinamide adenine dinucleotide (NAD$^+$) has emerged as a vital cofactor in the regulation of NAD$^+$-consuming enzymes such as sirtuins [29], several reports have arisen to try to understand the metabolic control of sirtuins and its modulation by small molecules, thus preventing multiple age-associated diseases.

The discovery that *SIR2* gene manipulation (*e.g.* increasing their amount) in yeast, worms, and flies prolongs life span stimulated the research on mammalian sirtuins. In mammals, there are seven sirtuin enzymes (SIRT1-7) categorized by their highly conserved central NAD$^+$-binding and catalytic domains, the sirtuin core domain [30]. Despite the relatively conserved nature of sirtuins, their N and C termini differ, which make sirtuins largely different regarding their biological function, their partners and subtracts as well as their distinct subcellular localization and expression patterns [31].

The subcellular localization of these proteins has been described in numerous compartments within the mammalian cell depending on cell type, stress status, and molecular interactions. SIRT1, SIRT6 and SIRT7 are predominantly located in the nucleus but it has been shown that SIRT1 can shuttle in and out of the nucleus [32 - 34]. This particularity of SIRT1 is due the presence of two primary amino acid nuclear export signals [34] in addition to the nuclear localization signals that SIRT6 and SIRT7 also display. Three sirtuins, SIRT3-5, contain N-terminal mitochondrial targeting sequences and are believed to localize at mitochondrial matrix [33, 35, 36]; however, two different studies have suggested that during cellular stress, SIRT3 may also translocate to the nucleus [37, 38]. SIRT2 are primarily cytosolic, regulating gene expression of transcription factors that shuttles from cytosol to nucleus [39], but SIRT2 was also found to localize in the nucleus and interact with nuclear proteins [40]. In summary, seems evident that sirtuins are highly distributed through the cell and that their localization may be dynamic, varying in tissue/cell type and depending on physiological conditions.

Apart from distinct subcellular localization, sirtuin family members also present differences in their enzymatic activity. Mechanistically, sirtuins use NAD$^+$ as cosubstrate to remove acetyl moieties from lysines on histones and proteins [41]. The reaction begins with an amide cleavage of NAD$^+$ realizing nicotinamide (NAM) and a covalent ADP-ribose peptide-imidate intermediate. The intermediate then is formed in O-acetyl-ADP-ribose and the deacetylated subtract is released [42 - 44]. The NAD$^+$ consumption during deacetylation is in this way what determines sirtuins as type III lysine deacetylases (KDACs) and divides them from type I, II, and IV KDACs. A strong deacetylase activity has been described for SIRT1, SIRT2, and SIRT3, comparing with weak activity of SIRT4, SIRT5, and SIRT6 [29, 36, 45, 46]. SIRT4 has been described as NAD$^+$-

dependent mono-ADP-ribosyl transferase along with SIRT6 [47, 48] and to have lipoamidase activity [49]. Furthermore, SIRT6 has also the ability to remove long-chain fatty acyl groups from lysine residues [50], whereas SIRT5 has been described to act as demalonylase, desuccinylase, and deglutarylase [51, 52]. Lastly, SIRT7 is proposed to be a NAD^+-dependent deacetylase with few known *in vivo* and *in vitro* substrates [53 - 55].

Physiological Role of Sirtuins in Metabolism

Sirtuins interact with all major preserved longevity pathways, such as AMPK [56], and insulin-IGF1 signaling, with targets including protein kinase A (PKA) [57], mTOR [58, 59], forkhead box O (FOXO) [60], PGC-1α [61], NF-kβ [62], p53 [46] and IGF1 [63]. During times of energy deficit and reduced carbohydrate energy sources, sirtuins prompt cellular adaptations improving metabolic efficiency. Fasting [61, 64], caloric restriction [65], exercise [66], or low glucose availability [67], increases SIRT1 enzymatic activity, the most studied member of the sirtuins family. Additionally, mitochondrial metabolism is stimulated in several tissues due to SIRT1-dependent deacetylation of transcription factors, cofactors, and histones [61, 64, 66, 68 - 71]. Fat and cholesterol catabolism in liver, skeletal muscle and adipose tissue are also stimulated by SIRT1 [72]. Animal models of SIRT1 overexpression have also been used to show the impact of SIRT1 in preventing metabolic age-related complications, such as obesity, insulin resistance, and hepatic steatosis [73 - 75]. High fat diet (HFD)-related lifespan reduction was also prevented after pharmacological activation of SIRT1 [76, 77]. Remarkably, a transgenic mouse model of SIRT1 overexpression exhibits several of the benefits of CR, including high metabolic activity, reduced blood lipid levels and improved glucose metabolism, but not increased lifespan [78]. Like SIRT1, overexpression of SIRT6 has also been shown to increase lifespan in mouse [79].

SIRT3 has been stated as a primary mediator of mitochondrial deacetylation after reports showing no significant changes in acetylation status in mice lacking SIRT4 and SIRT5 [80]. SIRT3 plays an important role in mitochondrial metabolism by targeting key metabolic enzymes and modulating tricarboxylic acid cycle, respiration chain, ketogenesis, and fatty acid β-oxidation [81]. Additional metabolic processes from acetate metabolism to BAT thermogenesis [82], as well as, activation of acetyl-CoA synthetase 2 (ACSS2) and glutamate dehydrogenase (GDH) are under regulation of SIRT3 [83, 84]. SIRT3 is also capable to manage NAD^+ levels, thus regulating mitochondrial function and preventing liver injury associated with fatty liver [85] as well as acute kidney injury [86]. SIRT3 expression is increased in the liver by fasting [87] as well as in the muscle by fasting, caloric restriction and exercise [88], while prolonged HFD-feeding has the opposite effect [89].

SIRT3 expression is regulated by PGC-1α, and estrogen-related receptor α (ERRα) [90, 91]. ERRα belongs to a family of estrogen-related receptors capable of promoting mitochondrial biogenesis, primary expressed in tissues with high oxidative metabolism [92]. ERRα DNA-binding-sites were mapped in many nuclear-encoded mitochondrial genes including OXPHOS, fatty acid oxidation, TCA cycle, as well as factors that regulate mitochondrial fission/fusion. ERRα is modulated by coactivators/corepressor complexes like PGC-1α/β, an efficacious activator of ERRα that promotes expression of mitochondrial genes [93 - 95]. PGC-1α and PGC-1β are sufficient to increase mitochondrial mass and expression of ROS scavenger enzymes, genes related with OXPHOS and mitochondrial dynamics, as well as sirtuins [96 - 100]. This is related to the activating action of PGC-1 proteins on transcription factors like ERRα.

Research on loss-of-function models has been performed over the years.SIRT1, SIRT3 and SIRT7 models have been linked with higher susceptibility for metabolic and age-related diseases and reduced lifespan [53, 54, 101, 102]. SIRT3-KO mice were reported to be prone to age-related disease such as metabolic syndrome [102]. Also SIRT3-KO mice fed a high cholesterol diet were unable to maintain superoxide dismutase 2 (SOD2) homeostasis and ROS levels, leading to mild endothelial dysfunction [103]. Experiments with SIRT6 model revealed high mortality within the first month of life associated with severe hypoglycemia [104, 105]. In contrast, SIRT-2 and SIRT5-deficient mice do not manifest altered metabolic phenotype in the basal state [106 - 108] while, contrarily to the most sirtuins, SIRT4 deficiency enhances oxidative metabolism [109].

Physiological Role of Sirtuins and Obesity and Metabolic Syndrome

An association between sirtuins, obesity and obesity-related disorders has been established in the past few years. Numerous independent studies have elucidated the regulatory role of sirtuins in metabolic pathways and its effects regarding the expression of adipocyte cytokines (adipokines), insulin secretion, variation of plasma glucose levels, cholesterol and lipid homeostasis, as well as mitochondrial energy efficiency [110]. SIRT1 seems to stimulate fatty acid oxidation by promoting adiponectin synthesis [111], is related to hypothalamic control of energy balance [112], plays a role in adipogenesis and has also been shown to respond to fasting by regulation of lipolysis and fatty acid mobilization [113]. Moreover, mice with deficiency in SIRT1 present hyperglycemia, oxidative damage and insulin resistance, resulting in obesity when fed HFD [114, 115].

Besides being a key mediator of metabolic adaptations in peripheral tissues to nutrient deprivation, SIRT1 is highly expressed in the hypothalamus and has been implicated as critical for normal body weight, energy homeostasis and the regulation of food intake [112, 116]. Hence fasting-induced SIRT1 has been shown altered in obese mice [116]. Additionally, models of pharmacological inhibition of SIRT1 in the hypothalamus have shown to decrease food intake and body weight gain [112], which can allow us to argue that hypothalamic inhibition of SIRT1 might be a strategy to suppress appetite.

Over the years, approaches with transgenic mice with SIRT1 over- and underexpression in different tissues have been linked SIRT1 and obesity. In adipose tissue of both *db/db* leptin resistant obese mice and HFD-induced obese mice, expression of SIRT1 was significantly low [117, 118]. Furthermore, experiments with white adipose tissue (WAT) specific SIRT1 knockout mice have shown enhanced adipogenesis and compromised WAT fatty acid mobilization while WAT SIRT1 overexpression attenuated adipogenesis and boosted lipolysis [113]. It was also observed that mice overexpressing SIRT1 display a characteristic leaner phenotype than littermate controls, with decreased levels of plasma cholesterol, insulin and fasting glucose, as well as, reduced adiposity [73, 78]. In another study, Paul Pfluger and colleagues [75], observed beneficial effects of SIRT1 overexpression in mice fed HFD such as less inflammation, improved glucose tolerance and protection against hepatic steatosis; however an anti-obesity effect was not observed. Like rodents, SIRT1 expression in obese pigs was shown to be lesser than in lean pigs [119].

The overload of lipids accumulated in adipose tissue is known to trigger inflammation and since obesity-related inflammation is documented as a major factor underlying the pathogenesis of diseases associated with metabolic syndrome [120], this field has been under study in order to identify potential targets for new strategies against obesity and its related complications. Two different studies have shown that whereas modest overexpression of SIRT1 results in suppression of inflammatory responses, SIRT1 deficient mice subjected to HFD present systemic inflammation [114, 121]. The beneficial effect of SIRT1 on metabolic syndrome has been correlated with its ability to repress NF-kβ activation, a key transcriptional factor related with inflammatory responses [122]. Paul Pfluger and colleagues [75] have observed that SIRT1 overexpression reduces IL-6 and TNF-α levels in the serum of the mice fed a HFD, as well as decreases TNF-α-induced NF-kβ activation in embryonic fibroblasts of the transgenic mice.

SIRT1 has been shown to deacetylate and consequently repress NF-kβ, causing a reduction in the production of pro-inflammatory cytokines [62]. Contrarily, inhibition of SIRT1 appears to be pro-inflammatory. Using small interference

RNA (siRNA) to knockdown SIRT1, Takeshi Yoshizaki and colleagues [123] described an increase in TNF-α-induced MCP-1 and other inflammatory-related genes in 3T3-L1 adipocytes. Moreover, in transgenic mice subjected to HFD, adipose tissue SIRT1-specific knockdown showed increased macrophage recruitment while overexpression of SIRT1 avoids macrophage accumulation [124]. However, it is interesting to note that an antagonistic cross talk may be present between SIRT1 and NF-kβ signaling in the regulation of obesity-related inflammatory responses. In addition to the regulatory inhibition of SIRT1 to NF-kβ, NF-kβ has been shown to downregulate SIRT1 activity through the expression of pro-inflammatory cytokines such as IFNγ [125]. Putting together these findings, we can argue that decreased SIRT1 activity is may be related with NF-kβ activation as well as with increases in transcription of pro-inflammatory mediators which can be important for a valuable translational application to treat obesity and its related diseases.

Inflammation of adipose tissue is also recognized has a hallmark of insulin resistance [126] and SIRT1 expression in different tissues has also been linked to insulin sensitivity. In adipocytes, for instance, SIRT1 has been shown to regulate insulin-stimulated glucose uptake as well as GLUT4 translocation, with increased SIRT1 activity attenuating insulin resistance [123]. SIRT1 activity has been shown reduced in highly insulin resistant cells, being insulin insensitivity attenuated by increasing SIRT1 expression [73]. In skeletal muscle, repression of protein tyrosine phosphatase 1B (PTP1B) by SIRT1, which is critical in insulin signaling, contributes to the improvement of insulin sensitivity [127]. Complementary experiments over the years, using transgenic mice as well as *in vitro* studies, have clarified the role of SIRT1 in the regulation of insulin secretion. Increasing expression of SIRT1 has been shown to improve insulin secretion and SIRT1 overexpression in pancreatic β-cells enhances glucose-stimulated insulin secretion and improves glucose tolerance [128]. This was also observed in aged animals and subjected to HFD [129, 130]. Additionally, SIRT1 transgenic mice exhibit improved glucose tolerance, with decreased hepatic glucose production as well as increased hepatic insulin sensitivity [73].

A decrease in SIRT3 content with obesity brought attention to a role of SIRT3 in the pathophysiology of obesity. SIRT3 deficient mice (SIRT3$^{-/-}$) exhibit increased mitochondrial protein hyperacetylation and accelerated development of metabolic syndrome when fed HFD [85, 102]. SIRT3 have also been described to regulate fatty acid oxidation and adaptive thermogenesis. Fatty acid oxidation disorders were shown to arise during fasting in SIRT3 knockdown mice. These mice also show intolerance to cold exposure during fasting, suggesting altered thermogenic response [82, 87]. SIRT3 expression was observed to increase in BAT and WAT during CR and decrease in genetically modified obese mice [82]. In another study,

Alrob and colleagues, have shown an increase in cardiac fatty acid oxidation in SIRT3-KO mice under HFD as consequence of increased acetylation of mitochondrial β-oxidation enzymes [131]. Additionally, Zeng and colleagues have also reported the importance of SIRT3 in preserving heart function and capillary density in obesity [132]. The impact of SIRT3 in maternal obese environment to oocytes was also studied. Using mice fed HFD, Zhang and colleagues have shown that SIRT3-dependent deacetylation of SOD2 plays a protective role against oxidative stress and meiotic defects in oocytes [133]. Finally, a recent work has reported the importance of SIRT3 as a target for the protection of pancreatic β-cells dysfunction due oxidative stress-induced cell damage in obesity and T2D [134].

Besides the extensive work done in SIRT1 and, in a lower extent in SIRT3, less research has been conducted regarding other members of the sirtuin family and their association with obesity. It has been shown that SIRT2 overexpression, which has been proposed as the most abundant sirtuin in adipocytes, can inhibit preadipocyte differentiation into adipocytes whereas SIRT2 downregulation promotes adipogenesis [39]. Additionally, a recent work has shown that SIRT2 regulates sepsis-related inflammation in *ob/ob* mice [135]. Regarding other mitochondrial sirtuins, SIRT4 expression β-cells may be linked to the mitochondrial regulation of insulin secretion [136]. Experiments based on altered SIRT6 expression have linked this sirtuin with glucose homeostasis, with SIRT6-deficient mouse developing lethal hypoglycaemia in early life [105]. On the other hand, mice overexpressing SIRT6 subjected to HFD presented significantly less visceral fat, enhanced glucose tolerance, and better glucose-stimulated insulin secretion when compared with controls [137]. Finally, regarding SIRT7, few research has been conducted over the years, however two recent papers have related the impact of SIRT7 modulation by microRNAs on obesity [138, 139]. Moreover, SIRT7 knockout animals were shown to be resistant to HFD-induced obesity, although the researchers have argued that these abnormalities may be the result of impaired PPARγ expression [140]. Also, interactions between SIRT1 and SIRT7 have been described *in vitro* and *in vivo*. Again, using SIRT7 knockout animals, SIRT1 protein content and enzymatic activity were increased in WAT [141, 142].

Contrary to animal studies, the number of human studies relating sirtuins and obesity is limited to weight loss analyses and caloric restriction approaches. SIRT1 transcription levels were shown to be significantly lower in obese individuals when compared with normal-weight controls. In these studies, the researchers have shown that SIRT1 transcription is restored by CR [143-148], which can be associated with the previously shown relationship between decreased SIRT1 expression, obesity-related inflammation and excessive fat accumulation in adipose tissue. In fact, it was observed that SIRT1 expression was lower in adipose tissue from obese patients when compared with controls [149, 150]. Moreover, studies with nondiabetic offspring of type 2 diabetes patients have shown that SIRT1 expression in adipose tissue seems to correlate with energy expenditure and insulin sensitivity [150]. Similarly, de Kreutzenberg and colleagues have also observed an association between insulin resistance and metabolic syndrome with decreased SIRT1 expression [151].

Regarding SIRT3, analyses of the effect of weight reduction in obese patients have shown increased SIRT3 expression in adipose tissue and liver, probably linked to reduced inflammation [143]. Vargas-Ortiz and colleagues have analysed the impact of aerobic training on overweight adolescents. In this study, the researchers found that aerobic training increased SIRT3 as well as PGC-1α expression in overweight or obese adolescents [152]. Notably, decreased PGC-1α content in HFD feeding conditions has been hypothesized as responsible for lower SIRT3 protein content in obesity [102]. The role of SIRT3 in endothelial insulin resistance and vascular dysfunction in obese human subjects was also investigated. It was found that SIRT3 positively regulates endothelial insulin sensitivity with SIRT3 deficiency contributing to vascular dysfunction in obesity [153]. Nevertheless, all these evidences must be better explored to make it clear if this negative relation between SIRT1 and/or SIRT3 expression and obesity relies on protection, resistance, or even in response to dietary, lifestyle and environmental factors.

Expression of other sirtuins in obese patients has also been addressed. Tarantino and colleagues found low levels of SIRT4 in serum from obese patients with non-alcoholic fatty liver disease, with the authors proposing that this decrease may occur as an adaptation to decrease fat oxidative capacity in response to caloric excess [154]. Furthermore, like in animal models, a negative correlation between SIRT1 and SIRT7 was also found in adipose tissue from obese patients [141].

Besides analyses of sirtuins expression in obese patients, studies with volunteers subjected to changes in caloric intake were also performed. Adipose tissue biopsies collected before and after six days of total fasting showed an increase in SIRT1 mRNA levels after fasting [146]. In another study, analysis of adipose tissue from obese woman placed on either moderate-fat (low-carbohydrate) or low-fat (high-carbohydrate) hypoenergetic diet for 10 weeks, showed that one thousand genes, including sirtuins, were regulated by diet-induced energy restriction. Particularly, SIRT3 gene was increased with moderate-fat diet [155].

Together, all these studies extend our knowledge about the varied possible actions of sirtuins in obesity and related issues. However, limitations of genetic manipulation are illustrated and due to this, a growing interest appeared over the years in a way to try to identify possible potent and selective sirtuin activators.

Sirtuins Activators for Therapy

Following their apparent role in the regulation of lipid and glucose metabolism, adipogenesis and appetite control, sirtuins have attracted significant interest as drug targets. Over the years, some activators and inhibitors have been described and potential clinical applications proposed, in the setting of diabetes, cardiovascular diseases, cancer or neurodegenerative diseases.

The search for sirtuins activators started in 2003 when Konrad Howitz through a high-throughput screen identified the first potent activators. Over ~18000 compounds were screened and more than 20 sirtuin activators were described [156]. Several plant-derived metabolites including flavones (for example, quercetin), stilbenes (for example, resveratrol), chalcones (for example, butein) and anthocyanidins were shown to directly activate SIRT1 *in vitro* by increasing their affinity to peptide substrates through allosteric mechanism that lowers the Michaelis-Menten constant (K_m) [156].

From all the natural SIRT1 activators described to date, resveratrol (RSV) (3,5,4'-trihydroxystilbene) is still the most powerful. This phytoalexin from the dried root of white hellebore *Veratrum grandiflorum* was described for the first time in 1940, and later was also shown to be present in Japanese knotweed *Polygonum sachalinense* [157]. However, in the 1990s, the interest in RSV increased when it was discovered as an active component of red wine. This discover lead many to propose an explanation for the unusual low rates of mortality from chronic heart diseases in French people, the so-called "French paradox", from regions with high consumption of this wine [158 - 160].

Nevertheless, over the years RSV was not a successful drug given its insolubility and poor bioavailability. The half-life was also low, between 12-15 min [160, 161], and the reached concentration in the low micromolar range after gram amounts administered orally [162, 163]. Surprisingly, Thomas Walle and colleagues observed that the half-life of RSV conjugates was much higher (~9h) when compared to its native form, which opened the possibility to use these conjugates *in vivo* to achieve greater pharmacokinetic effects [164]. Clinical trials have been conducted to explore the health impact of RSV in individuals with obesity, diabetes and cardiovascular diseases. In some cases, beneficial effects were shown upon RSV treatment regarding improved insulin sensitivity, neurocognition and amelioration of cardiovascular diseases [157, 165]. Additionally, the toxicity of RSV was also addressed and studies, both in human subjects and animals, have showed no serious effects after controlled administration of RSV [166 - 169]. However, side effects have been reported in the gastrointestinal tract [170, 171].

The discovery of natural compounds as activators of SIRT1, like RSV, blunted a search for new possible synthetic activators that could be more potent and efficacious, surpassing the bioavailability problems that RSV presented at the time. The search started with Sinclair and colleagues looking for RSV analogues. Some of these synthetic compounds were shown to be more powerful than RSV, and considering tri-acetyl-stilbene, the compound appeared to be more effective in extending life span [172]. In 2007 a new method was developed to identify new sirtuin activators structurally unrelated to RSV. The first synthetic sirtuin activators were chemically distinct from RSV and based on an imidazothiazole scaffold (*e.g.*, SRT1460, SRT1720, SRT2183) [173]. Like RSV, these molecules activated SIRT1 by a similar mechanism through the lowering of K_m for its substrates [173]. Later, synthetic compounds based on thiazolopyridines (for example, STAC-2), benzimidazole (for example, STAC-5), and bridged ureas (for example, STAC-9) were also described [174, 175].

Sirtuin Activators for Therapy in Obesity

The ability of sirtuin activators to prevent or reverse the effects of obesity has been under extensive study in the past years. Beneficial effects of RSV and synthetic sirtuin activators are associated with improvements in glucose homeostasis and insulin sensitivity in different models of obesity.

Regarding RSV, in 2006 it was shown the capacity of RSV to improve metabolism and protect against obesity and insulin resistance in mice fed HFD [76, 157, 176], which was correlated with longer lifespan. Also RSV prevented fatty liver and increased PGC-1α activity, the well-known regulator of mitochondrial biogenesis [76, 157]. Similarly RSV beneficial effects were also observed in rat models [177 - 179]. Rivera and colleagues showed that prolonged administration (8 weeks) of RSV to obese Zucker rats improved plasma triglycerides and free fatty acids when compared with animals without RSV treatment [179]. Regarding the central nervous system, administration of RSV was shown to limit consequences of high-caloric diet in mice [180]. Like *in vivo*, *in vitro* studies also support the beneficial effects of RSV in obesity. Reduction in both fatty acid synthesis and triglyceride accumulation in hepatocytes [178, 181] as well as inhibition of adipogenesis in isolated cells [182] have been described. The capacity of RSV to alleviate secondary phenotypes associated with diabetes, like diabetic nephropathy and tissue inflammation, was also described [183]. RSV enhanced metabolism in non-human primate's [184] and, in rhesus monkeys fed with high-fat, high-sugar diet, RSV improved adipose insulin signaling, as well as an anti-inflammatory effect of RSV in visceral WAT of the monkeys [185]. Additionally, chronic administration of moderate doses of RSV was reported to improve insulin sensitivity in both obese Zucker rats and mice subjected to HFD [76, 176, 180]. However *in vitro* studies have shown that RSV is capable of inhibiting insulin pathways such as Akt, MAPK, PI3K, and PKB [186, 187].

All of the aforementioned findings encouraged many companies to develop dietary supplements or foods containing small amounts of RSV. Supporting this, few clinical studies have been conducted with RSV with the goal to evaluate the possible beneficial effect of RSV on human metabolism. Foremost, a double-blind crossover study on obese but healthy males was performed. In this study the researchers treated the subjects with placebo or 150 mg/day RSV (dose comparable to what was used in previous animal study [76]) and after 30 days of RSV supplementation, it was observed increased insulin sensitivity, glucose tolerance, SIRT1 and PGC-1α levels, while decreased circulating levels of triglycerides and lipid content, mimicking CR [165]. Moreover, RSV-containing compositions were also produced showing greater bioavailability and RSV-specific activity stability. Longevinex® (composed by RSV supplemented with 5% quercetin and 5% rice bran phytate, a chelator, hyaluronic acid and/or vitamin D) showed capacity to upregulate survival/longevity genes to a greater extent than RSV alone or CR [188]. PGC-1α (controls energy metabolism and mitochondrial genes [61]) and pyruvate dehydrogenase (responsible for the regulation of fuel selection during fasting and promotion of fatty acid metabolism [189]) as well as uncoupling protein 3 [190] were upregulated by Longevinex®. Additionally, type 2 diabetes patients treated for 4 weeks with RSV, showed improved insulin sensitivity as well as decreased oxidative stress when compared with non-treated patients [191]. However a negative study with non-obese woman with normal glucose tolerance showed that 75 mg/day treatment with RSV for 12 weeks did not improve metabolic parameters [170].

In addition to RSV, several naturally occurring compounds with SIRT1 activating capacity and anti-obesity proprieties have been described [172]. Indole-3-carbinol (I3C), a natural occurring anti-obese agent of brassica vegetables such as broccoli and cabbage, has been shown to be a potent specific SIRT1 activator, acting like other SIRT1 activators by lowering the K_m value of the acetylated substrates and inhibiting adipocyte differentiation [192, 193]. Moreover, Fernández-Galilea and colleagues in a study with overweight/obese subjects observed the ability of α-Lipoic acid in the remodelling of white subcutaneous adipocytes by increasing mitochondrial biogenesis and fatty acid oxidation enzymes in a mechanism mediated by SIRT1/PGC-1α pathway [194]. Rutin (rutoside, quercetin-3-*O*-rutinoside and sophorin), a flavonoid glycoside composed of quercetin and disaccharide rutinose present in many plants, including buckwheat [195], was also described due to its anti-obesity proprieties [196]. Rutin-fed rats showed a high decrease in body weight without changes in foot intake, as well as decrease in adipocyte size, adipogenic expression of PPAR-γ, SREBP-1c, and aP2, a regarded marker of obesity. Also, since the rhizome of *Polygonatum sibiricum* Redoute (Liliaceae) has been used to treat diabetes-associated complications, Ko and colleagues tested the impact of an ethanol extract of *P. sibiricum* rhizomes (ID1216) on obesity [197]. The researchers showed that ID1216 administration to HFD-fed mice significantly decreased body weight, lipid accumulation in adipose tissue, as well plasmatic triglycerides and free fatty acids. Additionally, ID1216 regulated gene expression related with adipogenesis and fatty acid oxidation in 3T3-L1 cells and enhanced the expression of genes responsible for the regulation of energy homeostasis in C2C12 myocytes. These improvements in obesity were mediated through SIRT1/PGC-1α pathway.

Naturally occurring compounds with the ability to modulate SIRT3 activity in obesity-related conditions have also been described. Beberine, an isoquinoline alkaloid known by its anti-diabetic properties, has been shown to recover mitochondrial deficiency in HFD-fed rats. The improved mitochondrial function was accompanied by an increase in SIRT3 activity avoiding an energy deficiency state and impaired OXPHOS [9]. Additionally, Korean pine nut oil (PNO) has been shown to alter weight and lipid metabolism, which was proposed to involve PNO prevention of SIRT3 downregulation and consequently HFD-induced mitochondrial dysfunction [198]. Nitrite has also been tested in models of obesity. Lai and colleagues have shown that oral nitrite treatment improved hyperglycemia in obese ZSF1 rats in a process involving skeletal muscle SIRT3-AMPK-GLUT4 [199]. Additionally, in the same study, analysis of skeletal muscle biopsies from patients with metabolic syndrome showed increased activation of SIRT3 and AMPK after 12 weeks of oral sodium nitrite and nitrate treatment. Finally, the adipocyte-derived peptide apelin, has been described to contribute to cardiovascular and metabolic homeostasis in an obesity-like condition. Apelin treatment prevented mitochondrial damage and cardiac dysfunction in obesity-related heart failure, in a process that involves SIRT3 activation [200].

Besides natural compound, the capacity of sirtuins synthetic activators to ameliorate obesity-related disorders has also been evaluated. First, SRT1720 has been shown to have similar effects to RSV in obese mice, improving metabolic parameters related to glucose homeostasis and insulin sensitivity, as well as, decreasing oxidative stress markers [201, 202]. Additionally, SRT1720 has been described to extend life span of mice fed HFD or a standard chow diet [77, 202]. SRT2379 was tested in Zucker fa/fa rats with improvements in glucose tolerance, reduced hyperinsulinemia, as well as enhanced glucose uptake capacity [203]. Also, in the same study, reduced levels of inflammatory markers in adipose tissue as well as a reduction in inflammatory state of adipose tissue macrophages were observed. Another sirtuin activator, SRT2104, was shown to mimic CR aspects and to extend male mouse life span [204]. Sirtris Pharmaceuticals (Cambridge, MA, USA) has developed a RSV formulation, SRT501, with the ability to mimic CR by enhancing mitochondrial biogenesis, improving metabolic signaling pathways and blunting pro-inflammatory pathways in mice fed HDF [205]. Additionally, SRT501 was also shown to improve glucose and insulin homeostasis, again mimicking CR [206]. Moreover, Vu and colleagues, after synthetizing a series of compound derived from imidazo[1,2-b]thiazole, discovered that compound 29 showed oral antidiabetic activity in the *ob/ob* mouse model, the diet-induced obesity mouse model and the Zucker fa/fa rat model [207, 208]. Type 2 diabetic patients between 30 and 70 years old, supplemented for 28 days with SRT2104, showed improvements in lipid profiles, with lower LDL levels and increased HDL. However, in these patients improvements in glucose and insulin homeostasis were not observed [209]. Two additional clinical trials testing SRT2104 in elderly volunteers and healthy smokers, described a slight reduction in body weight, an improvement in cholesterol ratio as well as a decrease in triglyceride levels [210, 211]. Furthermore, again in type 2 diabetic patients, SRT501 was shown to improve glucose tolerance in the absence of any adverse side effect [212].

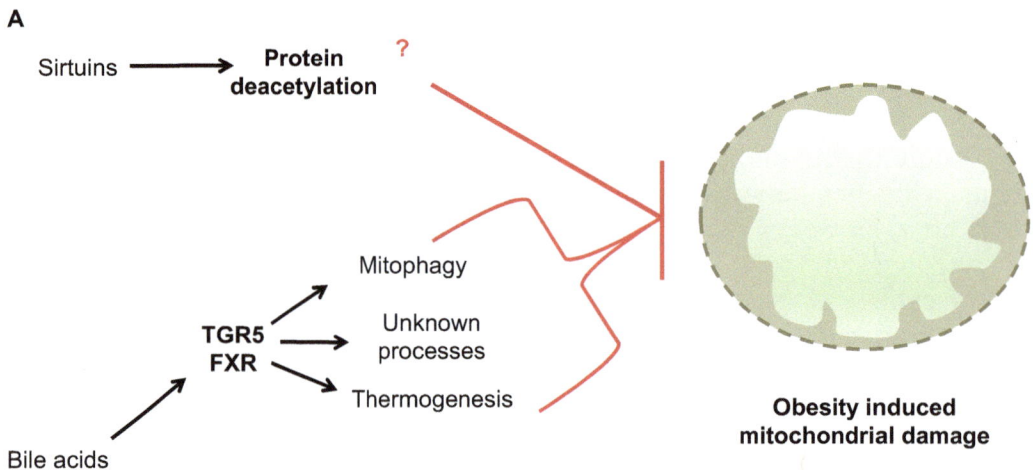

A

Sirtuins ⟶ **Protein deacetylation** ?

Mitophagy

TGR5 FXR ⟶ Unknown processes

Thermogenesis

Bile acids

Obesity induced mitochondrial damage

Fig. 1 cont.....

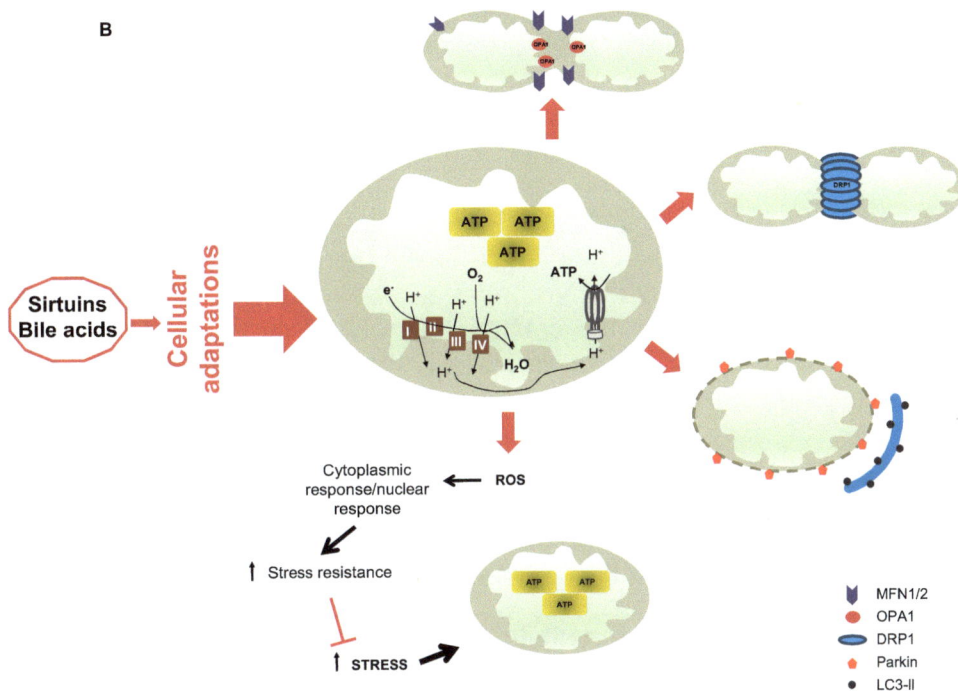

Fig. (1). (**A**) The possible role of Sirtuins and Bile Acids as a strategy against obesity. Although no concrete evidence exists so far regarding whether BA induce a response that might, at least partially, help to protect against obesity, sirtuins have a clear protective role against obesity-induced damage. (**B**) Additionally, BA and sirtuins may have a effect on mitochondrial biology. Whether through FXR, TGR5 or any other unknown receptor/effector, in the case of BA, and through sirtuins activity, different cellular adaptations may protect obesity-induced mitochondrial damage. Removal of mitochondria that are inefficient/damaged through mitophagy, regulation of mitochondrial dynamics (fusion and fission) as well as cytoplasmic/nuclear response through mitohormesis may be the mechanisms responsible for the protection of mitochondria on obesity-induced damage. This ultimately leads to a more potent and capable mitochondrial population, which in turn explains some of the effects of BA and Sirtuins on metabolic improvement.

Pharmaceutical companies are continuing to develop sirtuin activators with pharmaceutical proprieties, however, beneficial metabolic effects stimulated by these activators must be analysed with careful attention since side effects due to the extensive activation of sirtuins may cause serious damage in human patients. Additional studies with these activators are necessary.

NAD$^+$-boosting Compounds

Associated with the discoveries regarding the impact of sirtuin activity in several age-related diseases including obesity, studies on sirtuin regulating mechanisms, such as, the available NAD$^+$ within the cell, have also been conducted. The general decline in NAD^+ has arisen as a likely explanation for the association between decreased sirtuins activity and aging. The first evidence that NAD^+ could decline over age was shown in transgenic mice overexpressing SIRT1 in pancreatic β cells (BESTO mice) [130]. Young BESTO mice exhibit increased glucose-stimulated insulin secretion, a phenotype absent in older animals. Notably, treatment with nicotinamide mononucleotide (NMN), a key NAD^+ intermediate, restored the metabolic phenotype in old BESTO mice as well as insulin secretion in old wild type control mice. Three major molecules have been described to be involved in different NAD^+ biosynthetic pathways: the amino acid tryptophan (Trp), nicotinic acid (NA), and nicotinamide riboside (NR). NR as well as NMN have been shown to enhance mitochondrial function and improve glucose homeostasis in obese mice, in a SIRT1-dependent manner [8, 213, 214]. NMN has been shown to restore several key aspects in aged mice such as muscle type switching, insulin sensitivity, OXPHOS and gene expression [8]. Yoshino and colleagues have also shown that NMN is capable to restore NAD^+ levels thus preventing diet- and age-induced type 2 diabetes [214]. Thus, NAD^+-boosting molecules have been looked as a new class of sirtuin activators with the ability to restore NAD^+ levels and potentially activate or restore sirtuin activities.

Besides the focus on NAD^+ intermediate supplementation, attention has also been brought into the enzymes with impact on NAD^+ levels. NAMPT catalyses the formation of NMN from NAM, which is then converted to NAD^+ by nicotinamide mononucleotide adenylyltransferase 1 (NMNAT1), NMNAT2, and NMNAT3. Dahl and colleagues have hypothesize that decreased levels of NAD^+ in obesity may be due in part to the downregulation of NAMPT [215]. Another enzyme, nicotinamide riboside kinase (NRK) is responsible for NR and nicotinic acid riboside (NaR) entry in the salvage pathway after being converted to NMN and mononucleotide (NaMN), respectively. On the other side, CD38 and its homologue CD157 are glycohydrolases that degrade NAD^+, and poly(ADP-ribose) polymerases (PARPs), which have been intensely related with DNA repair, inflammation and cell death, catalyses the transfer of ADP-ribose subunits from NAD^+ to protein receptors.

Although we are in the beginning of this new approach regarding NAD^+ and its impact in diseases linked to impaired sirtuins activity, these so-called NAD^+-boosting molecules have shown interesting and effective effects in the treatment of metabolic dysfunction in animal models. NAD^+ supplementation as well as modulation of NAD^+-dependent enzymes appears to be a window for new studies in the field. However, a better understanding of how these different NAD^+ precursors are metabolized as well as an assessment of the bioavailability and effectiveness of these precursors is needed before stepping into human therapy.

BILE ACIDS, OBESITY AND MITOCHONDRIA

Bile Acid Receptors Discovery and Properties

For some time now, bile acids (BA) have been known to possess anti-obesity properties. First reported in obese patients with BA therapy for gallstone management as a curious side-effect [216], a receptor for BA was quickly identified, in the shape of NR1H4, better known as the Farnesoid X Receptor (FXR) [217].

FXR is a heterodimerizable receptor for BA that, when activated, promotes the transcription of the small heterodimer partner (SHP) gene [218]. SHP is primarily a repressor, binding and thus inactivating several transcription factors, such as the peroxisome proliferator-activated receptor gamma (PPARγ) [219], the liver X receptor (LXR) [220] or the liver receptor homolog 1 (LRH1), which provides the better known effect of FXR-SHP activation, the inhibition of the transcription of the cholesterol 7α-hydroxylase (CYP7A1), the rate-limiting enzyme of BA production [221]. Thus, BA regulates its own synthesis by a closed loop. Interestingly, due to the above-mentioned anti-obesity effects found by BA supplementation, FXR research yielded numerous works describing an impaired lipid metabolism, ranging from increased circulating free-fatty acids (FFA) [222] to elevated circulating triglycerides (TG) and HDL cholesterol [223], as well as elevated activity of fatty acid synthase [224]. Furthermore, the normalization of several adipokines by FXR agonism was also reported [225, 226]. Other key transcription factors involved in lipid metabolism, such as PPARα and PPARγ, were also shown to be regulated by FXR activity [227, 228]. In addition to the involvement in lipid metabolism, FXR also appeared to have a key role in regulating glucose metabolism [218]. In fact, FXR agonism induced the normalization of circulating glucose levels of both wild-type and genetically diabetic strains of animals [226, 229]. Accordingly, FXR agonism decreases the expression of phosphoenolpyruvate carboxykinase (PEPCK) and glucose-6-phosphatase (G6P), two key enzymes in the gluconeogenic process, resulting in diminished circulating glucose levels [230, 231]. Concomitantly, FXR-*null* mice are peripherally insulin resistant [222, 226]. Also, FXR agonism appears to elevate glucose storage as glycogen, thus contributing to the removal of excess glucose from circulation [232]. Given the central role of mitochondria in energetic metabolism, it is unsurprising to assume that FXR activation will lead to alterations in mitochondrial activity. In fact, FXR agonism leads to increased mitochondrial mass and activity, by a process dubbed mitochondrial biogenesis [233 - 235], which might explain some (if not all) of the effects of BA in improving and normalizing metabolism in obese and diabetic conditions [218].

However, despite this intense study on the matter, the role of FXR has been questioned. Some works demonstrate that by using synthetic, more specific, agonists of FXR, obesity and metabolic alterations are in fact exacerbated. A seminal work by Watanabe and collaborators [236], which was followed by the work of the same group [237] and others [238], highlighted that it was not FXR the mediator of BA effects, but instead the Takeda G protein-coupled receptor 5 (TGR5) bile acid receptor. This receptor (unlike FXR, which is a soluble nuclear receptor) is a typical membrane-bound G protein-coupled receptor, which upon activation (in this case, by BA) leads to the intracellular production of cyclic AMP (cAMP), a known secondary messenger. This, in turn, activates protein kinase A (PKA) that phosphorylates and activates the cAMP response element-binding protein (CREB), a known transcription factor. From here, there is induction of the transcription of several genes [239]. Of particular importance for the story conveyed by Watanabe and collaborators is the fact that TGR5 activation in brown adipose tissue (BAT), leads to the induction of a biogenic (resulting in more mitochondria due to the induction of the PPARγ co-activator 1α, or PGC-1α) and a thermogenic process (due to the transcription of the *Dio2* gene, resulting in elevated quantities of the deiodinase 2 enzyme, D2). This enzyme is responsible for the intracellular conversion of thyroxine (T4) into triiodothyronine (T3), the much more active form of the thyroid hormone. T3 results in a known biogenic process (due to the agonism of the thyroid hormone receptor (TR) [240], but also in a thermogenic one, since it causes the elevation of the levels of the mitochondrial Uncoupling protein 1 (UCP1), a known and powerful thermogenic inducer [241]. Thus, through various studies [236, 242, 243], to name a few, BA have been shown to result in enhanced brown adipose tissue activity in mice, small animals which are highly dependent in non-shivering thermogenesis for maintenance of body core temperature. Furthermore, despite being conducted in lean subjects, it has also been shown that BA also activates BAT UCP1 in humans [244].

As such, it would appear that TGR5 is universally accepted as the sole receptor and pathway conductor for BA effects on obesity. However, this is far from the truth, since TGR5's role has also been extensively questioned. The most powerful natural BA, chenodeoxycholic acid (CDCA), has been reported to be a not very powerful TGR5 activator, whilst being the most potent natural FXR agonist [243, 245].

Furthermore, the work that established TGR5 against FXR [236] also demonstrates that CDCA is a more potent inducer of *Dio2* expression than cholic acid (CA), which the authors use presumably because it is not as potent as CDCA as a FXR activator [246]. The same work also reports a systemic increase of T3 in response to CA supplementation, raising questions regarding the role of intracellular T3 production. Finally, we have recently shown that CDCA also possesses a powerful anti-obesity activity in cultured, differentiated murine 3T3-L1 white adipocytes [235]. Interestingly, we demonstrate an acceleration of catabolism in adipocytes exposed to CDCA, an effect highly pronounced if the cells were also exposed to elevated concentrations of glucose. Associated with this, there is a clear elevation of mitochondrial activity and upstream pathways, which appears to indicate that, in fact, there is an increase of energy expenditure caused by BA in white adipocytes, and not just brown adipocytes as the *in vivo* studies seem to indicate. We have not assessed the expression levels of UCP1 on these samples, since it not only could provide a false interpretation of the results [247], but also since we are dealing with cultured cells, the amount of T4 hormone is probably low, deriving exclusively from the cell culture serum. We thus propose that BA activate other mechanisms of energy waste, whether by futile cycling or other unconsidered means. Furthermore, various FXR or TGR5 activators are not specific. In fact, most bile acids are dual agonists of both receptors. Most synthetic ones are too, despite some initial claims of specificity. For example, the better-known FXR "specific" synthetic agonist, GW4064, has also been shown to activate several classes of G-coupled receptors, albeit not TGR5 [248]. Also Guggulsterone, a claimed FXR specific antagonist also binds and alters the function of various corticoid-type receptors [249]. As such, much is yet to be understood, for no universally accepted mechanism is sufficiently demonstrated and future claims of direct effects of one of these receptors should be carefully examined. In fact, it is better to assume that there is dual agonism of both receptors (or, even possibly, other/others not identified) when discussing bile acids or similar molecular behaviour compounds. In conclusion, it is safe to assume that the mechanisms of BA activity are far from understood.

BA Effects and Mitochondria

Assuming that the axis TGR5-D2-T3-UCP1 is the main source of energy expenditure promoted by BA (or, with greater probability, not discarding FXR contribution or any other class of receptors), there is a major player on which these effects hinge: mitochondria. Since TR activation by T3 results in UCP1 gene expression and PGC-1α induction of a mitochondrial biogenic program [239, 240], it is safe to assume that BA effects are dependent on increased mitochondrial mass and activity. However, it has been extensively shown that high-fat dieting, obesity, diabetes and other metabolic pathologies have a striking common feature: mitochondrial dysfunction [5, 6, 9, 235, 250 - 252]. As such, it is safe to assume that, despite a surprising lack of data on the major works on the field, mitochondrial activity is not compromised in these studies where BA have restored metabolic normality. Furthermore, since new mitochondria arise from the growth and fission of preexisting ones [253], one can infer that an elevation of mitochondrial mass and activity is dependent on functional mitochondria. This means that BA are probably creating an environment of mitochondrial recovery and repair. We theorize that this is primarily possible by the induction of a program of removal of damaged mitochondria by autophagy and restoration (or, in this case, elevation) of mitochondrial numbers by replication of the remaining, little to not affected mitochondrial population. This process is known as mitophagy [254], a process of mitochondrial population and activity restoration, whose imbalance in the pathogenesis of countless diseases, ranging from obesity and diabetes, to aging and neurodegeneration is a key factor.

The mitophagic process is primarily dependent on the action of two key effectors, Parkin and PINK1. These proteins are largely involved in promoting the quality control of the mitochondrial population, being directly involved in the processes of mitochondrial fission and fusion. And, as their name implies, they are heavily implied in the development and progression of Parkinson's Disease [255]. Briefly, when a mitochondrion needs to be targeted for mitophagy (for example, when its membrane potential is severely diminished), it no longer can deactivate and remove units of PINK1 that are constantly binding to its membrane (conversely, viable mitochondria are able to remove PINK1, thus preventing mitophagy on themselves). This signals Parkin, an E3 ubiquitin ligase, to start to ubiquitinate outer mitochondrial membrane proteins, which are a signal for the recruitment of autophagy machinery [255]. If indeed BA have the capacity to improve the function of the mitochondrial population of a cell, this will be true for all situations where the mitochondrial activity is compromised, not just in obesity and diabetes. As such, there are already some reports which appear to point in that direction, albeit few in number.

Going back to Parkinson's disease, it has been shown that the BA ursodeoxycholic acid can restore mitochondrial activity by elevating mitochondrially-generated ATP levels [256]. A variation of this BA, tauroUDCA (TUDCA), has also very strong protective effects on a genetic model of Parkinsonian *Caenorhabditis elegans* against the toxicity of the known mitochondrial toxicants, rotenone or paraquat [257]. On another process that is highly dependent on mitochondrial senescence (aging), a work published in 2010 revealed the BA litocholic acid (LCA), amongst other species of BA, is an anti-aging compound in yeast grown in normal conditions and exposed to calorie restriction, and related this effect to an improved mitochondrial function [258]. The same group, a few years later, published a follow-up study, where they demonstrate that the effects of LCA on life extension are dependent on an increase of the rates of mitophagy [259]. Finally, a recent report links BA to the elevation of the rates of autophagy (granted, this is not just mitophagy, but some parallels can be traced [260], and the concession of protection against hepatic injury [261].

It has similarly been shown that FXR is involved in the regulation of autophagic processes, since its agonism with GW4064 induced the expression of p62/Sqstm1, an essential protein for selective autophagy [262], or of FOXO3a, a protein involved in oxidative stress response [263]. This same work demonstrated that, in FXR-*null* animals' livers, mitophagy is impaired, despite elevated BA levels due to unchecked CYP7A1 activity, which seems to reduce the importance (at least, at the liver) of the TGR5 receptor for these processes. In contrast, two other works are in contradiction to this concept, which clearly indicates that the role of FXR (and of BA, for that matter) is still far from being totally understood. Seok and collaborators studied FXR's role in different nutritional status of both normal and FXR-*null* animals and concluded that FXR is a repressor of mitophagy, even in fasted livers [264]. A similar conclusion was reached by Lee and collaborators where it was found that FXR competes with the peroxisome proliferator-activated receptor α (PPARα) for access to mitophagy-related DNA binding sites [265].

As such, it is reasonable to assume that BA have the capacity to modulate mitochondrial function, which is still probably true in obesity. Understanding this process, and particularly, how it happens, could provide an immense contribution towards the understanding of how BA reverse obesity and diabetes and potentially contribute to the development of the study of other unrelated pathologies.

CONCLUDING REMARKS

Mitochondrial dysfunction involving decreased mitochondrial mass, defects in the mitochondrial OXPHOS system, decreased rate of ATP synthesis and increased ROS formation, is associated with the development of obesity, one of the most important and costly problems affecting the world's population and health care systems. Stimulation of mitochondrial metabolism and maintenance of mitochondrial homeostasis (Fig. **1**) appears as an efficient therapeutic strategy to manage the increased flux of reduced substrates to the electron transport chain that occurs with obesity. On one hand, sirtuin-activating compounds, by stimulating mitochondrial biogenesis, have been shown to boost metabolism. On the other hand, stimulation of energy expenditure by bile acids action on adipose tissue appears as a potential candidate against obesity.

CONSENT FOR PUBLICATION

Not applicable.

CONFLICT OF INTEREST

The authors declare no conflict of interest.

ACKNOWLEDGEMENTS

This work was financed by the European Regional Development Fund (ERDF), through the Centro 2020 Regional Operational Programme: project CENTRO-0--0145-FEDER-000012-HealthyAging2020, the Portugal 2020 - Operational Programme for Competitiveness and Internationalisation, and the Portuguese national funds *via* FCT – Fundação para a Ciência e a Tecnologia, I.P.: project POCI-01-0145-FEDER-016770, as well as by UID/NEU/04539/2013 (CNC.IBILI Consortium strategic project). JST and JAA are recipients of scholarships from FCT (SFRH/BPD/ 94036//2013 and PD/BD/114173/2016, respectively).

REFERENCES

[1]   World Health Organization. http://www.who.int/gho/ncd/risk_factors/obesity_text/en/

[2]   Apovian CM. Obesity: definition, comorbidities, causes, and burden. Am J Manag Care 2016; 22(7) (Suppl.): s176-85.
[PMID: 27356115]

[3]   López-Lluch G. Mitochondrial activity and dynamics changes regarding metabolism in ageing and obesity. Mech Ageing Dev 2017; 162: 108-21.
[http://dx.doi.org/10.1016/j.mad.2016.12.005] [PMID: 27993601]

[4]   Wang W, Karamanlidis G, Tian R. Novel targets for mitochondrial medicine. Sci Transl Med 2016; 8(326): 326rv3.
[http://dx.doi.org/10.1126/scitranslmed.aac7410] [PMID: 26888432]

[5]   Teodoro JS, Rolo AP, Duarte FV, Simões AM, Palmeira CM. Differential alterations in mitochondrial function induced by a choline-deficient diet: understanding fatty liver disease progression. Mitochondrion 2008; 8(5-6): 367-76.
[http://dx.doi.org/10.1016/j.mito.2008.07.008] [PMID: 18765303]

[6]   Gomes AP, Duarte FV, Nunes P, *et al.* Berberine protects against high fat diet-induced dysfunction in muscle mitochondria by inducing SIRT1-dependent mitochondrial biogenesis. Biochim Biophys Acta 2012; 1822(2): 185-95.
[http://dx.doi.org/10.1016/j.bbadis.2011.10.008] [PMID: 22027215]

[7]   James AM, Collins Y, Logan A, Murphy MP. Mitochondrial oxidative stress and the metabolic syndrome. Trends Endocrinol Metab 2012; 23(9): 429-34.
[http://dx.doi.org/10.1016/j.tem.2012.06.008] [PMID: 22831852]

[8]   Gomes AP, Price NL, Ling AJ, *et al.* Declining NAD(+) induces a pseudohypoxic state disrupting nuclear-mitochondrial communication during aging. Cell 2013; 155(7): 1624-38.
[http://dx.doi.org/10.1016/j.cell.2013.11.037] [PMID: 24360282]

[9]   Teodoro JS, Duarte FV, Gomes AP, *et al.* Berberine reverts hepatic mitochondrial dysfunction in high-fat fed rats: a possible role for SirT3 activation. Mitochondrion 2013; 13(6): 637-46.
[http://dx.doi.org/10.1016/j.mito.2013.09.002] [PMID: 24041461]

[10]   Schatz G. Mitochondria: beyond oxidative phosphorylation. Biochim Biophys Acta 1995; 1271(1): 123-6.
[http://dx.doi.org/10.1016/0925-4439(95)00018-Y] [PMID: 7599197]

[11]   Cheng Z, Ristow M. Mitochondria and metabolic homeostasis. Antioxid Redox Signal 2013; 19(3): 240-2.
[http://dx.doi.org/10.1089/ars.2013.5255] [PMID: 23432475]

[12]   Murphy MP. How mitochondria produce reactive oxygen species. Biochem J 2009; 417(1): 1-13.
[http://dx.doi.org/10.1042/BJ20081386] [PMID: 19061483]

[13]   Brand MD. The sites and topology of mitochondrial superoxide production. Exp Gerontol 2010; 45(7-8): 466-72.
[http://dx.doi.org/10.1016/j.exger.2010.01.003] [PMID: 20064600]

[14]   Skulachev VP. Role of uncoupled and non-coupled oxidations in maintenance of safely low levels of oxygen and its one-electron reductants. Q Rev Biophys 1996; 29(2): 169-202.
[http://dx.doi.org/10.1017/S0033583500005795] [PMID: 8870073]

[15]   Raffaella C, Francesca B, Italia F, Marina P, Giovanna L, Susanna I. Alterations in hepatic mitochondrial compartment in a model of obesity and insulin resistance. Obesity (Silver Spring) 2008; 16(5): 958-64.
[http://dx.doi.org/10.1038/oby.2008.10] [PMID: 18277391]

[16]   Anderson EJ, Lustig ME, Boyle KE, *et al.* Mitochondrial H2O2 emission and cellular redox state link excess fat intake to insulin resistance in both rodents and humans. J Clin Invest 2009; 119(3): 573-81.
[http://dx.doi.org/10.1172/JCI37048] [PMID: 19188683]

[17]   Ruggiero C, Ehrenshaft M, Cleland E, Stadler K. High-fat diet induces an initial adaptation of mitochondrial bioenergetics in the kidney despite evident oxidative stress and mitochondrial ROS production. Am J Physiol Endocrinol Metab 2011; 300(6): E1047-58.
[http://dx.doi.org/10.1152/ajpendo.00666.2010] [PMID: 21386058]

[18]   Ploumi C, Daskalaki I, Tavernarakis N. Mitochondrial biogenesis and clearance: a balancing act. FEBS J 2017; 284(2): 183-95.
[http://dx.doi.org/10.1111/febs.13820] [PMID: 27462821]

[19]   Palikaras K, Lionaki E, Tavernarakis N. Balancing mitochondrial biogenesis and mitophagy to maintain energy metabolism homeostasis. Cell Death Differ 2015; 22(9): 1399-401.
[http://dx.doi.org/10.1038/cdd.2015.86] [PMID: 26256515]

[20]   Handschin C, Spiegelman BM. Peroxisome proliferator-activated receptor gamma coactivator 1 coactivators, energy homeostasis, and metabolism. Endocr Rev 2006; 27(7): 728-35.
[http://dx.doi.org/10.1210/er.2006-0037] [PMID: 17018837]

[21]   Austin S, St-Pierre J. PGC1α and mitochondrial metabolism--emerging concepts and relevance in ageing and neurodegenerative disorders. J Cell Sci 2012; 125(Pt 21): 4963-71.
[http://dx.doi.org/10.1242/jcs.113662] [PMID: 23277535]

[22]   Sinclair DA, Guarente L. Extrachromosomal rDNA circles - A cause of aging in yeast. Cell 1997; 91(7): 1033-42.

[23]   Kaeberlein M, Mcvey M, Guarente L. Saccharomyces cerevisiae by two different mechanisms promote longevity in Saccharomyces cerevisiae by two different mechanisms. Genes Dev 1999; 13(19): 2570-80.
[http://dx.doi.org/10.1101/gad.13.19.2570] [PMID: 10521401]

[24]   Friedman DB, Johnson TE. Three mutants that extend both mean and maximum life span of the nematode, Caenorhabditis elegans, define the age-1 gene. J Gerontol 1988; 43(4): B102-9.
[http://dx.doi.org/10.1093/geronj/43.4.B102] [PMID: 3385139]

[25]   Friedman DB, Johnson TE. A mutation in the age-1 gene in Caenorhabditis elegans lengthens life and reduces hermaphrodite fertility. Genetics 1988; 118(1): 75-86.
[PMID: 8608934]

[26]   Kennedy BK, Austriaco NR Jr, Zhang J, Guarente L. Mutation in the silencing gene SIR4 can delay

aging in S. cerevisiae. Cell 1995; 80(3): 485-96.
[http://dx.doi.org/10.1016/0092-8674(95)90499-9] [PMID: 7859289]

[27]   Kenyon C, Chang J, Gensch E, Rudner A, Tabtiang R. A C. elegans mutant that lives twice as long as wild type. Nature 1993; 366(6454): 461-4.
[http://dx.doi.org/10.1038/366461a0] [PMID: 8247153]

[28]   Sinclair DA, Guarente L. Unlocking the secrets of longevity genes. Sci Am 2006; 294(3): 48-51, 54-57.
[http://dx.doi.org/10.1038/scientificamerican0306-48] [PMID: 16502611]

[29]   Imai S, Armstrong CM, Kaeberlein M, Guarente L. Transcriptional silencing and longevity protein Sir2 is an NAD-dependent histone deacetylase. Nature 2000; 403(6771): 795-800.
[http://dx.doi.org/10.1038/35001622] [PMID: 10693811]

[30]   Frye RA. A polymorphism in the growth hormone (GH)-releasing hormone (GHRH) receptor gene is associated with elevated response to GHRH by human pituitary somatotrophinomas *in vitro.* Biochem Biophys Res Commun 2000; 273: 793-8.
[http://dx.doi.org/10.1006/bbrc.2000.3000] [PMID: 10873683]

[31]   Haigis MC, Guarente LP. Mammalian sirtuins--emerging roles in physiology, aging, and calorie restriction. Genes Dev 2006; 20(21): 2913-21.
[http://dx.doi.org/10.1101/gad.1467506] [PMID: 17079682]

[32]   Michan S, Sinclair D. Sirtuins in mammals: insights into their biological function. Biochem J 2007; 404(1): 1-13.
[http://dx.doi.org/10.1042/BJ20070140] [PMID: 17447894]

[33]   Michishita E, Park JY, Burneskis JM, Barrett JC, Horikawa I. Evolutionarily conserved and nonconserved cellular localizations and functions of human SIRT proteins. Mol Biol Cell 2005; 16(10): 4623-35.
[http://dx.doi.org/10.1091/mbc.e05-01-0033] [PMID: 16079181]

[34]   Tanno M, Sakamoto J, Miura T, Shimamoto K, Horio Y. Nucleocytoplasmic shuttling of the NAD+-dependent histone deacetylase SIRT1. J Biol Chem 2007; 282(9): 6823-32.
[http://dx.doi.org/10.1074/jbc.M609554200] [PMID: 17197703]

[35]   Onyango P, Celic I, McCaffery JM, Boeke JD, Feinberg AP. SIRT3, a human SIR2 homologue, is an NAD-dependent deacetylase localized to mitochondria. Proc Natl Acad Sci USA 2002; 99(21): 13653-8.
[http://dx.doi.org/10.1073/pnas.222538099] [PMID: 12374852]

[36]   Schwer B, North BJ, Frye RA, Ott M, Verdin E. The human silent information regulator (Sir)2 homologue hSIRT3 is a mitochondrial nicotinamide adenine dinucleotide-dependent deacetylase. J Cell Biol 2002; 158(4): 647-57.
[http://dx.doi.org/10.1083/jcb.200205057] [PMID: 12186850]

[37]   Nakamura Y, Ogura M, Tanaka D, Inagaki N. Localization of mouse mitochondrial SIRT proteins: shift of SIRT3 to nucleus by co-expression with SIRT5. Biochem Biophys Res Commun 2008; 366(1): 174-9.
[http://dx.doi.org/10.1016/j.bbrc.2007.11.122] [PMID: 18054327]

[38]   Scher MB, Vaquero A, Reinberg D. SirT3 is a nuclear NAD+-dependent histone deacetylase that translocates to the mitochondria upon cellular stress. Genes Dev 2007; 21(8): 920-8.
[http://dx.doi.org/10.1101/gad.1527307] [PMID: 17437997]

[39]   Jing E, Gesta S, Kahn CR. SIRT2 regulates adipocyte differentiation through FoxO1 acetylation/deacetylation. Cell Metab 2007; 6(2): 105-14.
[http://dx.doi.org/10.1016/j.cmet.2007.07.003] [PMID: 17681146]

[40]   North BJ, Verdin E. Interphase nucleo-cytoplasmic shuttling and localization of SIRT2 during mitosis. PLoS One 2007; 2(8): e784.

[http://dx.doi.org/10.1371/journal.pone.0000784] [PMID: 17726514]

[41] Houtkooper RH, Cantó C, Wanders RJ, Auwerx J. The secret life of NAD+: an old metabolite controlling new metabolic signaling pathways. Endocr Rev 2010; 31(2): 194-223.
[http://dx.doi.org/10.1210/er.2009-0026] [PMID: 20007326]

[42] Sauve AA, Celic I, Avalos J, Deng H, Boeke JD, Schramm VL. Chemistry of gene silencing: the mechanism of NAD+-dependent deacetylation reactions. Biochemistry 2001; 40(51): 15456-63.
[http://dx.doi.org/10.1021/bi011858j] [PMID: 11747420]

[43] Schmidt MT, Smith BC, Jackson MD, Denu JM. Coenzyme specificity of Sir2 protein deacetylases: implications for physiological regulation. J Biol Chem 2004; 279(38): 40122-9.
[http://dx.doi.org/10.1074/jbc.M407484200] [PMID: 15269219]

[44] Borra MT, Langer MR, Slama JT, Denu JM. Substrate Specificity and Kinetic Mechanism of the Sir2 Family of Deacetylases. Biochemistry 2004; 43(30): 9877-87.
[http://dx.doi.org/10.1021/bi049592e] [PMID: 15274642]

[45] North BJ, Marshall BL, Borra MT, Denu JM, Verdin E. The human Sir2 ortholog, SIRT2, is an NAD+-dependent tubulin deacetylase. Mol Cell 2003; 11(2): 437-44.
[http://dx.doi.org/10.1016/S1097-2765(03)00038-8] [PMID: 12620231]

[46] Vaziri H, Dessain SK, Ng Eaton E, *et al.* hSIR2(SIRT1) functions as an NAD-dependent p53 deacetylase. Cell 2001; 107(2): 149-59.
[http://dx.doi.org/10.1016/S0092-8674(01)00527-X] [PMID: 11672523]

[47] Haigis MC, Mostoslavsky R, Haigis KM, *et al.* SIRT4 inhibits glutamate dehydrogenase and opposes the effects of calorie restriction in pancreatic beta cells. Cell 2006; 126(5): 941-54.
[http://dx.doi.org/10.1016/j.cell.2006.06.057] [PMID: 16959573]

[48] Liszt G, Ford E, Kurtev M, Guarente L. Mouse Sir2 homolog SIRT6 is a nuclear ADP-ribosyltransferase. J Biol Chem 2005; 280(22): 21313-20.
[http://dx.doi.org/10.1074/jbc.M413296200] [PMID: 15795229]

[49] Mathias RA, Greco TM, Oberstein A, *et al.* Sirtuin 4 is a lipoamidase regulating pyruvate dehydrogenase complex activity. Cell 2014; 159(7): 1615-25.
[http://dx.doi.org/10.1016/j.cell.2014.11.046] [PMID: 25525879]

[50] Jiang H, Khan S, Wang Y, *et al.* SIRT6 regulates TNF-α secretion through hydrolysis of long-chain fatty acyl lysine. Nature 2013; 496(7443): 110-3.
[http://dx.doi.org/10.1038/nature12038] [PMID: 23552949]

[51] Du J, Zhou Y, Su X, *et al.* Sirt5 is a NAD-dependent protein lysine demalonylase and desuccinylase. Science 2011; 334(6057): 806-9.
[http://dx.doi.org/10.1126/science.1207861] [PMID: 22076378]

[52] Tan M, Peng C, Anderson KA, *et al.* Lysine glutarylation is a protein posttranslational modification regulated by SIRT5. Cell Metab 2014; 19(4): 605-17.
[http://dx.doi.org/10.1016/j.cmet.2014.03.014] [PMID: 24703693]

[53] Ryu D, Jo YS, Lo Sasso G, *et al.* A SIRT7-dependent acetylation switch of GABPβ1 controls mitochondrial function. Cell Metab 2014; 20(5): 856-69.
[http://dx.doi.org/10.1016/j.cmet.2014.08.001] [PMID: 25200183]

[54] Vakhrusheva O, Smolka C, Gajawada P, *et al.* Sirt7 increases stress resistance of cardiomyocytes and prevents apoptosis and inflammatory cardiomyopathy in mice. Circ Res 2008; 102(6): 703-10.
[http://dx.doi.org/10.1161/CIRCRESAHA.107.164558] [PMID: 18239138]

[55] Chen S, Seiler J, Santiago-Reichelt M, Felbel K, Grummt I, Voit R. Repression of RNA polymerase I upon stress is caused by inhibition of RNA-dependent deacetylation of PAF53 by SIRT7. Mol Cell 2013; 52(3): 303-13.
[http://dx.doi.org/10.1016/j.molcel.2013.10.010] [PMID: 24207024]

[56]   Wang Y, Liang Y, Vanhoutte PM. SIRT1 and AMPK in regulating mammalian senescence: a critical review and a working model. FEBS Lett 2011; 585(7): 986-94.
[http://dx.doi.org/10.1016/j.febslet.2010.11.047] [PMID: 21130086]

[57]   Gerhart-Hines Z, Dominy JE Jr, Blättler SM, *et al.* The cAMP/PKA pathway rapidly activates SIRT1 to promote fatty acid oxidation independently of changes in NAD(+). Mol Cell 2011; 44(6): 851-63.
[http://dx.doi.org/10.1016/j.molcel.2011.12.005] [PMID: 22195961]

[58]   Armour SM, Baur JA, Hsieh SN, Land-Bracha A, Thomas SM, Sinclair DA. Inhibition of mammalian S6 kinase by resveratrol suppresses autophagy. Aging (Albany NY) 2009; 1(6): 515-28.
[http://dx.doi.org/10.18632/aging.100056] [PMID: 20157535]

[59]   Liu M, Liu F. Resveratrol inhibits mTOR signaling by targeting DEPTOR. Commun Integr Biol 2011; 4(4): 382-4.
[http://dx.doi.org/10.4161/cib.15309] [PMID: 21966552]

[60]   Mouchiroud L, Houtkooper RH, Moullan N, *et al.* The NAD+/sirtuin pathway modulates longevity through activation of mitochondrial UPR and FOXO signaling. Cell 2013; 154(2): 430-41.
[http://dx.doi.org/10.1016/j.cell.2013.06.016] [PMID: 23870130]

[61]   Rodgers JT, Lerin C, Haas W, Gygi SP, Spiegelman BM, Puigserver P. Nutrient control of glucose homeostasis through a complex of PGC-1alpha and SIRT1. Nature 2005; 434(7029): 113-8.
[http://dx.doi.org/10.1038/nature03354] [PMID: 15744310]

[62]   Yeung F, Hoberg JE, Ramsey CS, *et al.* Modulation of NF-kappaB-dependent transcription and cell survival by the SIRT1 deacetylase. EMBO J 2004; 23(12): 2369-80.
[http://dx.doi.org/10.1038/sj.emboj.7600244] [PMID: 15152190]

[63]   Longo VD. Linking sirtuins, IGF-I signaling, and starvation. Exp Gerontol 2009; 44(1-2): 70-4.
[http://dx.doi.org/10.1016/j.exger.2008.06.005] [PMID: 18638538]

[64]   Cantó C, Jiang LQ, Deshmukh AS, *et al.* Interdependence of AMPK and SIRT1 for metabolic adaptation to fasting and exercise in skeletal muscle. Cell Metab 2010; 11(3): 213-9.
[http://dx.doi.org/10.1016/j.cmet.2010.02.006] [PMID: 20197054]

[65]   Chen D, Bruno J, Easlon E, *et al.* Tissue-specific regulation of SIRT1 by calorie restriction. Genes Dev 2008; 22(13): 1753-7.
[http://dx.doi.org/10.1101/gad.1650608] [PMID: 18550784]

[66]   Cantó C, Gerhart-Hines Z, Feige JN, *et al.* AMPK regulates energy expenditure by modulating NAD+ metabolism and SIRT1 activity. Nature 2009; 458(7241): 1056-60.
[http://dx.doi.org/10.1038/nature07813] [PMID: 19262508]

[67]   Fulco M, Cen Y, Zhao P, *et al.* Glucose restriction inhibits skeletal myoblast differentiation by activating SIRT1 through AMPK-mediated regulation of Nampt. Dev Cell 2008; 14(5): 661-73.
[http://dx.doi.org/10.1016/j.devcel.2008.02.004] [PMID: 18477450]

[68]   Boily G, Seifert EL, Bevilacqua L, *et al.* SirT1 regulates energy metabolism and response to caloric restriction in mice. PLoS One 2008; 3(3): e1759.
[http://dx.doi.org/10.1371/journal.pone.0001759] [PMID: 18335035]

[69]   Feige JN, Lagouge M, Canto C, *et al.* Specific SIRT1 activation mimics low energy levels and protects against diet-induced metabolic disorders by enhancing fat oxidation. Cell Metab 2008; 8(5): 347-58.
[http://dx.doi.org/10.1016/j.cmet.2008.08.017] [PMID: 19046567]

[70]   Menzies KJ, Singh K, Saleem A, Hood DA. Sirtuin 1-mediated effects of exercise and resveratrol on mitochondrial biogenesis. J Biol Chem 2013; 288(10): 6968-79.
[http://dx.doi.org/10.1074/jbc.M112.431155] [PMID: 23329826]

[71]   Price NL, Gomes AP, Ling AJ, *et al.* SIRT1 is required for AMPK activation and the beneficial effects of resveratrol on mitochondrial function. Cell Metab 2012; 15(5): 675-90.
[http://dx.doi.org/10.1016/j.cmet.2012.04.003] [PMID: 22560220]

[72]   Silva JP, Wahlestedt C. Role of Sirtuin 1 in metabolic regulation. Drug Discov Today 2010; 15(17-18): 781-91.
       [http://dx.doi.org/10.1016/j.drudis.2010.07.001] [PMID: 20621197]

[73]   Banks AS, Kon N, Knight C, *et al.* SirT1 gain of function increases energy efficiency and prevents diabetes in mice. Cell Metab 2008; 8(4): 333-41.
       [http://dx.doi.org/10.1016/j.cmet.2008.08.014] [PMID: 18840364]

[74]   Herranz D, Muñoz-Martin M, Cañamero M, *et al.* Sirt1 improves healthy ageing and protects from metabolic syndrome-associated cancer. Nat Commun 2010; 1: 3.
       [http://dx.doi.org/10.1038/ncomms1001] [PMID: 20975665]

[75]   Pfluger PT, Herranz D, Velasco-Miguel S, Serrano M, Tschöp MH. Sirt1 protects against high-fat diet-induced metabolic damage. Proc Natl Acad Sci USA 2008; 105(28): 9793-8.
       [http://dx.doi.org/10.1073/pnas.0802917105] [PMID: 18599449]

[76]   Baur JA, Pearson KJ, Price NL, *et al.* Resveratrol improves health and survival of mice on a high-calorie diet. Nature 2006; 444(7117): 337-42.
       [http://dx.doi.org/10.1038/nature05354] [PMID: 17086191]

[77]   Minor RK, Baur JA, Gomes AP, *et al.* SRT1720 improves survival and healthspan of obese mice. Sci Rep 2011; 1: 70.
       [http://dx.doi.org/10.1038/srep00070] [PMID: 22355589]

[78]   Bordone L, Cohen D, Robinson A, *et al.* SIRT1 transgenic mice show phenotypes resembling calorie restriction. Aging Cell 2007; 6(6): 759-67.
       [http://dx.doi.org/10.1111/j.1474-9726.2007.00335.x] [PMID: 17877786]

[79]   Kanfi Y, Naiman S, Amir G, *et al.* The sirtuin SIRT6 regulates lifespan in male mice. Nature 2012; 483(7388): 218-21.
       [http://dx.doi.org/10.1038/nature10815] [PMID: 22367546]

[80]   Lombard DB, Alt FW, Cheng H-L, *et al.* Mammalian Sir2 homolog SIRT3 regulates global mitochondrial lysine acetylation. Mol Cell Biol 2007; 27(24): 8807-14.
       [http://dx.doi.org/10.1128/MCB.01636-07] [PMID: 17923681]

[81]   Giralt A, Villarroya F. SIRT3, a pivotal actor in mitochondrial functions: metabolism, cell death and aging. Biochem J 2012; 444(1): 1-10.
       [http://dx.doi.org/10.1042/BJ20120030] [PMID: 22533670]

[82]   Shi T, Wang F, Stieren E, Tong Q. SIRT3, a mitochondrial sirtuin deacetylase, regulates mitochondrial function and thermogenesis in brown adipocytes. J Biol Chem 2005; 280(14): 13560-7.
       [http://dx.doi.org/10.1074/jbc.M414670200] [PMID: 15653680]

[83]   Hallows WC, Lee S, Denu JM. Sirtuins deacetylate and activate mammalian acetyl-CoA synthetases. Proc Natl Acad Sci USA 2006; 103(27): 10230-5.
       [http://dx.doi.org/10.1073/pnas.0604392103] [PMID: 16790548]

[84]   Schlicker C, Gertz M, Papatheodorou P, Kachholz B, Becker CF, Steegborn C. Substrates and regulation mechanisms for the human mitochondrial sirtuins Sirt3 and Sirt5. J Mol Biol 2008; 382(3): 790-801.
       [http://dx.doi.org/10.1016/j.jmb.2008.07.048] [PMID: 18680753]

[85]   Kendrick AA, Choudhury M, Rahman SM, *et al.* Fatty liver is associated with reduced SIRT3 activity and mitochondrial protein hyperacetylation. Biochem J 2011; 433(3): 505-14.
       [http://dx.doi.org/10.1042/BJ20100791] [PMID: 21044047]

[86]   Morigi M, Perico L, Rota C, *et al.* Sirtuin 3-dependent mitochondrial dynamic improvements protect against acute kidney injury. J Clin Invest 2015; 125(2): 715-26.
       [http://dx.doi.org/10.1172/JCI77632] [PMID: 25607838]

[87]   Hirschey MD, Shimazu T, Goetzman E, *et al.* SIRT3 regulates mitochondrial fatty-acid oxidation by

reversible enzyme deacetylation. Nature 2010; 464(7285): 121-5.
[http://dx.doi.org/10.1038/nature08778] [PMID: 20203611]

[88] Hokari F, Kawasaki E, Sakai A, Koshinaka K, Sakuma K, Kawanaka K. Muscle contractile activity regulates Sirt3 protein expression in rat skeletal muscles. J Appl Physiol 2010; 109(2): 332-40.
[http://dx.doi.org/10.1152/japplphysiol.00335.2009] [PMID: 20413424]

[89] Palacios OM, Carmona JJ, Michan S, *et al.* Diet and exercise signals regulate SIRT3 and activate AMPK and PGC-1alpha in skeletal muscle. Aging (Albany NY) 2009; 1(9): 771-83.
[http://dx.doi.org/10.18632/aging.100075] [PMID: 20157566]

[90] Giralt A, Hondares E, Villena JA, *et al.* Peroxisome proliferator-activated receptor-gamma coactivator-1alpha controls transcription of the Sirt3 gene, an essential component of the thermogenic brown adipocyte phenotype. J Biol Chem 2011; 286(19): 16958-66.
[http://dx.doi.org/10.1074/jbc.M110.202390] [PMID: 21454513]

[91] Kong X, Wang R, Xue Y, *et al.* Sirtuin 3, a new target of PGC-1alpha, plays an important role in the suppression of ROS and mitochondrial biogenesis. PLoS One 2010; 5(7): e11707.
[http://dx.doi.org/10.1371/journal.pone.0011707] [PMID: 20661474]

[92] Eichner LJ, Giguère V. Estrogen related receptors (ERRs): a new dawn in transcriptional control of mitochondrial gene networks. Mitochondrion 2011; 11(4): 544-52.
[http://dx.doi.org/10.1016/j.mito.2011.03.121] [PMID: 21497207]

[93] Mootha VK, Handschin C, Arlow D, *et al.* Erralpha and Gabpa/b specify PGC-1α-dependent oxidative phosphorylation gene expression that is altered in diabetic muscle. Proc Natl Acad Sci USA 2004; 101(17): 6570-5.
[http://dx.doi.org/10.1073/pnas.0401401101] [PMID: 15100410]

[94] Schreiber SN, Emter R, Hock MB, *et al.* The estrogen-related receptor α (ERRalpha) functions in PPARgamma coactivator 1α (PGC-1α)-induced mitochondrial biogenesis. Proc Natl Acad Sci USA 2004; 101(17): 6472-7.
[http://dx.doi.org/10.1073/pnas.0308686101] [PMID: 15087503]

[95] Cartoni R, Léger B, Hock MB, *et al.* Mitofusins 1/2 and ERRalpha expression are increased in human skeletal muscle after physical exercise. J Physiol 2005; 567(Pt 1): 349-58.
[http://dx.doi.org/10.1113/jphysiol.2005.092031] [PMID: 15961417]

[96] Mootha VK, Lindgren CM, Eriksson KF, *et al.* PGC-1α-responsive genes involved in oxidative phosphorylation are coordinately downregulated in human diabetes. Nat Genet 2003; 34(3): 267-73.
[http://dx.doi.org/10.1038/ng1180] [PMID: 12808457]

[97] Uldry M, Yang W, St-Pierre J, Lin J, Seale P, Spiegelman BM. Complementary action of the PGC-1 coactivators in mitochondrial biogenesis and brown fat differentiation. Cell Metab 2006; 3(5): 333-41.
[http://dx.doi.org/10.1016/j.cmet.2006.04.002] [PMID: 16679291]

[98] Cunningham JT, Rodgers JT, Arlow DH, Vazquez F, Mootha VK, Puigserver P. mTOR controls mitochondrial oxidative function through a YY1-PGC-1alpha transcriptional complex. Nature 2007; 450(7170): 736-40.
[http://dx.doi.org/10.1038/nature06322] [PMID: 18046414]

[99] Rasbach KA, Gupta RK, Ruas JL, *et al.* PGC-1α regulates a HIF2α-dependent switch in skeletal muscle fiber types. Proc Natl Acad Sci USA 2010; 107(50): 21866-71.
[http://dx.doi.org/10.1073/pnas.1016089107] [PMID: 21106753]

[100] Handschin C, Spiegelman BM. PGC-1 coactivators and the regulation of skeletal muscle fiber-type determination. Cell Metab 2011; 13(4): 351.
[http://dx.doi.org/10.1016/j.cmet.2011.03.008] [PMID: 21459315]

[101] Boutant M, Cantó C. SIRT1 metabolic actions: Integrating recent advances from mouse models. Mol Metab 2013; 3(1): 5-18.
[http://dx.doi.org/10.1016/j.molmet.2013.10.006] [PMID: 24567900]

[102]   Hirschey MD, Shimazu T, Jing E, *et al.* SIRT3 deficiency and mitochondrial protein hyperacetylation accelerate the development of the metabolic syndrome. Mol Cell 2011; 44(2): 177-90.
[http://dx.doi.org/10.1016/j.molcel.2011.07.019] [PMID: 21856199]

[103]   Winnik S, Gaul DS, Siciliani G, *et al.* Mild endothelial dysfunction in Sirt3 knockout mice fed a high-cholesterol diet: protective role of a novel C/EBP-β-dependent feedback regulation of SOD2. Basic Res Cardiol 2016; 111(3): 33.
[http://dx.doi.org/10.1007/s00395-016-0552-7] [PMID: 27071400]

[104]   Mostoslavsky R, Chua KF, Lombard DB, *et al.* Genomic instability and aging-like phenotype in the absence of mammalian SIRT6. Cell 2006; 124(2): 315-29.
[http://dx.doi.org/10.1016/j.cell.2005.11.044] [PMID: 16439206]

[105]   Zhong L, D'Urso A, Toiber D, *et al.* The histone deacetylase Sirt6 regulates glucose homeostasis *via* Hif1alpha. Cell 2010; 140(2): 280-93.
[http://dx.doi.org/10.1016/j.cell.2009.12.041] [PMID: 20141841]

[106]   Beirowski B, Gustin J, Armour SM, *et al.* Sir-two-homolog 2 (Sirt2) modulates peripheral myelination through polarity protein Par-3/atypical protein kinase C (aPKC) signaling. Proc Natl Acad Sci USA 2011; 108(43): E952-61.
[http://dx.doi.org/10.1073/pnas.1104969108] [PMID: 21949390]

[107]   Bobrowska A, Donmez G, Weiss A, Guarente L, Bates G. SIRT2 ablation has no effect on tubulin acetylation in brain, cholesterol biosynthesis or the progression of Huntington's disease phenotypes *in vivo.* PLoS One 2012; 7(4): e34805.
[http://dx.doi.org/10.1371/journal.pone.0034805] [PMID: 22511966]

[108]   Yu J, Sadhukhan S, Noriega LG, *et al.* Metabolic characterization of a Sirt5 deficient mouse model. Sci Rep 2013; 3: 2806.
[http://dx.doi.org/10.1038/srep02806] [PMID: 24076663]

[109]   Laurent G, German NJ, Saha AK, *et al.* SIRT4 coordinates the balance between lipid synthesis and catabolism by repressing malonyl CoA decarboxylase. Mol Cell 2013; 50(5): 686-98.
[http://dx.doi.org/10.1016/j.molcel.2013.05.012] [PMID: 23746352]

[110]   Liang F, Kume S, Koya D. SIRT1 and insulin resistance. Nat Rev Endocrinol 2009; 5(7): 367-73.
[http://dx.doi.org/10.1038/nrendo.2009.101] [PMID: 19455179]

[111]   Iwabu M, Yamauchi T, Okada-Iwabu M, *et al.* Adiponectin and AdipoR1 regulate PGC-1alpha and mitochondria by Ca(2+) and AMPK/SIRT1. Nature 2010; 464(7293): 1313-9.
[http://dx.doi.org/10.1038/nature08991] [PMID: 20357764]

[112]   Cakir I, Perello M, Lansari O, Messier NJ, Vaslet CA, Nillni EA. Hypothalamic Sirt1 regulates food intake in a rodent model system. PLoS One 2009; 4(12): e8322.
[http://dx.doi.org/10.1371/journal.pone.0008322] [PMID: 20020036]

[113]   Picard F, Kurtev M, Chung N, *et al.* Sirt1 promotes fat mobilization in white adipocytes by repressing PPAR-gamma. Nature 2004; 429(6993): 771-6.
[http://dx.doi.org/10.1038/nature02583] [PMID: 15175761]

[114]   Purushotham A, Xu Q, Li X. Systemic SIRT1 insufficiency results in disruption of energy homeostasis and steroid hormone metabolism upon high-fat-diet feeding. FASEB J 2012; 26(2): 656-67.
[http://dx.doi.org/10.1096/fj.11-195172] [PMID: 22006157]

[115]   Wang RH, Kim HS, Xiao C, Xu X, Gavrilova O, Deng CX. Hepatic Sirt1 deficiency in mice impairs mTorc2/Akt signaling and results in hyperglycemia, oxidative damage, and insulin resistance. J Clin Invest 2011; 121(11): 4477-90.
[http://dx.doi.org/10.1172/JCI46243] [PMID: 21965330]

[116]   Ramadori G, Lee CE, Bookout AL, *et al.* Brain SIRT1: anatomical distribution and regulation by energy availability. J Neurosci 2008; 28(40): 9989-96.
[http://dx.doi.org/10.1523/JNEUROSCI.3257-08.2008] [PMID: 18829956]

[117] Qiao L, Shao J. SIRT1 regulates adiponectin gene expression through Foxo1-C/enhancer-binding protein alpha transcriptional complex. J Biol Chem 2006; 281(52): 39915-24.
[http://dx.doi.org/10.1074/jbc.M607215200] [PMID: 17090532]

[118] Chalkiadaki A, Guarente L. High-fat diet triggers inflammation-induced cleavage of SIRT1 in adipose tissue to promote metabolic dysfunction. Cell Metab 2012; 16(2): 180-8.
[http://dx.doi.org/10.1016/j.cmet.2012.07.003] [PMID: 22883230]

[119] Pang W, Wang Y, Wei N, *et al.* Sirt1 inhibits akt2-mediated porcine adipogenesis potentially by direct protein-protein interaction. PLoS One 2013; 8(8): e71576.
[http://dx.doi.org/10.1371/journal.pone.0071576] [PMID: 23951196]

[120] Hotamisligil GS. Inflammation, metaflammation and immunometabolic disorders. Nature 2017; 542(7640): 177-85.
[http://dx.doi.org/10.1038/nature21363] [PMID: 28179656]

[121] Xu F, Gao Z, Zhang J, *et al.* Lack of SIRT1 (Mammalian Sirtuin 1) activity leads to liver steatosis in the SIRT1+/- mice: a role of lipid mobilization and inflammation. Endocrinology 2010; 151(6): 2504-14.
[http://dx.doi.org/10.1210/en.2009-1013] [PMID: 20339025]

[122] Kauppinen A, Suuronen T, Ojala J, Kaarniranta K, Salminen A. Antagonistic crosstalk between NF-κB and SIRT1 in the regulation of inflammation and metabolic disorders. Cell Signal 2013; 25(10): 1939-48.
[http://dx.doi.org/10.1016/j.cellsig.2013.06.007] [PMID: 23770291]

[123] Yoshizaki T, Milne JC, Imamura T, *et al.* SIRT1 exerts anti-inflammatory effects and improves insulin sensitivity in adipocytes. Mol Cell Biol 2009; 29(5): 1363-74.
[http://dx.doi.org/10.1128/MCB.00705-08] [PMID: 19103747]

[124] Gillum MP, Kotas ME, Erion DM, *et al.* SirT1 regulates adipose tissue inflammation. Diabetes 2011; 60(12): 3235-45.
[http://dx.doi.org/10.2337/db11-0616] [PMID: 22110092]

[125] Li P, Zhao Y, Wu X, *et al.* Interferon gamma (IFN-γ) disrupts energy expenditure and metabolic homeostasis by suppressing SIRT1 transcription. Nucleic Acids Res 2012; 40(4): 1609-20.
[http://dx.doi.org/10.1093/nar/gkr984] [PMID: 22064865]

[126] Shoelson SE, Lee J, Goldfine AB. Inflammation and insulin resistance. J Clin Invest 2006; 116(7): 1793-801.
[http://dx.doi.org/10.1172/JCI29069] [PMID: 16823477]

[127] Sun C, Zhang F, Ge X, *et al.* SIRT1 improves insulin sensitivity under insulin-resistant conditions by repressing PTP1B. Cell Metab 2007; 6(4): 307-19.
[http://dx.doi.org/10.1016/j.cmet.2007.08.014] [PMID: 17908559]

[128] Bordone L, Motta MC, Picard F, *et al.* Sirt1 regulates insulin secretion by repressing UCP2 in pancreatic beta cells. PLoS Biol 2006; 4(2): e31.
[http://dx.doi.org/10.1371/journal.pbio.0040031] [PMID: 16366736]

[129] Moynihan KA, Grimm AA, Plueger MM, *et al.* Increased dosage of mammalian Sir2 in pancreatic β cells enhances glucose-stimulated insulin secretion in mice. Cell Metab 2005; 2(2): 105-17.
[http://dx.doi.org/10.1016/j.cmet.2005.07.001] [PMID: 16098828]

[130] Ramsey KM, Mills KF, Satoh A, Imai S. Age-associated loss of Sirt1-mediated enhancement of glucose-stimulated insulin secretion in beta cell-specific Sirt1-overexpressing (BESTO) mice. Aging Cell 2008; 7(1): 78-88.
[http://dx.doi.org/10.1111/j.1474-9726.2007.00355.x] [PMID: 18005249]

[131] Alrob OA, Sankaralingam S, Ma C, *et al.* Obesity-induced lysine acetylation increases cardiac fatty acid oxidation and impairs insulin signalling. Cardiovasc Res 2014; 103(4): 485-97.
[http://dx.doi.org/10.1093/cvr/cvu156] [PMID: 24966184]

[132] Zeng H, Vaka VR, He X, Booz GW, Chen JX. High-fat diet induces cardiac remodelling and dysfunction: assessment of the role played by SIRT3 loss. J Cell Mol Med 2015; 19(8): 1847-56.
[http://dx.doi.org/10.1111/jcmm.12556] [PMID: 25782072]

[133] Zhang L, Han L, Ma R, *et al.* Sirt3 prevents maternal obesity-associated oxidative stress and meiotic defects in mouse oocytes. Cell Cycle 2015; 14(18): 2959-68.
[http://dx.doi.org/10.1080/15384101.2015.1026517] [PMID: 25790176]

[134] Zhou Y, Chung ACK, Fan R, *et al.* Sirt3 Deficiency Increased the Vulnerability of Pancreatic Beta Cells to Oxidative Stress-Induced Dysfunction. Antioxid Redox Signal 2017; 27(13): 962-76.
[http://dx.doi.org/10.1089/ars.2016.6859] [PMID: 28375738]

[135] Wang X, Buechler NL, Martin A, *et al.* Sirtuin-2 regulates sepsis inflammation in ob/ob mice. PLoS One 2016; 11(8): e0160431.
[http://dx.doi.org/10.1371/journal.pone.0160431] [PMID: 27500833]

[136] Ahuja N, Schwer B, Carobbio S, *et al.* Regulation of insulin secretion by SIRT4, a mitochondrial ADP-ribosyltransferase. J Biol Chem 2007; 282(46): 33583-92.
[http://dx.doi.org/10.1074/jbc.M705488200] [PMID: 17715127]

[137] Kanfi Y, Peshti V, Gil R, *et al.* SIRT6 protects against pathological damage caused by diet-induced obesity. Aging Cell 2010; 9(2): 162-73.
[http://dx.doi.org/10.1111/j.1474-9726.2009.00544.x] [PMID: 20047575]

[138] Cioffi M, Vallespinos-Serrano M, Trabulo SM, *et al.* MiR-93 Controls Adiposity *via* Inhibition of Sirt7 and Tbx3. Cell Reports 2015; 12(10): 1594-605.
[http://dx.doi.org/10.1016/j.celrep.2015.08.006] [PMID: 26321631]

[139] Kurylowicz A, Owczarz M, Polosak J, *et al.* SIRT1 and SIRT7 expression in adipose tissues of obese and normal-weight individuals is regulated by microRNAs but not by methylation status. Int J Obes 2016; 40(11): 1635-42.
[http://dx.doi.org/10.1038/ijo.2016.131] [PMID: 27480132]

[140] Yoshizawa T, Karim MF, Sato Y, *et al.* SIRT7 controls hepatic lipid metabolism by regulating the ubiquitin-proteasome pathway. Cell Metab 2014; 19(4): 712-21.
[http://dx.doi.org/10.1016/j.cmet.2014.03.006] [PMID: 24703702]

[141] Shin J, He M, Liu Y, *et al.* SIRT7 represses Myc activity to suppress ER stress and prevent fatty liver disease. Cell Reports 2013; 5(3): 654-65.
[http://dx.doi.org/10.1016/j.celrep.2013.10.007] [PMID: 24210820]

[142] Bober E, Fang J, Smolka C, *et al.* Sirt7 promotes adipogenesis by binding to and inhibiting Sirt1. BMC Proc 2012; 6 (Suppl. 3): 57.
[http://dx.doi.org/10.1186/1753-6561-6-S3-P57]

[143] Moschen AR, Wieser V, Gerner RR, *et al.* Adipose tissue and liver expression of SIRT1, 3, and 6 increase after extensive weight loss in morbid obesity. J Hepatol 2013; 59(6): 1315-22.
[http://dx.doi.org/10.1016/j.jhep.2013.07.027] [PMID: 23928404]

[144] Crujeiras AB, Parra D, Goyenechea E, Martínez JA. Sirtuin gene expression in human mononuclear cells is modulated by caloric restriction. Eur J Clin Invest 2008; 38(9): 672-8.
[http://dx.doi.org/10.1111/j.1365-2362.2008.01998.x] [PMID: 18837744]

[145] Clark SJ, Falchi M, Olsson B, *et al.* Association of sirtuin 1 (SIRT1) gene SNPs and transcript expression levels with severe obesity. Obesity (Silver Spring) 2012; 20(1): 178-85.
[http://dx.doi.org/10.1038/oby.2011.200] [PMID: 21760635]

[146] Pedersen SB, Ølholm J, Paulsen SK, Bennetzen MF, Richelsen B. Low Sirt1 expression, which is upregulated by fasting, in human adipose tissue from obese women. Int J Obes 2008; 32(8): 1250-5.
[http://dx.doi.org/10.1038/ijo.2008.78] [PMID: 18560370]

[147] Dong Y, Guo T, Traurig M, *et al.* SIRT1 is associated with a decrease in acute insulin secretion and a

sex specific increase in risk for type 2 diabetes in Pima Indians. Mol Genet Metab 2011; 104(4): 661-5.
[http://dx.doi.org/10.1016/j.ymgme.2011.08.001] [PMID: 21871827]

[148] Song YS, Lee SK, Jang YJ, *et al.* Association between low SIRT1 expression in visceral and subcutaneous adipose tissues and metabolic abnormalities in women with obesity and type 2 diabetes. Diabetes Res Clin Pract 2013; 101(3): 341-8.
[http://dx.doi.org/10.1016/j.diabres.2013.07.002] [PMID: 23876548]

[149] Costa CdosS, Hammes TO, Rohden F, *et al.* SIRT1 transcription is decreased in visceral adipose tissue of morbidly obese patients with severe hepatic steatosis. Obes Surg 2010; 20(5): 633-9.
[http://dx.doi.org/10.1007/s11695-009-0052-z] [PMID: 20033348]

[150] Rutanen J, Yaluri N, Modi S, *et al.* SIRT1 mRNA expression may be associated with energy expenditure and insulin sensitivity. Diabetes 2010; 59(4): 829-35.
[http://dx.doi.org/10.2337/db09-1191] [PMID: 20107110]

[151] de Kreutzenberg SV, Ceolotto G, Papparella I, *et al.* Downregulation of the longevity-associated protein sirtuin 1 in insulin resistance and metabolic syndrome: potential biochemical mechanisms. Diabetes 2010; 59(4): 1006-15.
[http://dx.doi.org/10.2337/db09-1187] [PMID: 20068143]

[152] Vargas-Ortiz K, Perez-Vazquez V, Diaz-Cisneros FJ, *et al.* Aerobic training increases expression levels of SIRT3 and PGC-1α in skeletal muscle of overweight adolescents without change in caloric intake. Pediatr Exerc Sci 2015; 27(2): 177-84.
[http://dx.doi.org/10.1123/pes.2014-0112] [PMID: 25680002]

[153] Yang L, Zhang J, Xing W, *et al.* SIRT3 deficiency induces endothelial insulin resistance and blunts endothelial-dependent vasorelaxation in mice and human with obesity 2016.

[154] Tarantino G, Finelli C, Scopacasa F, *et al.* Circulating levels of sirtuin 4, a potential marker of oxidative metabolism, related to coronary artery disease in obese patients suffering from NAFLD, with normal or slightly increased liver enzymes. Oxid Med Cell Longev 2014; 2014: 920676.
[http://dx.doi.org/10.1155/2014/920676] [PMID: 25045415]

[155] Capel F, Viguerie N, Vega N, *et al.* Contribution of energy restriction and macronutrient composition to changes in adipose tissue gene expression during dietary weight-loss programs in obese women. J Clin Endocrinol Metab 2008; 93(11): 4315-22.
[http://dx.doi.org/10.1210/jc.2008-0814] [PMID: 18782868]

[156] Howitz KT, Bitterman KJ, Cohen HY, *et al.* Small molecule activators of sirtuins extend Saccharomyces cerevisiae lifespan. Nature 2003; 425(6954): 191-6.
[http://dx.doi.org/10.1038/nature01960] [PMID: 12939617]

[157] Baur JA, Sinclair DA. Therapeutic potential of resveratrol: the *in vivo* evidence. Nat Rev Drug Discov 2006; 5(6): 493-506.
[http://dx.doi.org/10.1038/nrd2060] [PMID: 16732220]

[158] Frankel EN, Waterhouse AL, Kinsella JE. Inhibition of human LDL oxidation by resveratrol. Lancet 1993; 341(8852): 1103-4.
[http://dx.doi.org/10.1016/0140-6736(93)92472-6] [PMID: 8097009]

[159] Renaud S, de Lorgeril M. Wine, alcohol, platelets, and the French paradox for coronary heart disease. Lancet 1992; 339(8808): 1523-6.
[http://dx.doi.org/10.1016/0140-6736(92)91277-F] [PMID: 1351198]

[160] Richard JL. [Coronary risk factors. The French paradox]. Arch Mal Coeur Vaiss 1987; 80(Spec No): 17-21. [Coronary risk factors. The French paradox].
[PMID: 3113393]

[161] Asensi M, Medina I, Ortega A, *et al.* Inhibition of cancer growth by resveratrol is related to its low bioavailability. Free Radic Biol Med 2002; 33(3): 387-98.

[http://dx.doi.org/10.1016/S0891-5849(02)00911-5] [PMID: 12126761]

[162] Marier JF, Vachon P, Gritsas A, Zhang J, Moreau JP, Ducharme MP. Metabolism and disposition of resveratrol in rats: extent of absorption, glucuronidation, and enterohepatic recirculation evidenced by a linked-rat model. J Pharmacol Exp Ther 2002; 302(1): 369-73.
[http://dx.doi.org/10.1124/jpet.102.033340] [PMID: 12065739]

[163] Subramanian L, Youssef S, Bhattacharya S, Kenealey J, Polans AS, van Ginkel PR. Resveratrol: challenges in translation to the clinic--a critical discussion. Clin Cancer Res 2010; 16(24): 5942-8.
[http://dx.doi.org/10.1158/1078-0432.CCR-10-1486] [PMID: 21045084]

[164] Walle T, Hsieh F, DeLegge MH, Oatis JE Jr, Walle UK. High absorption but very low bioavailability of oral resveratrol in humans. Drug Metab Dispos 2004; 32(12): 1377-82.
[http://dx.doi.org/10.1124/dmd.104.000885] [PMID: 15333514]

[165] Timmers S, Konings E, Bilet L, *et al.* Calorie restriction-like effects of 30 days of resveratrol supplementation on energy metabolism and metabolic profile in obese humans. Cell Metab 2011; 14(5): 612-22.
[http://dx.doi.org/10.1016/j.cmet.2011.10.002] [PMID: 22055504]

[166] Pearson KJ, Baur JA, Lewis KN, *et al.* Resveratrol delays age-related deterioration and mimics transcriptional aspects of dietary restriction without extending life span. Cell Metab 2008; 8(2): 157-68.
[http://dx.doi.org/10.1016/j.cmet.2008.06.011] [PMID: 18599363]

[167] Crowell JA, Korytko PJ, Morrissey RL, Booth TD, Levine BS. Resveratrol-associated renal toxicity. Toxicol Sci 2004; 82(2): 614-9.
[http://dx.doi.org/10.1093/toxsci/kfh263] [PMID: 15329443]

[168] Juan ME, Vinardell MP, Planas JM. The daily oral administration of high doses of trans-resveratrol to rats for 28 days is not harmful. J Nutr 2002; 132(2): 257-60.
[http://dx.doi.org/10.1093/jn/132.2.257] [PMID: 11823587]

[169] Brown VA, Patel KR, Viskaduraki M, *et al.* Repeat dose study of the cancer chemopreventive agent resveratrol in healthy volunteers: safety, pharmacokinetics, and effect on the insulin-like growth factor axis. Cancer Res 2010; 70(22): 9003-11.
[http://dx.doi.org/10.1158/0008-5472.CAN-10-2364] [PMID: 20935227]

[170] Yoshino J, Conte C, Fontana L, *et al.* Resveratrol supplementation does not improve metabolic function in nonobese women with normal glucose tolerance. Cell Metab 2012; 16(5): 658-64.
[http://dx.doi.org/10.1016/j.cmet.2012.09.015] [PMID: 23102619]

[171] Yang H, Baur JA, Chen A, *et al.* Design and synthesis of compounds that extend yeast replicative lifespan. Aging Cell 2007; 6(1): 35-43.
[http://dx.doi.org/10.1111/j.1474-9726.2006.00259.x] [PMID: 17156081]

[172] Milne JC, Lambert PD, Schenk S, *et al.* Small molecule activators of SIRT1 as therapeutics for the treatment of type 2 diabetes. Nature 2007; 450(7170): 712-6.
[http://dx.doi.org/10.1038/nature06261] [PMID: 18046409]

[173] Hubbard BP, Sinclair DA. Small molecule SIRT1 activators for the treatment of aging and age-related diseases. Trends Pharmacol Sci 2014; 35(3): 146-54.
[http://dx.doi.org/10.1016/j.tips.2013.12.004] [PMID: 24439680]

[174] Dai H, Kustigian L, Carney D, *et al.* SIRT1 activation by small molecules: kinetic and biophysical evidence for direct interaction of enzyme and activator. J Biol Chem 2010; 285(43): 32695-703.
[http://dx.doi.org/10.1074/jbc.M110.133892] [PMID: 20702418]

[175] Lagouge M, Argmann C, Gerhart-Hines Z, *et al.* Resveratrol improves mitochondrial function and protects against metabolic disease by activating SIRT1 and PGC-1alpha. Cell 2006; 127(6): 1109-22.
[http://dx.doi.org/10.1016/j.cell.2006.11.013] [PMID: 17112576]

[176] Aubin MC, Lajoie C, Clément R, Gosselin H, Calderone A, Perrault LP. Female rats fed a high-fat diet

were associated with vascular dysfunction and cardiac fibrosis in the absence of overt obesity and hyperlipidemia: therapeutic potential of resveratrol. J Pharmacol Exp Ther 2008; 325(3): 961-8.
[http://dx.doi.org/10.1124/jpet.107.135061] [PMID: 18356487]

[177] Shang J, Chen LL, Xiao FX, Sun H, Ding HC, Xiao H. Resveratrol improves non-alcoholic fatty liver disease by activating AMP-activated protein kinase. Acta Pharmacol Sin 2008; 29(6): 698-706.
[http://dx.doi.org/10.1111/j.1745-7254.2008.00807.x] [PMID: 18501116]

[178] Rocha KK, Souza GA, Ebaid GX, Seiva FR, Cataneo AC, Novelli EL. Resveratrol toxicity: effects on risk factors for atherosclerosis and hepatic oxidative stress in standard and high-fat diets. Food Chem Toxicol 2009; 47(6): 1362-7.
[http://dx.doi.org/10.1016/j.fct.2009.03.010] [PMID: 19298841]

[179] Rivera L, Morón R, Zarzuelo A, Galisteo M. Long-term resveratrol administration reduces metabolic disturbances and lowers blood pressure in obese Zucker rats. Biochem Pharmacol 2009; 77(6): 1053-63.
[http://dx.doi.org/10.1016/j.bcp.2008.11.027] [PMID: 19100718]

[180] Ramadori G, Gautron L, Fujikawa T, Vianna CR, Elmquist JK, Coppari R. Central administration of resveratrol improves diet-induced diabetes. Endocrinology 2009; 150(12): 5326-33.
[http://dx.doi.org/10.1210/en.2009-0528] [PMID: 19819963]

[181] Gnoni GV, Paglialonga G. Resveratrol inhibits fatty acid and triacylglycerol synthesis in rat hepatocytes. Eur J Clin Invest 2009; 39(3): 211-8.
[http://dx.doi.org/10.1111/j.1365-2362.2008.02077.x] [PMID: 19260951]

[182] Fischer-Posovszky P, Kukulus V, Tews D, *et al.* Resveratrol regulates human adipocyte number and function in a Sirt1-dependent manner. Am J Clin Nutr 2010; 92(1): 5-15.
[http://dx.doi.org/10.3945/ajcn.2009.28435] [PMID: 20463039]

[183] Jiang B, Guo L, Li BY, *et al.* Resveratrol attenuates early diabetic nephropathy by down-regulating glutathione s-transferases Mu in diabetic rats. J Med Food 2013; 16(6): 481-6.
[http://dx.doi.org/10.1089/jmf.2012.2686] [PMID: 23767859]

[184] Fiori JL, Shin YK, Kim W, *et al.* Resveratrol prevents β-cell dedifferentiation in nonhuman primates given a high-fat/high-sugar diet. Diabetes 2013; 62(10): 3500-13.
[http://dx.doi.org/10.2337/db13-0266] [PMID: 23884882]

[185] Jimenez-Gomez Y, Mattison JA, Pearson KJ, *et al.* Resveratrol improves adipose insulin signaling and reduces the inflammatory response in adipose tissue of rhesus monkeys on high-fat, high-sugar diet. Cell Metab 2013; 18(4): 533-45.
[http://dx.doi.org/10.1016/j.cmet.2013.09.004] [PMID: 24093677]

[186] Zhang J. Resveratrol inhibits insulin responses in a SirT1-independent pathway. Biochem J 2006; 397(3): 519-27.
[http://dx.doi.org/10.1042/BJ20050977] [PMID: 16626303]

[187] Fröjdö S, Cozzone D, Vidal H, Pirola L. Resveratrol is a class IA phosphoinositide 3-kinase inhibitor. Biochem J 2007; 406(3): 511-8.
[http://dx.doi.org/10.1042/BJ20070236] [PMID: 17550345]

[188] Resveratrol Partners Dietary supplement and method of processing same. 2005.WO2005099761

[189] Pilegaard H, Neufer PD. Transcriptional regulation of pyruvate dehydrogenase kinase 4 in skeletal muscle during and after exercise. Proc Nutr Soc 2004; 63(2): 221-6.
[http://dx.doi.org/10.1079/PNS2004345] [PMID: 15294034]

[190] Barger JL, Kayo T, Pugh TD, Prolla TA, Weindruch R. Short-term consumption of a resveratrol-containing nutraceutical mixture mimics gene expression of long-term caloric restriction in mouse heart. Exp Gerontol 2008; 43(9): 859-66.
[http://dx.doi.org/10.1016/j.exger.2008.06.013] [PMID: 18657603]

[191] Brasnyó P, Molnár GA, Mohás M, *et al.* Resveratrol improves insulin sensitivity, reduces oxidative

stress and activates the Akt pathway in type 2 diabetic patients. Br J Nutr 2011; 106(3): 383-9.
[http://dx.doi.org/10.1017/S0007114511000316] [PMID: 21385509]

[192] Choi Y, Kim Y, Park S, Lee KW, Park T. Indole-3-carbinol prevents diet-induced obesity through modulation of multiple genes related to adipogenesis, thermogenesis or inflammation in the visceral adipose tissue of mice. J Nutr Biochem 2012; 23(12): 1732-9.
[http://dx.doi.org/10.1016/j.jnutbio.2011.12.005] [PMID: 22569347]

[193] Choi Y, Um SJ, Park T. Indole-3-carbinol directly targets SIRT1 to inhibit adipocyte differentiation. Int J Obes 2013; 37(6): 881-4.
[http://dx.doi.org/10.1038/ijo.2012.158] [PMID: 22986685]

[194] Fernández-Galilea M, Pérez-Matute P, Prieto-Hontoria PL, *et al.* α-Lipoic acid treatment increases mitochondrial biogenesis and promotes beige adipose features in subcutaneous adipocytes from overweight/obese subjects. Biochim Biophys Acta 2015; 1851(3): 273-81.
[http://dx.doi.org/10.1016/j.bbalip.2014.12.013] [PMID: 25542506]

[195] Kurisawa M, Chung JE, Uyama H, Kobayashi S. Enzymatic synthesis and antioxidant properties of poly(rutin). Biomacromolecules 2003; 4(5): 1394-9.
[http://dx.doi.org/10.1021/bm034136b] [PMID: 12959611]

[196] Seo S, Lee MS, Chang E, *et al.* Rutin Increases Muscle Mitochondrial Biogenesis with AMPK Activation in High-Fat Diet-Induced Obese Rats. Nutrients 2015; 7(9): 8152-69.
[http://dx.doi.org/10.3390/nu7095385] [PMID: 26402699]

[197] Ko JH, Kwon HS, Yoon JM, *et al.* Effects of Polygonatum sibiricum rhizome ethanol extract in high-fat diet-fed mice. Pharm Biol 2015; 53(4): 563-70.
[http://dx.doi.org/10.3109/13880209.2014.932393] [PMID: 25327577]

[198] Park S, Shin S, Lim Y, Shin JH, Seong JK, Han SN. Korean pine nut oil attenuated hepatic triacylglycerol accumulation in high-fat diet-induced obese mice. Nutrients 2016; 8(1): E59.
[http://dx.doi.org/10.3390/nu8010059] [PMID: 26805879]

[199] Lai YC, Tabima DM, Dube JJ, *et al.* SIRT3-AMP-Activated Protein Kinase Activation by Nitrite and Metformin Improves Hyperglycemia and Normalizes Pulmonary Hypertension Associated With Heart Failure With Preserved Ejection Fraction. Circulation 2016; 133(8): 717-31.
[http://dx.doi.org/10.1161/CIRCULATIONAHA.115.018935] [PMID: 26813102]

[200] Alfarano C, Foussal C, Lairez O, *et al.* Transition from metabolic adaptation to maladaptation of the heart in obesity: role of apelin. Int J Obes 2015; 39(2): 312-20.
[http://dx.doi.org/10.1038/ijo.2014.122] [PMID: 25027224]

[201] Yamazaki Y, Usui I, Kanatani Y, *et al.* Treatment with SRT1720, a SIRT1 activator, ameliorates fatty liver with reduced expression of lipogenic enzymes in MSG mice. Am J Physiol Endocrinol Metab 2009; 297(5): E1179-86.
[http://dx.doi.org/10.1152/ajpendo.90997.2008] [PMID: 19724016]

[202] Mitchell SJ, Martin-Montalvo A, Mercken EM, *et al.* The SIRT1 activator SRT1720 extends lifespan and improves health of mice fed a standard diet. Cell Reports 2014; 6(5): 836-43.
[http://dx.doi.org/10.1016/j.celrep.2014.01.031] [PMID: 24582957]

[203] Yoshizaki T, Schenk S, Imamura T, *et al.* SIRT1 inhibits inflammatory pathways in macrophages and modulates insulin sensitivity. Am J Physiol Endocrinol Metab 2010; 298(3): E419-28.
[http://dx.doi.org/10.1152/ajpendo.00417.2009] [PMID: 19996381]

[204] Mercken EM, Mitchell SJ, Martin-Montalvo A, *et al.* SRT2104 extends survival of male mice on a standard diet and preserves bone and muscle mass. Aging Cell 2014; 13(5): 787-96.
[http://dx.doi.org/10.1111/acel.12220] [PMID: 24931715]

[205] Sirtris Pharma. Methods and related compositions for treating or preventing obesity, insulin resistance disorders, and mitochondrial-associated disorders. 2007.WO2007008548

[206] Smith JJ, Kenney RD, Gagne DJ, *et al.* Small molecule activators of SIRT1 replicate signaling

pathways triggered by calorie restriction *in vivo.* BMC Syst Biol 2009; 3: 31.
[http://dx.doi.org/10.1186/1752-0509-3-31] [PMID: 19284563]

[207]   Vu CB, Bemis JE, Disch JS, *et al.* Discovery of imidazo[1,2-b]thiazole derivatives as novel SIRT1
        activators. J Med Chem 2009; 52(5): 1275-83.
        [http://dx.doi.org/10.1021/jm8012954] [PMID: 19199480]

[208]   Sirtris Pharma. Pharma S. Imidazo [2, 1-b] thiazole derivatives as sirtuin modulating compounds.
        2007.WO20070193

[209]   Baksi A, Kraydashenko O, Zalevkaya A, *et al.* A phase II, randomized, placebo-controlled, double-
        blind, multi-dose study of SRT2104, a SIRT1 activator, in subjects with type 2 diabetes. Br J Clin
        Pharmacol 2014; 78(1): 69-77.
        [http://dx.doi.org/10.1111/bcp.12327] [PMID: 24446723]

[210]   Libri V, Brown AP, Gambarota G, *et al.* A pilot randomized, placebo controlled, double blind phase I
        trial of the novel SIRT1 activator SRT2104 in elderly volunteers. PLoS One 2012; 7(12): e51395.
        [http://dx.doi.org/10.1371/journal.pone.0051395] [PMID: 23284689]

[211]   Venkatasubramanian S, Noh RM, Daga S, *et al.* Cardiovascular effects of a novel SIRT1 activator,
        SRT2104, in otherwise healthy cigarette smokers. J Am Heart Assoc 2013; 2(3): e000042.
        [http://dx.doi.org/10.1161/JAHA.113.000042] [PMID: 23770971]

[212]   Smoliga JM, Baur JA, Hausenblas HA. Resveratrol and health--a comprehensive review of human
        clinical trials. Mol Nutr Food Res 2011; 55(8): 1129-41.
        [http://dx.doi.org/10.1002/mnfr.201100143] [PMID: 21688389]

[213]   Cantó C, Houtkooper RH, Pirinen E, *et al.* The NAD(+) precursor nicotinamide riboside enhances
        oxidative metabolism and protects against high-fat diet-induced obesity. Cell Metab 2012; 15(6): 838-
        47.
        [http://dx.doi.org/10.1016/j.cmet.2012.04.022] [PMID: 22682224]

[214]   Yoshino J, Mills KF, Yoon MJ, Imai S. Nicotinamide mononucleotide, a key NAD(+) intermediate,
        treats the pathophysiology of diet- and age-induced diabetes in mice. Cell Metab 2011; 14(4): 528-36.
        [http://dx.doi.org/10.1016/j.cmet.2011.08.014] [PMID: 21982712]

[215]   Dahl TB, Haukeland JW, Yndestad A, *et al.* Intracellular nicotinamide phosphoribosyltransferase
        protects against hepatocyte apoptosis and is down-regulated in nonalcoholic fatty liver disease. J Clin
        Endocrinol Metab 2010; 95(6): 3039-47.
        [http://dx.doi.org/10.1210/jc.2009-2148] [PMID: 20392873]

[216]   Angelin B, Einarsson K, Hellström K, Leijd B. Effects of cholestyramine and chenodeoxycholic acid
        on the metabolism of endogenous triglyceride in hyperlipoproteinemia. J Lipid Res 1978; 19(8): 1017-
        24.
        [PMID: 731123]

[217]   Makishima M, Okamoto AY, Repa JJ, *et al.* Identification of a nuclear receptor for bile acids. Science
        1999; 284(5418): 1362-5.
        [http://dx.doi.org/10.1126/science.284.5418.1362] [PMID: 10334992]

[218]   Teodoro JS, Rolo AP, Palmeira CM. Hepatic FXR: key regulator of whole-body energy metabolism.
        Trends Endocrinol Metab 2011; 22(11): 458-66.
        [http://dx.doi.org/10.1016/j.tem.2011.07.002] [PMID: 21862343]

[219]   Nishizawa H, Yamagata K, Shimomura I, *et al.* Small heterodimer partner, an orphan nuclear receptor,
        augments peroxisome proliferator-activated receptor gamma transactivation. J Biol Chem 2002;
        277(2): 1586-92.
        [http://dx.doi.org/10.1074/jbc.M104301200] [PMID: 11696534]

[220]   Brendel C, Schoonjans K, Botrugno OA, Treuter E, Auwerx J. The small heterodimer partner interacts
        with the liver X receptor alpha and represses its transcriptional activity. Mol Endocrinol 2002; 16(9):
        2065-76.

[http://dx.doi.org/10.1210/me.2001-0194] [PMID: 12198243]

[221] Goodwin B, Jones SA, Price RR, *et al.* A regulatory cascade of the nuclear receptors FXR, SHP-1, and LRH-1 represses bile acid biosynthesis. Mol Cell 2000; 6(3): 517-26.
[http://dx.doi.org/10.1016/S1097-2765(00)00051-4] [PMID: 11030332]

[222] Ma K, Saha PK, Chan L, Moore DD. Farnesoid X receptor is essential for normal glucose homeostasis. J Clin Invest 2006; 116(4): 1102-9.
[http://dx.doi.org/10.1172/JCI25604] [PMID: 16557297]

[223] Lambert G, Amar MJ, Guo G, Brewer HB Jr, Gonzalez FJ, Sinal CJ. The farnesoid X-receptor is an essential regulator of cholesterol homeostasis. J Biol Chem 2003; 278(4): 2563-70.
[http://dx.doi.org/10.1074/jbc.M209525200] [PMID: 12421815]

[224] Matsukuma KE, Bennett MK, Huang J, Wang L, Gil G, Osborne TF. Coordinated control of bile acids and lipogenesis through FXR-dependent regulation of fatty acid synthase. J Lipid Res 2006; 47(12): 2754-61.
[http://dx.doi.org/10.1194/jlr.M600342-JLR200] [PMID: 16957179]

[225] Abdelkarim M, Caron S, Duhem C, *et al.* The farnesoid X receptor regulates adipocyte differentiation and function by promoting peroxisome proliferator-activated receptor-γ and interfering with the Wnt/β-catenin pathways. J Biol Chem 2010; 285(47): 36759-67.
[http://dx.doi.org/10.1074/jbc.M110.166231] [PMID: 20851881]

[226] Cariou B, van Harmelen K, Duran-Sandoval D, *et al.* The farnesoid X receptor modulates adiposity and peripheral insulin sensitivity in mice. J Biol Chem 2006; 281(16): 11039-49.
[http://dx.doi.org/10.1074/jbc.M510258200] [PMID: 16446356]

[227] Pineda Torra I, Claudel T, Duval C, Kosykh V, Fruchart JC, Staels B. Bile acids induce the expression of the human peroxisome proliferator-activated receptor alpha gene *via* activation of the farnesoid X receptor. Mol Endocrinol 2003; 17(2): 259-72.
[http://dx.doi.org/10.1210/me.2002-0120] [PMID: 12554753]

[228] Rizzo G, Disante M, Mencarelli A, *et al.* The farnesoid X receptor promotes adipocyte differentiation and regulates adipose cell function *in vivo.* Mol Pharmacol 2006; 70(4): 1164-73.
[http://dx.doi.org/10.1124/mol.106.023820] [PMID: 16778009]

[229] Yang ZX, Shen W, Sun H. Effects of nuclear receptor FXR on the regulation of liver lipid metabolism in patients with non-alcoholic fatty liver disease. Hepatol Int 2010; 4(4): 741-8.
[http://dx.doi.org/10.1007/s12072-010-9202-6] [PMID: 21286345]

[230] Borgius LJ, Steffensen KR, Gustafsson JA, Treuter E. Glucocorticoid signaling is perturbed by the atypical orphan receptor and corepressor SHP. J Biol Chem 2002; 277(51): 49761-6.
[http://dx.doi.org/10.1074/jbc.M205641200] [PMID: 12324453]

[231] Stayrook KR, Bramlett KS, Savkur RS, *et al.* Regulation of carbohydrate metabolism by the farnesoid X receptor. Endocrinology 2005; 146(3): 984-91.
[http://dx.doi.org/10.1210/en.2004-0965] [PMID: 15564327]

[232] Zhang Y, Lee FY, Barrera G, *et al.* Activation of the nuclear receptor FXR improves hyperglycemia and hyperlipidemia in diabetic mice. Proc Natl Acad Sci USA 2006; 103(4): 1006-11.
[http://dx.doi.org/10.1073/pnas.0506982103] [PMID: 16410358]

[233] Zhang Y, Castellani LW, Sinal CJ, Gonzalez FJ, Edwards PA. Peroxisome proliferator-activated receptor-γ coactivator 1α (PGC-1α) regulates triglyceride metabolism by activation of the nuclear receptor FXR. Genes Dev 2004; 18(2): 157-69.
[http://dx.doi.org/10.1101/gad.1138104] [PMID: 14729567]

[234] Fang S, Suh JM, Reilly SM, *et al.* Intestinal FXR agonism promotes adipose tissue browning and reduces obesity and insulin resistance. Nat Med 2015; 21(2): 159-65.
[http://dx.doi.org/10.1038/nm.3760] [PMID: 25559344]

[235] Teodoro JS, Rolo AP, Jarak I, Palmeira CM, Carvalho RA. The bile acid chenodeoxycholic acid

directly modulates metabolic pathways in white adipose tissue *in vitro*: insight into how bile acids decrease obesity. NMR Biomed 2016; 29(10): 1391-402.
[http://dx.doi.org/10.1002/nbm.3583] [PMID: 27488269]

[236] Watanabe M, Houten SM, Mataki C, *et al.* Bile acids induce energy expenditure by promoting intracellular thyroid hormone activation. Nature 2006; 439(7075): 484-9.
[http://dx.doi.org/10.1038/nature04330] [PMID: 16400329]

[237] Watanabe M, Horai Y, Houten SM, *et al.* Lowering bile acid pool size with a synthetic farnesoid X receptor (FXR) agonist induces obesity and diabetes through reduced energy expenditure. J Biol Chem 2011; 286(30): 26913-20.
[http://dx.doi.org/10.1074/jbc.M111.248203] [PMID: 21632533]

[238] Prawitt J, Abdelkarim M, Stroeve JH, *et al.* Farnesoid X receptor deficiency improves glucose homeostasis in mouse models of obesity. Diabetes 2011; 60(7): 1861-71.
[http://dx.doi.org/10.2337/db11-0030] [PMID: 21593203]

[239] Fiorucci S, Mencarelli A, Palladino G, Cipriani S. Bile-acid-activated receptors: targeting TGR5 and farnesoid-X-receptor in lipid and glucose disorders. Trends Pharmacol Sci 2009; 30(11): 570-80.
[http://dx.doi.org/10.1016/j.tips.2009.08.001] [PMID: 19758712]

[240] Weitzel JM, Iwen KA, Seitz HJ. Regulation of mitochondrial biogenesis by thyroid hormone. Exp Physiol 2003; 88(1): 121-8.
[http://dx.doi.org/10.1113/eph8802506] [PMID: 12552316]

[241] Cannon B, Nedergaard J. Brown adipose tissue: function and physiological significance. Physiol Rev 2004; 84(1): 277-359.
[http://dx.doi.org/10.1152/physrev.00015.2003] [PMID: 14715917]

[242] Watanabe M, Houten SM, Wang L, *et al.* Bile acids lower triglyceride levels *via* a pathway involving FXR, SHP, and SREBP-1c. J Clin Invest 2004; 113(10): 1408-18.
[http://dx.doi.org/10.1172/JCI21025] [PMID: 15146238]

[243] Teodoro JS, Zouhar P, Flachs P, *et al.* Enhancement of brown fat thermogenesis using chenodeoxycholic acid in mice. Int J Obes 2014; 38(8): 1027-34.
[http://dx.doi.org/10.1038/ijo.2013.230] [PMID: 24310401]

[244] Broeders EP, Nascimento EB, Havekes B, *et al.* The Bile Acid Chenodeoxycholic Acid Increases Human Brown Adipose Tissue Activity. Cell Metab 2015; 22(3): 418-26.
[http://dx.doi.org/10.1016/j.cmet.2015.07.002] [PMID: 26235421]

[245] Katona BW, Cummins CL, Ferguson AD, *et al.* Synthesis, characterization, and receptor interaction profiles of enantiomeric bile acids. J Med Chem 2007; 50(24): 6048-58.
[http://dx.doi.org/10.1021/jm0707931] [PMID: 17963371]

[246] Ding L, Yang L, Wang Z, Huang W. Bile acid nuclear receptor FXR and digestive system diseases. Acta Pharm Sin B 2015; 5(2): 135-44.
[http://dx.doi.org/10.1016/j.apsb.2015.01.004] [PMID: 26579439]

[247] Nedergaard J, Cannon B. UCP1 mRNA does not produce heat. Biochim Biophys Acta 2013; 1831(5): 943-9.
[http://dx.doi.org/10.1016/j.bbalip.2013.01.009] [PMID: 23353596]

[248] Singh N, Yadav M, Singh AK, *et al.* Synthetic FXR agonist GW4064 is a modulator of multiple G protein-coupled receptors. Mol Endocrinol 2014; 28(5): 659-73.
[http://dx.doi.org/10.1210/me.2013-1353] [PMID: 24597548]

[249] Burris TP, Montrose C, Houck KA, *et al.* The hypolipidemic natural product guggulsterone is a promiscuous steroid receptor ligand. Mol Pharmacol 2005; 67(3): 948-54.
[http://dx.doi.org/10.1124/mol.104.007054] [PMID: 15602004]

[250] Teodoro JS, Rolo AP, Palmeira CM. The NAD ratio redox paradox: why does too much reductive power cause oxidative stress? Toxicol Mech Methods 2013; 23(5): 297-302.

[http://dx.doi.org/10.3109/15376516.2012.759305] [PMID: 23256455]

[251]   Teodoro JS, Varela AT, Rolo AP, Palmeira CM. High-fat and obesogenic diets: current and future strategies to fight obesity and diabetes. Genes Nutr 2014; 9(4): 406.
[http://dx.doi.org/10.1007/s12263-014-0406-6] [PMID: 24842072]

[252]   Teodoro JS, Gomes AP, Varela AT, Duarte FV, Rolo AP, Palmeira CM. Hepatic and skeletal muscle mitochondrial toxicity of chitosan oligosaccharides of normal and diabetic rats. Toxicol Mech Methods 2016; 26(9): 650-7.
[http://dx.doi.org/10.1080/15376516.2016.1222643] [PMID: 27790925]

[253]   Youle RJ, van der Bliek AM. Mitochondrial fission, fusion, and stress. Science 2012; 337(6098): 1062-5.
[http://dx.doi.org/10.1126/science.1219855] [PMID: 22936770]

[254]   Ding WX, Yin XM. Mitophagy: mechanisms, pathophysiological roles, and analysis. Biol Chem 2012; 393(7): 547-64.
[http://dx.doi.org/10.1515/hsz-2012-0119] [PMID: 22944659]

[255]   Scarffe LA, Stevens DA, Dawson VL, Dawson TM. Parkin and PINK1: much more than mitophagy. Trends Neurosci 2014; 37(6): 315-24.
[http://dx.doi.org/10.1016/j.tins.2014.03.004] [PMID: 24735649]

[256]   Mortiboys H, Furmston R, Bronstad G, Aasly J, Elliott C, Bandmann O. UDCA exerts beneficial effect on mitochondrial dysfunction in LRRK2(G2019S) carriers and in vivo. Neurology 2015; 85(10): 846-52.
[http://dx.doi.org/10.1212/WNL.0000000000001905] [PMID: 26253449]

[257]   Ved R, Saha S, Westlund B, *et al.* Similar patterns of mitochondrial vulnerability and rescue induced by genetic modification of alpha-synuclein, parkin, and DJ-1 in Caenorhabditis elegans. J Biol Chem 2005; 280(52): 42655-68.
[http://dx.doi.org/10.1074/jbc.M505910200] [PMID: 16239214]

[258]   Goldberg AA, Richard VR, Kyryakov P, *et al.* Chemical genetic screen identifies lithocholic acid as an anti-aging compound that extends yeast chronological life span in a TOR-independent manner, by modulating housekeeping longevity assurance processes. Aging (Albany NY) 2010; 2(7): 393-414.
[http://dx.doi.org/10.18632/aging.100168] [PMID: 20622262]

[259]   Richard VR, Leonov A, Beach A, *et al.* Macromitophagy is a longevity assurance process that in chronologically aging yeast limited in calorie supply sustains functional mitochondria and maintains cellular lipid homeostasis. Aging (Albany NY) 2013; 5(4): 234-69.
[http://dx.doi.org/10.18632/aging.100547] [PMID: 23553280]

[260]   Zhang J. Autophagy and Mitophagy in Cellular Damage Control. Redox Biol 2013; 1(1): 19-23.
[http://dx.doi.org/10.1016/j.redox.2012.11.008] [PMID: 23946931]

[261]   Tang Y, Fickert P, Trauner M, Marcus N, Blomenkamp K, Teckman J. Autophagy induced by exogenous bile acids is therapeutic in a model of α-1-AT deficiency liver disease. Am J Physiol Gastrointest Liver Physiol 2016; 311(1): G156-65.
[http://dx.doi.org/10.1152/ajpgi.00143.2015] [PMID: 27102560]

[262]   Williams JA, Thomas AM, Li G, *et al.* Tissue specific induction of p62/Sqstm1 by farnesoid X receptor. PLoS One 2012; 7(8): e43961.
[http://dx.doi.org/10.1371/journal.pone.0043961] [PMID: 22952826]

[263]   Manley S, Ni HM, Williams JA, *et al.* Farnesoid X receptor regulates forkhead Box O3a activation in ethanol-induced autophagy and hepatotoxicity. Redox Biol 2014; 2: 991-1002.
[http://dx.doi.org/10.1016/j.redox.2014.08.007] [PMID: 25460735]

[264]   Seok S, Fu T, Choi SE, *et al.* Transcriptional regulation of autophagy by an FXR-CREB axis. Nature 2014; 516(7529): 108-11.
[http://dx.doi.org/10.1038/nature13949] [PMID: 25383523]

[265] Lee JM, Wagner M, Xiao R, *et al.* Nutrient-sensing nuclear receptors coordinate autophagy. Nature 2014; 516(7529): 112-5.
[http://dx.doi.org/10.1038/nature13961] [PMID: 25383539]

CHAPTER 4

Development and Characterization of Calcium Silicate Based Formulations for Anti-Obesity Therapy: Orlistat

Sunil K. Jain[*]

Institute of Pharmaceutical Sciences, Guru Ghasidas Vishwavidyalaya, Bilaspur, Chhattisgarh, India

Abstract: On health front, today's generation is struggling with increasing rate of obesity which is undisputedly reckoned as a leading cause for a number of pathological conditions *e.g.* coronary heart disease (CHD), high blood pressure, stroke, abnormal blood fats, metabolic syndrome, cancer, osteoarthritis, sleep apnea, obesity hypoventilation syndrome, reproductive problems, gallstones, and type 2 diabetes *etc.* In recent research, calcium silicate based two formulations *i.e.,* floating microspheres and floating granules have been developed for anti-obesity drug *i.e.,* orlistat, to deliver the incorporated therapeutic agent in effective concentrations and extended therapeutic course of time. Floating characteristic over the gastric content of such formulations is capable to provide prolonged retention in gastric region. Formulation of microspheres with incorporation of calcium silicate increases the effectiveness of this granular formulation to matchup the desired release pattern with buoyancy. The developed formulations of orlistat are found to be safer and more effective which is the need of day in pharmaceutical industry as an alternative drug delivery system for a highly prevalent and chronic disease like obesity.

Keywords: BMI, Buoyancy, Calcium silicate, Floating granules, Floating microspheres, Gamma scintigraphy, Gastro-retention, *In vitro* drug release, Obesity, Orlistat, Pharmacokinetics.

INTRODUCTION

Obesity is a disorder related to the accumulation of extra body fat to an extent which triggers health risks in terms of different diseases. It also leads to the reduction in life expectancy with or without stimulating any health complications [1]. Body mass index (BMI) is generally used for the assessment of obesity. BMI is first introduced by Belgian statistician and anthropometrist, Adolphe Quetelet

---
[*] **Corresponding author Sunil K. Jain:** Institute of Pharmaceutical Sciences, Guru Ghasidas Vishwavidyalaya, Bilaspur, Chhattisgarh, India; Tel: +91 9425452174; E-mail: suniljain25in@yahoo.com

Atta-ur-Rahman & M. Iqbal Choudhary (Eds.)

in 19th century [2]. It provides an accurate prediction of fat proportion in the body of most of the peoples. BMI is calculated by the mathematical relationship between body weight and height of the subject under consideration. This mathematical relationship is given by the equation:

$$BMI = \frac{Body\ Weight\ (Kg)}{Height\ (m^2)}$$

According to WHO, BMI value of obese individuals are equal to or greater than 30 kg/m^2. The studies for the European and American continent reveals the fact that mortality risk is lowermost in non-smokers having BMI between 20–25 kg/m^2 [3, 4] over smokers with BMI value 24–27 kg/m^2, however risk is increasing owing to variations [5, 6]. A value of BMI greater than 32 kg/m^2 is found to be associated with a twofold increase in mortality rate in women aging above 16-year [7].

Another study published in medical journal Lancet claims that India is just behind US and China in this global hazard list of top 10 countries facing health issues associated with obesity [1]. The statistical data shows that the number of overweight and obese people globally increased from 857 million in 1980 to 2.1 billion in 2013 which is approximately equivalent to 1/3rd of human population on this earth. In a study of 2014 it was found that more than 1.9 billion adults ($\geq$ 18 years) were overweight and out of these over 600 million were obese. Among 39% of adults aged 18 years and over (38% of men and 40% of women) were overweight. The mortality data of countries where most of the world's population lives shows that overweight and obesity kills more people than underweight [8].

To provide a uniform measure for the assessment of obesity, World Health Organization (WHO) has established a classification by providing range of BMI values (Table **1**) [2]. Class III type of obesity is also classified in to different categories. Further, few specific bodies have made some amendments in these values however accurate values are still unclear (Table **2**) [9]. The effect of obesity on human health is prominent as it decreases the average life expectancy by 6 to 7 years [1, 10]. More precisely, a BMI of 30–35 kg/m^2 reduces life expectancy by 2 to 4 years, while severe obesity with BMI > 40 kg/m^2 decreases the life expectancy by 10 years.

Table 1. Classification of BMI according to WHO.

BMI	Classification
< 18.5	Underweight
18.5–24.9	normal weight
25.0–29.9	Overweight
30.0–34.9	class I obesity
35.0–39.9	class II obesity
≥ 40.0	class III obesity

Table 2. Sub classification of class III.

BMI	Classification
≥ 35 or 40	Severe obesity
≥ 35 or 40–44.9 or 49.9	Morbid obesity
≥ 45 or 50	Super obese

The numbers of diseases associated with obesity are constantly rising; particularly type 2 diabetes and cardiac diseases, specific type of cancer, osteoarthritis and disruptive sleep apnea [1]. Among the numerous causes of obesity, prominent ones include (a) intake of high-calorie food, (b) lack of physical work-out, and (c) hereditary susceptibility. Obesity is one of the far most serious disorders of 21st century. It is responsible for a large number of avertable deaths taking place worldwide [11].

A vast variety of anti-obesity drugs is available to combat obesity *e.g.* orlistat (OT), lorcaserin, rimonabant, metformin, exenatide *etc.* Lorcaserin is generally used for weight loss for long term in obese persons [12]. Despite mass loss, some common side effects are associated with it, which are considered benign. Rimonabant acts centrally as an antagonist for cannabinoid (CB1) receptor and therefore decrease appetite [13]. It could also act peripherally by enhancing energy expenditure by increasing thermogenesis. However, it is considered to be less effective than other available mass-loss medication [13]. Metformin causes decrease in mass in individuals with type 2 diabetes [14]. It restricts the quantity of glucose produced by liver to decrease glucose level and increases the consumption of glucose by muscles. In response to the presence of food intestine secrete exenatide (an analogue of the hormone GLP-1) which delays the gastric emptying and supports a sensation of satiety. Obese peoples are particularly deficient for GLP-1, and dieting further decreases GLP-1 [15].

OT, a lipase inhibitor employed for obesity management which acts by inhibiting the absorption of dietary fats. OT has short half-life (<2 h), unstable at alkaline pH and requires administration 3 times in a day. It mainly acts at stomach and pancreas [16]. The properties of OT *e.g.* short half-life, high dosing frequency, and undue gastric side effects at high concentration, makes it a potential candidate for the development of floating controlled release system. In clinical trials for OT, about 54.8% of subject has attained ≥5% fall in body mass. However, an obese population treated with OT exhibited decreased incidence (6.2%) of type 2 diabetes over placebo (9.0%) after 4 years [17]. In addition, persistent use of OT also leads to a modest decrease in blood pressure (systolic; 2.5 mmHg and diastolic; 1.9 mmHg) [18]. Only some adverse-effects including frequent movements of oily bowel (steatorrhea) were observed, which can be improved by the adoption of fat free diet. Among the 40 million OT users globally, 13 cases have been reported with severe liver damage [19].

Numerous approaches have been employed for the development of intra-gastric floating and sustained release preparations to achieve prolonged therapeutic effect in the stomach along with enhanced retention time for better absorption in the upper part of small intestine. Floating drug delivery systems (FDDS) or Hydro dynamically balanced systems (HBS) are among the several approaches that have been developed in order to increase the gastric residence time (GRT) of incorporated therapeutic agent [20, 21]. Floating drug delivery systems are preferred for drugs that (a) act locally in the stomach; (b) have penchant absorption window in the stomach; (c) have poor solubility at alkaline pH values; (d) have a narrow window of absorption; and (e) are unstable in the intestinal or colonic environment [22]. To inculcate good floating behavior in the stomach, the density of the delivery system should be less than that of the gastric contents (≈ 1.004 g/cm^3).

The combination of intra-gastric floating delivery with anti-obesity drug could be an important tool to achieve sustained release action. Recent reports over these floating systems with prolonged drug effects in the upper part of small intestine proved the effectiveness of this approach for the development of a formulation, which have lower density than gastric fluids so that it remains buoyant in stomach [23 - 28]. Furthermore, such floating systems containing anti-obesity agents offer several merits over conventional delivery systems [23, 29]. The utilization of floating microparticles also results into reduced mucosal irritancy caused by the incorporated therapeutic agent [30].

Recently, scientists have explored a scientific resolution to overcome the limitations associated with oral delivery of anti-obesity agents. Sangwai *et al,.* [31] developed a nanoemulsion of OT and its successive conversion into multi-unit pellet system (MUPS) for enhanced oral delivery of poorly water-soluble drug. The comparative *in vivo* dissolution studies demonstrated significant improvement in dissolution over pure OT and marketed formulation (Xenical capsules 120 mg). Comparison for *in vivo* bovine porcine pancreatic lipase inhibition showed 13.57 and 2.41 time greater values over pure OT and marketed product, respectively. Another orlistat loaded self-micro-emulsifying drug delivery system (SMEDDS) consisting orlistat (7.9% w/w), Propylene glycol monocaprylate (18.42% w/w), Propylene glycol laurate (49.21% w/w) and Polysorbate 80 (24.47% w/w) was successfully developed which offers increased solubility, increased dissolution rate resulting in enhanced bioavailability of OT when compared with the conventional oral formulation [32].

Dolenc *et al,.* [33] developed a nanosuspension containing OT to obtain uniform particle size and to get dry product, they used lactose as filler and spray to obtain final powder. This developed nano-suspension provides significantly greater *in vivo* lipase inhibition. To improve the bioavailability of incorporated drug, a nano-emulsified water-soluble system of conjugated linoleic acid (N-CLA) was developed, and evaluated for *in vitro* and *in vivo* studies. The anti-obesity effect of N-CLA was observed on male Sprague-Dawley rats, N-CLA exhibited a better lipolytic effect on differentiated 3T3-L1 adipocytes over normal CLA [34]. Metformin hydrochloride, having good absorption in upper intestine, developed as a floating (buoyant) matrix tablet using sodium bicarbonate and a gel forming hydrophilic polymer (hydroxypropyl methylcellulose) and optimized for floating ability and *in vitro* drug release profile. They showed gradual and near complete drug release with buoyancy and suggested controlled and sustained release (96-99%) of metformin hydrochloride over a period of 8 h [35].

Calcium silicate (CS), due to its characteristic porous structure with many pores exhibits a large pore volume. Such intrinsic properties of CS make it capable to be employed as a sustained release carrier. Its floating ability is owed to entrapment of air within its pores when covered with a polymer [36]. Our research group first utilized CS as floating and sustained release carrier for the development of floating microspheres and floating granules [24, 37]. These developed formulations were subjected to evaluation for their gastro-retentive behavior using gamma scintigraphy and pharmacokinetic parameters [26].

Two formulations consisting OT were prepared with the aim: (a) to develop and evaluate floating microspheres using Eudragit® S (ES) as a polymer and a highly porous carrier material like calcium silicate (CS), which is capable of floating on gastric fluid and delivering the therapeutic agent over an extended period of time, and (b) to develop and evaluate a floating granular drug delivery system composed of CS with matrix forming polymers such as hydroxypropyl methylcellulose K4M, ethyl cellulose and Carbopol 934. Such granules are capable of floating on gastric fluid.

FLOATING MICROSPHERES

Preparation of OT Absorbed CS

CS (1.0 g) was dispersed in 10 ml ethanolic solution of OT (50 mg) and prepared slurry was ultrasonicated for 10 min in an ice bath at 40% voltage frequency using a probe sonicator (Soniweld, Imeco Ultrasonics, India) to allow the drug entrapment inside the pores of porous carrier. Then the excess ethanolic content was removed by filtration followed by drying in vacuum to get OT absorbed CS powder (Fig. **1**).

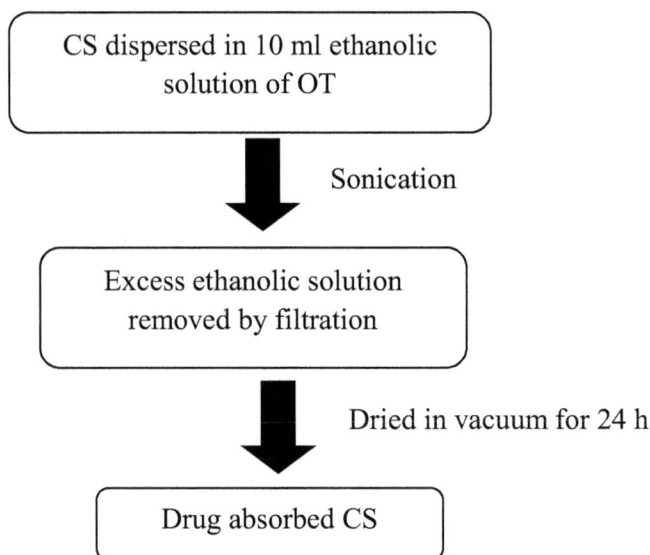

Fig. (1). Schematic of preparation of drug absorbed CS.

Preparation of Floating Microspheres

A modified emulsion solvent diffusion technique was employed for the preparation of floating microspheres [38]. The OT absorbed CS was added to Eudragit S100 (ES) (1g) solution in ethanol and dichloromethane (DCM) (2:1) followed by sonication by probe sonicator. The resulting suspension was poured into a 200 ml aqueous solution of polyvinyl alcohol (PVA) (0.75%w/v) in a 500 ml beaker at 40°C. Then obtained emulsion/suspension stirred at 500 rpm with a twin blade propeller type agitator (Remi, India) for 3 h. For the separation of prepared microspheres, the resulting solution was filtered through Whatmann filter paper (No. 41) and dried at room temperature in a desiccator for 24 h.

Similarly, microspheres of OT without CS (WC) were also prepared for comparative study. Schematic presentation of calcium silicate based floating microspheres is shown in Fig. (2).

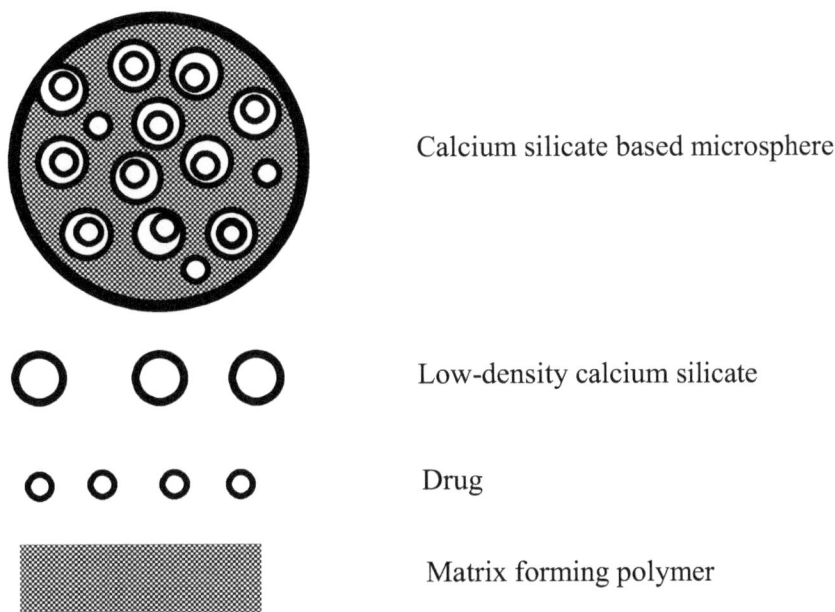

Calcium silicate based microsphere

Low-density calcium silicate

Drug

Matrix forming polymer

Fig. (2). Schematic presentation of calcium silicate based floating microspheres. [Adopted from: J Control Rel., Jain *et al,.*, 2005]

Characterization of Floating Microspheres

Micromeritic Properties and Morphology

Micromeritic properties *i.e.,* particle size, true density, tapped density, compressibility index and flow properties of prepared microspheres were studied [39]. The morphology of prepared microspheres and CS was explored by scanning electron microscopy (SEM).

The mean particle size of CS powder alone was found to be 142±02 μm while microsphere formulations containing CS in the range of 50-250 mg were measured 550±05, 610±08, 648±12, 720±10, and 828±12 μm, respectively. The particle size of microsphere formulation without CS powder was found to be 180±08 μm. The tapped density values for different formulations were ranged between 0.43±0.04 to 0.68±0.06 g/cm³, while their true densities were ranged between 1.66±0.12 to 1.94±0.10 g/cm³. This significant difference in the densities might be due to the presence of low-density CS particles in the microspheres. The porosity of all the microsphere formulations was ranged between 60.6±2.5 to 80.0±4.0%. However, microspheres showed compressibility index ranging between 25.0±2.2 to 34.6±3.1%. These observations conferred the excellent flow ability of prepared formulations which was further supported with the values of angle of repose (<40°) except formulation CS5, probably due to the greater proportion of CS. The better flow property of prepared microspheres indicates non-aggregated formulations.

The SEM photomicrographs of CS based Eudragit microspheres confirm the spherical shape and porous nature of the developed formulation (Fig. **3**). A large population of microspheres in the optimized formulation exists in spherical shape.

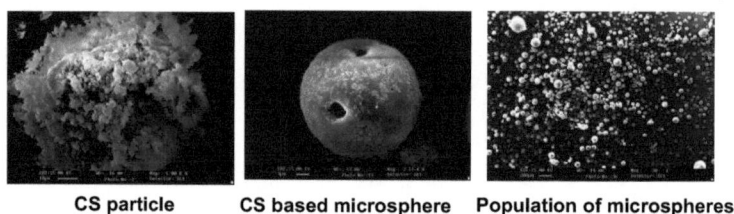

CS particle   CS based microsphere   Population of microspheres

Fig. (3). Scanning electron photomicrographs.
[Adopted from: AAPS PharmSciTech, Jain *et al*,., 2006]

Percentage Buoyancy and Drug Entrapment

For the determination of percentage buoyancy of developed floating microspheres, approximately 50 mg of the floating microspheres were placed in 100 ml of the simulated gastric fluid (SGF, pH 2.0) containing 0.02%w/v Tween 20. Then the content was stirred at 100 rpm with a magnetic stirrer. After 8 h, the layer of buoyant microspheres pipetted and separated by filtration. Particles in the sinking particulate layer are separated by filtration. Then both types of particles were dried to a constant weight in a desiccator. Both the fractions of microspheres were weighed and buoyancy was calculated by the weight ratio of floating particles to the sum of floating and sinking particles.

$$\text{Buoyancy (\%)} = \frac{W_f}{\left(W_f + W_s\right)} X100$$

Where, W_f and W_s are the weights of the floating and settled micro particles, respectively.

In order to determine the OT content in microspheres, 50 mg formulation was dispersed in 10 ml of ethanol followed by agitation with a magnetic stirrer for 12 h to allow the dissolution of polymer leading to drug extraction. The resulting dispersion was filtered through a 0.25 μm membrane filter (Millipore) and the OT content was determined in filtrate using LC/MS/MS method.

Ideal *in vivo* percentage buoyancy observed for all the developed microsphere formulations (Table **3**). This buoyant behavior may be attributed to the low tapped density of the microspheres owed to the entrapment of low density CS within the microsphere system [25, 40]. Microspheres formulation CS4 containing 200 mg CS showed the best floating ability (88±4% buoyancy) in SGF. The floating ability of microspheres up to 8 h may be considered satisfactory for desired therapeutic performance of the prepared formulations. The percent entrapment of OT was good for all the formulations. The high entrapment efficiency of OT in microspheres may be attributed to its poor aqueous solubility. The extent of drug loading influenced the particle size distribution of microspheres *i.e.,* when the loading is high; the proportion of larger particles is also high. With 80% drug entrapment, most of the particles were in the size range of 600-1200 μm, which are suitable for oral administration. During the determination of experimental yields it was revealed that about 35% microspheres does not contain any porous carrier. This may be due to the difference in particle size of microspheres. During the sieving step microspheres with variable size were observed as the microspheres without porous carrier and carrier particles are much smaller in size (100 to 200 μm) when compared to microspheres-containing carrier (500 to 800 μm).

Table 3. Buoyancy and drug entrapment of different floating microspheres.

Formulation Code	CS Content (mg)	Buoyancy (%)	Drug Entrapment (%)
WC	0	70 ± 3	70 ± 2.5
CS1	50	77 ± 2	78 ± 2.4
CS2	100	80 ± 4	82 ± 1.4
CS3	150	83 ± 2	82 ± 3.0
CS4	200	88 ± 4	84 ± 2.8
CS5	250	82 ± 5	80 ± 1.4

WC- Floating microspheres of orlistat without carrier; CS_{1-5} - Floating microspheres of orlistat with calcium silicate (n = 3). [Adopted from: AAPS PharmSciTech, Jain *et al,.,* 2006]

In vivo Drug Release of Floating Microspheres

USP XXIII basket type dissolution apparatus was used for the determination of release rate of OT from developed floating microspheres. A weighed amount of floating microspheres equivalent to 50 mg drug was filled in a hard gelatin capsule (# 0) and placed in the basket of dissolution apparatus. Five hundred ml of the SGF containing 0.02%w/v of Tween 20 was used as dissolution medium. The dissolution fluid maintained at 37±1°C with basket rotation speed of 100 rpm.

Perfect sink conditions were prevailed during the drug release study. Samples (5 ml) were withdrawn at each 30 min interval, passed through a 0.25 µm membrane filter (Millipore), and analyzed for OT content using LC/MS/MS method to determine the concentration of OT present in the dissolution medium. The initial volume of the dissolution fluid was maintained by adding 5 ml of fresh pre-warmed dissolution fluid after each sample withdrawal.

Release of OT from CS based microspheres was determined in SGF (pH 2.0). Since, acrylic polymer does not solubilize at acidic pH and it normally starts to dissolve above pH 7, therefore the release of OT from developed microspheres can be govern only by diffusion in SGF (pH 2.0). Furthermore, the low solubility of OT at acidic pH also add up to the slow dissolution of drug. No burst effect was observed from any of the developed formulations. The release of OT from different formulations was observed in following order: WC > CS1 > CS2 > CS3 > CS4 > CS5. This order also provides an idea about the effect of CS content on drug release from the microspheres as it was observed that the higher CS content in microspheres leads to lower drug release (Fig. **4**). The release mechanism of OT from floating microspheres was also evaluated based on theoretical dissolution equations *i.e.,* zero order, first order, Higuchi matrix, Peppas-Korsmeyer, and Hixon-Crowell kinetic models. The regression coefficients and rate constants obtained from *in vivo* release profiles of OT in SGF were calculated with PCP Disso v3 software (Table **4**). Drug release pattern from all the floating microspheres in SGF (pH 2.0) followed Higuchi matrix model and Peppas-Korsmeyer model. Earlier reports by Desai & Bolton [41] and Khattar *et al,*. [42] acknowledged that non-effervescent floating systems obeyed the Higuchi model indicating drug release *via* a diffusion mechanism.

Table 4. The regression coefficients and rate constants for release of OT from floating microspheres in SGF (pH 2.0).

Formulation	Zero order model		First order model		H-M model		P-K model		H-C model	
	r	k_1	r	k_2	r	k_3	r	k_4	r	k_5
WC	0.8762	10.6842	0.9799	-0.1641	0.9902	24.6715	0.9782	24.5398	0.9589	-0.0469
CS1	0.8523	8.4173	0.9564	-0.1140	0.9931	19.4937	0.9807	20.7807	0.9313	-0.0342
CS2	0.8652	7.3073	0.9488	-0.0939	0.9953	16.9078	0.9868	17.0995	0.9270	-0.0287
CS3	0.8674	6.7540	0.9457	-0.0849	0.9924	15.6110	0.9787	16.3321	0.9249	-0.0261
CS4	0.8629	6.1582	0.9362	-0.0755	0.9898	14.2356	0.9736	15.1140	0.9163	-0.0235
CS5	0.8563	5.5036	0.9247	-0.0657	0.9924	12.7386	0.9807	13.4997	0.9053	-0.0206

WC- Floating microspheres of orlistat without carrier; CS_{1-5} - Floating microspheres of orlistat with calcium silicate; r-Correlation coefficient; k_1, k_2, k_3, k_4 and k_5 -Rate constants of zero order, first order, Higuchi matrix (H-M), Peppas-Korsmeyer (P-K) and Hixon-Crowell (H-C) model, respectively.
[Adopted from: AAPS PharmSciTech, Jain *et al,*., 2006]

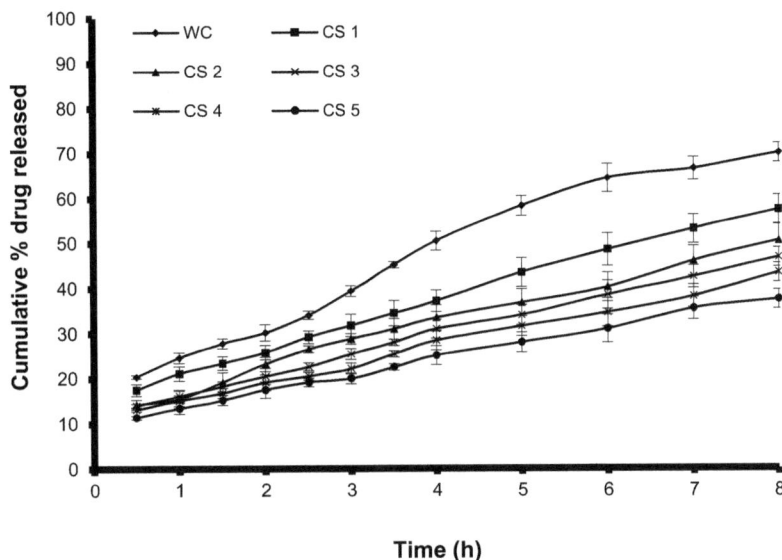

Fig. (4). *In vitro* release of OT from various floating microspheres in SGF (pH 2.0) (n = 3). [Adopted from: AAPS PharmSciTech, Jain *et al,.*, 2006]

Gamma Scintigraphy

For imaging studies, 500 mg of both *i.e.,* optimized formulation (CS4) and non-floating microspheres (NFM) loaded with $SnCl_2$ and OT were taken in a test tube containing 10 ml of normal saline (0.9% NaCl) and kept aside for 15 min. A small amount of sodium pertechnetate solution equivalent to radioactivity of 40 mBq in a sterile vial obtained from a technetium generator was added to the test tube and mixed intermittently for 15 min on a vortex shaker (Superfit, India). Then the supernatant was removed and the radiolabeled microspheres were recovered by filtration through Whatmann filter paper (No. 41) followed by washing thoroughly with deionized water. Then microspheres were dried in air for 15 min.

Male albino rabbits (1 yr old, 12) were employed to monitor the *in vivo* transit behavior of optimized floating and non-floating microspheres. These rabbits were divided into two groups *i.e.,* group I and group II. None of them had symptoms or a history of gastrointestinal (GI) disease. In order to standardize the conditions of GI motility, all the animals were kept on fasting for 12 h prior to commencement of each experiment. Radiolabeled CS4 (100 mg) was administered orally as suspension to group I and radiolabeled NFM to group II followed by sufficient volume of drinking water. All four legs of the rabbit were tied over a piece of plywood (20 X 20 inch) and then location of formulation in the stomach was monitored by keeping them in front of gamma camera. The gamma camera had a field view of 40 cm and was fitted with a medium energy parallel-hole collimator. The 140 keV gamma rays emitted by ^{99m}Tc were imaged. Specific stomach site (anterior) were imaged by E-Cam Single Head gamma camera at definite time intervals and activity counts were recorded for 5 min period to calculate the counts per minute (CPM). The gamma images were recorded using an online computer system (Macscnsetch, Germany), and stored on magnetic disk and analyzed to determine the distribution of activity in the oral cavity, stomach, and intestinal region. In between the gamma scanning, the animals were freed and allowed to move and carry out normal activities but are not allowed to take any food or water until the formulation had emptied from the stomach completely [43].

The optimized formulation (CS4) showed good *in vitro* buoyancy and controlled release behavior and were selected for *in vivo* study *i.e.,* gamma scintigraphy and the results were compared with that of NFM, prepared using the identical polymers. Gamma scintigraphic images of the ^{99m}Tc-labeled CS4 and NFM are shown in Fig. (**5** and **6**). Examination of the sequential gamma scintigraphic images clearly indicated that the CS4 remained buoyant with uniform distribution in gastric contents over a study period of 6 h. Prolonged GRT upto 6 h was observed in all the rabbits for the CS4, which remained buoyant in the stomach during entire test period. In contrast, NFM showed GRT of comparatively very shorter duration *i.e.,* less than 2 h. Following the oral administration, the floating microspheres tend to float over the stomach content. This floating behavior might be owed to the presence of porous low density CS and hollow cavity within the microspheres. Measurable number of counts of ^{99m}Tc-tagged CS4 for 6 h study period established very good gastro-retentive propensity of administered microspheres which remained in floating state with uniform distribution over the stomach contents for the overall study period of 6 h. In case of NFM, the radioactive counts decreased considerably after 2 h. Gamma scintigraphy was performed for 6 h duration which corresponds to the half-life of ^{99m}Tc [44].

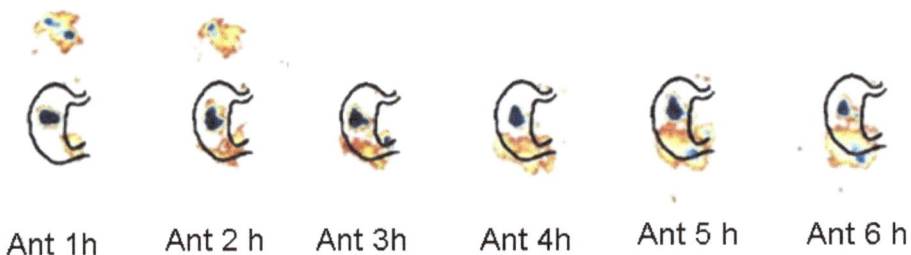

Ant 1h   Ant 2 h   Ant 3h   Ant 4h   Ant 5 h   Ant 6 h

Fig. (5). Gamma scintigraphic images of CS4 in albino rabbits.
[Adopted from: AAPS PharmSciTech, Jain *et al,*., 2006]

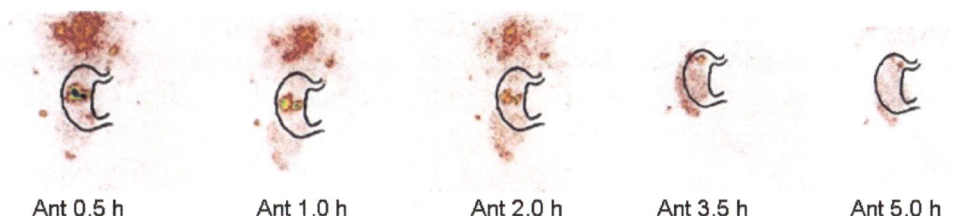

| Ant 0.5 h | Ant 1.0 h | Ant 2.0 h | Ant 3.5 h | Ant 5.0 h |

Fig. (6). Gamma scintigraphic images of NFM in albino rabbits.
[Adopted from: AAPS PharmSciTech, Jain *et al,*., 2006]

Pharmacokinetic Studies

The *in vivo* experiments were performed on healthy male albino rabbits weighing between 2.2-2.5 kg. All rabbits were kept in animal house for one week to acclimatize them and fed on fixed standard diet. For the experimental setup, twelve rabbits divided into two groups of six each and kept in fasting condition for 24 h. The first group fed with Xenical capsule (marketed product) equivalent to 12 mg of OT, while CS4 equivalent to 12 mg of OT was given to the second group of animals with *ad libitum* access to water during fasting and throughout the experiment. The rabbits were not anaesthetized during or prior to the treatment and the formulations were administered orally with a cannula. Blood samples (2 ml) were collected from the marginal ear vein into heparinized centrifuge tubes just before dosing and at 0.5, 1, 1.5, 2, 3, 4, 5, 6, 8, 10, 12, and 24 h during the study. All the blood samples were transferred to a series of graduated centrifuge tubes containing 0.4 ml of 2.5% w/v sodium citrate solution and centrifuged at 2500 rpm for 5 min. Then the separated plasma was transferred into another set of sample tubes and frozen until assayed. One undosed plasma sample was used as blank. For the analysis of OT concentration, all the samples were filtered through 0.25µm membrane filter (Millipore) and subjected to LC/MS/MS method for drug concentration measurement.

The peak plasma concentration (C_{max}) of OT with floating microspheres remained nearly unchanged when compared to marketed preparation (Xenical) as they showed the plasma concentrations of 9.4 ng/ml and 9.2 ng/ml, respectively (Table **5** and Fig. **6**). While time to attain peak plasma concentration (t_{max}) was increased to 8 h from 4 h with corresponding increase in area under the curve (AUC) from 69.0 ng.h/ml to 113.3 ng.h/ml (nearly 1.6 times). Elimination half-life ($t_{1/2}$) was increased by about 1.5 times (4.08 h) for the CS4 when compared to the Xenical capsule. The values of C_{max} and t_{max} indicated insignificant increased absorption of OT in GI tract, when given as floating formulations (Fig. **7**). It took 8 h in comparison to Xenical (4 h) to reach maximum concentration of OT in blood indicating delay in absorption and extending its localized concentration in the stomach and duodenum, the desired site of action for the inhibition of lipase enzyme. The *in vivo* study of selected floating formulation confirmed its ability to modify the pharmacokinetic behavior of OT in the desired manner. These results clearly indicated the controlled and sustained release of OT from developed gastro-retentive floating formulations. It may be concluded that the elongated elimination half-life observed during gamma scintigraphic study was due to the floating nature of these developed formulations.

Table 5. Pharmacokinetic parameters of OT formulations after oral administration in rabbits (n=6).

S. No.	Pharmacokinetic parameter	Marketed Preparation (Xenical)	Floating Microspheres (CS4)
1.	Peak plasma concentration C_{max} (ng/ ml)	9.2 ± 0.42	9.4 ± 0.62
2.	Time to reach peak plasma concentration t_{max} (h)	4	8
3.	Area under the curve AUC $_{0-24}$ (ng.h/ ml)	69.0	113.3
4.	Absorption rate constant K_a (h^{-1})	0.58	0.54
5.	Elimination rate constant K_e (h^{-1})	0.26	0.17
6.	Elimination half-life ($t_{1/2}$) (h)	2.67	4.08
7.	Lag time (min)	50	45
8.	Relative Bioavailability	1.00	1.64

[Adopted from: AAPS PharmSciTech, Jain *et al,.*, 2006]

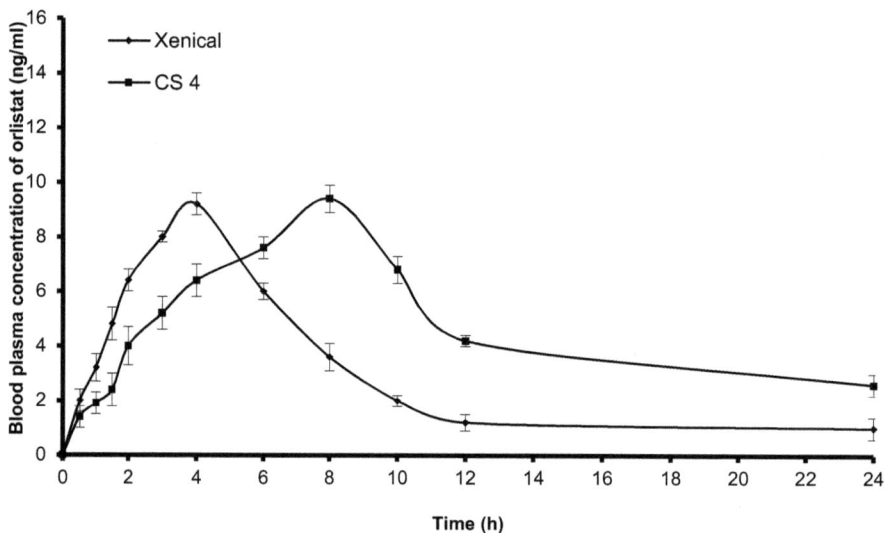

Fig. (7). Mean plasma concentration of OT following oral administration of its floating formulation and the marketed product (n = 6).
[Adopted from: AAPS PharmSciTech, Jain *et al,.*, 2006]

FLOATING GRANULES

Preparation of Floating Granules

Polymeric solutions (2%w/v) of hydroxypropyl methylcellulose (HPMC) and ethylcellulose (EC) (as primary coating solution) and of EC, CP, HPMC (as secondary coating solution) in different ratios were prepared in ethanol with mild heating and their viscosity was measured to test the solution using a Viscometer. OT absorbed CS powder was placed in a sigma blade mixer and sufficient amount of HPMC/EC solution (2%w/v in ethanol) was added drop wise with constant stirring at 100 rpm to form a wet mass of desired consistency. Maximum mixing allowed upto 30 min, then wet mass was passed through a screen (# 22) and dried in a forced air oven at 50°C for 3 h. These granules were designated as PCG's (primary coated granules of OT). Among these primary coated granules, PCG-5 (HPMC: EC ratio 25:75) were further coated with polymer solution of HPMC, EC and CP (2%w/v in ethanol) following the same procedure. The coated granules were dried at 50°C for 3 h and thus the secondary coated granules containing OT (SCG's) were obtained (Table **6**).

Table 6. Formulation code and ratio of polymers used in secondary coating of different formulations EC- Ethyl cellulose, HPMC- Hydroxypropyl methylcellulose K4M, CP- Carbopol 940, SCG_{1-9} - Secondary coated granules.

Formulation code	Ratio of EC: CP: HPMC
SCG-1	90: 10: 0
SCG-2	80: 10: 10
SCG-3	70: 10: 20
SCG-4	60: 10: 30
SCG-5	50: 10: 40
SCG-6	90: 0: 10
SCG-7	70: 20: 10
SCG-8	60: 30: 10
SCG-9	50: 40: 10

[Adopted from: PDA J Pharm Sci Tech, Jain *et al,*., 2008]

Characterization of Floating Granules

Drug Content and Floating Ability

An accurately weighed 100 mg of granular formulation of OT was digested with 10 ml ethanol (95%) for 1 h. Then the digested heterogenate granular mass was subjected to centrifugation (Remi, India) at 3000 rpm for 3 min and then supernatant was decanted off. The separated residue was re-digested with another 10 ml of ethanol for 15 min and again centrifuged for 3 min. After filtration through a Whatmann filter paper (# 41), the saturated solution of 2, 4-dinitrophenyl hydrazine (DNPH) in ethanol was mixed with the filtrate followed by heating for 10 min at 40°C. OT concentration in the ethanolic phase was then determined spectrophotometrically at 366.4 nm in a GBC Cintra-10 UV/Vis spectrometer.

The floating test for each formulation was carried out using dissolution apparatus USP XXIII method II [45]. The granules weighing 300 mg were immersed in 900 ml simulated gastric fluid (SGF, pH 2.0) containing Tween 20 (0.02% w/v), maintained at 37°C, which was agitated by a paddle at a speed of 100 rpm. The paddle blades were positioned at the surface of dissolution medium. The granules floating on the surface of SGF were recovered with a sieve (# 60) at 1 h time interval up to 8 h from these dissolution apparatus, such that first sample of floating granules was collected at 1 h from first DR apparatus, second sample after 2 h from second apparatus and so on. The granules so collected were dried and weighed.

The percentage content of OT in primary and secondary coated granules was found to be 80±4% in all the formulations. Good *in vitro* floating behavior was observed for all the prepared formulations. Tween 20 (0.02%w/v) was added to SGF to counteract the downward pulling at the liquid surface by lowering surface tension of SGF and increasing the surface area at the air fluid interface. In contrast to most conventional floating systems (including gas-generating ones), these granules floated immediately upon contact with the release medium showing no lag time in floating behavior because the low density prevailed from the beginning (t=0). The effect of polymer ratio (used for coating of granules) on the floating property of granules was also studied. High-viscosity grade (K4M and E4M) HPMC showed slightly better floating properties than low-viscosity grade (E5LV) HPMC. The floating study also suggested that the granules coated with higher proportion of HPMC in polymer solution were more floatable than those with lower proportion. The floating capacity or percentage buoyancy of SCG was higher than that of PCG. The floating study of granular formulations suggests that it is possible to attribute a high floating property in the secondary coated granular formulation through swelling of HPMC in the coating of granules. In order to evaluate the effect of CP on the floating property of granules, it was incorporated in floating granules in different ratios with HPMC and EC. CP played an important role for the drug release and buoyancy of SCG-5, when used in combination with HPMC K4M and EC. In the present formulation, carbopol was added to coating solution to control the drug release in the view of the fact that carbopol is insoluble in water and artificial gastric fluid. The swelling of HPMC in gastric fluid might have contributed partially to the floating behavior of these granular formulations. The floating behavior of secondary coated granules in SGF increased in the rank order SCG-5> SCG-4> SCG-2> SCG-3> SCG-6> SCG-7> SCG-8> SCG-9 >SCG-1 (Fig. **8**). With these results it was concluded that CP appeared to have a negative effect with respect to floating behavior of granules. Assessment of floating ability of granules for 8 h considered satisfactory for the performance of developed systems. Furthermore, it was also noticed that granules of bigger size showed longer floating time.

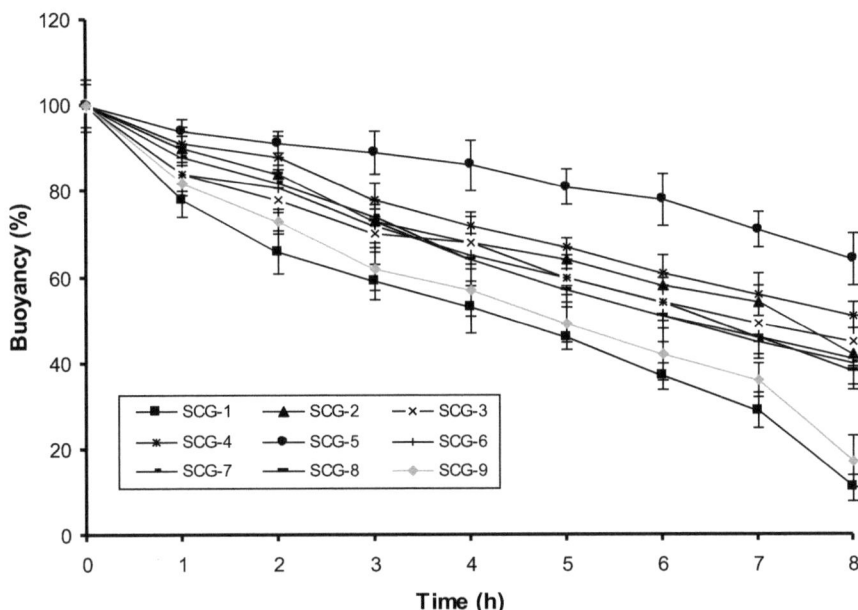

Fig. (8). Percent buoyancy of different granules (secondary coated) of Orlistat (SCG_{1-9}) in SGF (pH 2.0). Values are mean ± S.D. (n = 3).
[Adopted from: PDA J Pharm Sci Tech, Jain *et al,*., 2008]

In vitro Drug Release of Floating Granules

The drug release pattern from these floating granular formulations can be determined in simulated GI fluid using dissolution apparatus (USP XXIII basket type). Briefly, weighed amount of floating granules equivalent to 50 mg OT filled into a capsule (# 0) and it was placed in the basket of dissolution rate apparatus. The dissolution medium, SGF (pH 2.0) (500 ml) containing 0.02%w/v of Tween 20 was maintained at 37±1°C at 100 rpm. A sample of 5 ml was withdrawn at each 30 min interval and mixed with 1 ml saturated solution of 2, 4-D--nitrophenylhydrazine (DNPH) in ethanol followed by heating for 10 min at 40°C. After that, samples were filtered through Whatmann filter paper (# 41) and OT concentration was determined spectrophotometrically at 366.4 nm using GBC

Cintra-10 UV/Vis spectrometer. After each withdrawal, the initial volume of the dissolution fluid was replenished by addition of equivalent volume of fresh pre-warmed dissolution fluid. Perfect sink condition was prevailed during the drug release study. Similar process was adopted for the assessment of *in vivo* drug release in SGF from marketed product of OT *i.e.,* Xenical capsule.

Out of the primary coated five granular formulations of OT, formulation PCG-5 showed relatively better-controlled release of OT and buoyancy pattern in SGF (pH 2.0). Thus, the formulation PCG-5 was re-coated with polymer solution comprised of different ratios of EC, CP and HPMC and coded as SCG-1, SCG-2, to SCG-9. Insoluble EC might have played an important role to control the release of OT from PCG. In case of secondary coated granules, drug release in SGF (pH 2.0) followed the order as SCG-6> SCG-1 > SCG-2> SCG-7 > SCG-8 > SCG-9 > SCG-3> SCG-5 ≥ SCG-4 (Fig. **9**). The overall results of the study suggested that the initial high percent of release of OT from primary and secondary coated granules might be attributed to the dissolution of OT from those pores that are not covered with polymer. CP is a cross-linked polymer with high molecular weight (~2 X 10^6 Da) and viscosity; and, when exposed to water, it becomes viscous and thus tends to bind the mixed polymeric system together, resulting in reduced erosion of floating granules. Hence, formulations without CP exhibited faster release due to erosion of HPMC and EC present in the coating. It was clear from comparison of *in vivo* release of OT from secondary coated granules that as the ratio of HPMC decreased, the drug release was also increased. This may be due to the decrease in density of the swollen hydrogel network with reduction in amount of HPMC, offering lower hindrance to drug diffusion and hence the drug release. From drug release studies in GI fluids, it was concluded that the drug release depends on polymer concentration, amount of adsorbed polymer as well as the ratio of HPMC and CP in the polymer solution.

The release mechanism of OT from these primary and secondary coated granules was evaluated based on theoretical dissolution equations including zero order, first order, Higuchi matrix, Peppas-Korsmeyer, and Hixon-Crowell kinetic models. OT release from secondary coated granules in pH 2.0 followed Higuchi matrix, Peppas-Korsmeyer, and first order models (Table **7**). The *in vivo* drug release from optimized formulations SCG-4 and SCG-5 corresponds to highest regression coefficient values for Higuchi's model, indicating diffusion to be the predominant mechanism of drug release. Desai & Bolton [41] and Khattar *et al,*. [42] reported that non-effervescent floating systems obeyed the Higuchi model indicating drug release *via* a diffusion mechanism.

Table 7. The kinetic parameters for release of OT from secondary coated floating granules at 37°C in the SGF (pH 2.0), r-Correlation coefficient; k_1, k_2, k_3, k_4, and k_5 -Rate constants of zero order, first order, Higuchi matrix (HM), Peppas-Korsmeyer (P-K) and Hixon-Crowell (H-C) model, respectively.

Model → Formulation ↓	Zero order		First order		HM		P-K		H-C		Best fit model
	r	k_1	r	k_2	r	k_3	r	k_4	r	k_5	
SCG-1	0.9649	10.4535	0.9741	-0.1737	0.9789	24.9592	0.9880	20.8793	0.9850	-0.0481	P-K
SCG-2	0.8774	10.2454	0.9743	-0.1602	0.9976	24.8867	0.9970	26.1396	0.9547	-0.0455	HM
SCG-3	0.9534	7.4990	0.9886	-0.1006	0.9889	17.9804	0.9914	15.7903	0.9812	-0.0303	P-K
SCG-4	0.9336	6.6587	0.9665	-0.0860	0.9758	15.9827	0.9933	15.6665	0.9597	-0.0262	HM
SCG-5	0.9147	7.1497	0.9698	-0.0936	0.9970	17.2757	0.9941	17.0757	0.9554	-0.0284	HM
SCG-6	0.9685	12.6759	0.8890	-0.2958	0.9776	30.2341	0.9832	25.1866	0.9592	-0.0697	P-K
SCG-7	0.9336	9.6325	0.9845	-0.1470	0.9887	23.1723	0.9772	22.6094	0.9780	-0.0421	HM
SCG-8	0.9611	9.0108	0.9913	-0.1325	0.9831	21.5496	0.9853	18.1787	0.9881	-0.0385	1st order
SCG-9	0.9023	8.5285	0.9720	-0.1201	0.9921	20.6282	0.9710	21.4697	0.9553	-0.0355	HM

[Adopted from: PDA J Pharm Sci Tech, Jain *et al*,., 2008]

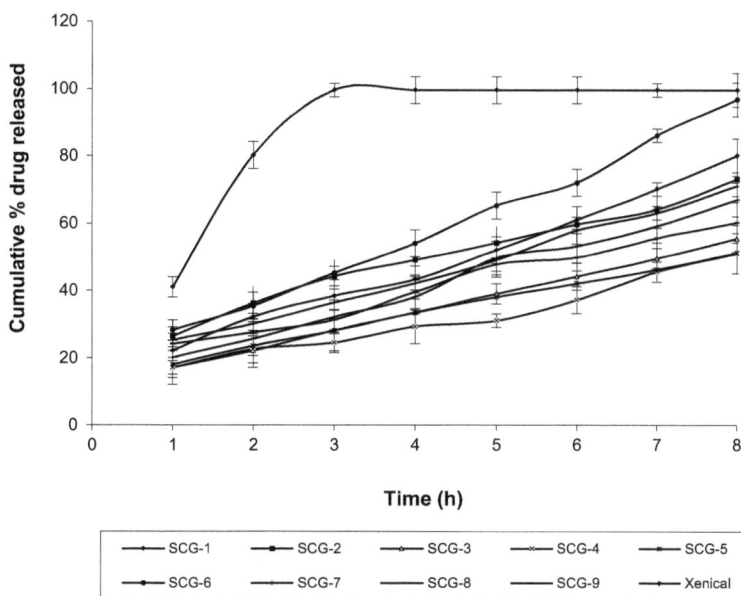

Fig. (9). *In vitro* Orlistat release profile of Xenical capsule and secondary coated floating granules (OTSCG$_{1-9}$) in SGF (pH 2.0). Xenical (Capsule) contains 120 mg Orlistat. Values are mean ± S.D. (n = 3). [Adopted from: PDA J Pharm Sci Tech, Jain *et al*,., 2008]

CONCLUSION

The results for different evaluation parameters clearly indicate the superiority of developed system with controlled and sustained release of OT from gastro-retentive floating microspheres and granules. The CS based floating multiparticulate delivery system radiolabeled with ^{99m}Tc was successfully visualized scintigraphically to establish gastro-retentive performance in the rabbit. The floating ability of the granules and the release rate of the drug (OT) from the granules can be controlled by changing the polymer type as well as the ratio of composition of HPMC, EC and CP in the polymer solution. It was observed that the optimized formulations followed the Higuchi matrix model for drug release. These designed systems presents the excellent combination of buoyancy with suitable drug release pattern and offers clear advantages in terms of enhanced bioavailability of OT. Further, these developed microspheres and granules could be compressed into tablets, filled into capsules, or may be formulated as oral suspension for reconstitution.

CONSENT FOR PUBLICATION

Not applicable.

CONFLICT OF INTEREST

The author (editor) declares no conflict of interest, financial or otherwise.

ACKNOWLEDGEMENTS

Dr. Jain acknowledges M/s F. Hoffmann-La Roche Ltd. Basel, Switzerland for the supply of Orlistat as a gift sample. The author also wish to thank Dr. D.C. Prasad, Jawaharlal Nehru Cancer Hospital and Research Centre, Bhopal, India and Dr. Rajesh Pathania, All India Institute of Medical Sciences, New Delhi, India for extending Gamma scintigraphy and SEM facilities, respectively.

REFERENCES

[1]   Haslam DW, James WP. Obesity. Lancet 2005; 366: 1197-209.
       [http://dx.doi.org/10.1016/S0140-6736(05)67483-1]

[2]   WHO. Obesity: preventing and managing the global epidemic Report of a WHO Consultation. WHO Technical Report Series 894 2000.

[3]   Berrington de Gonzalez A, Hartge P, Cerhan JR, *et al.* Body-mass index and mortality among 1.46 million white adults. N Engl J Med 2010; 363: 2211-9.
       [http://dx.doi.org/10.1056/NEJMoa1000367]

[4]   Whitlock G, Lewington S, Sherliker P, *et al.* Body-mass index and cause-specific mortality in 900 000 adults: collaborative analyses of 57 prospective studies. Lancet 2009; 373: 1083-96.
       [http://dx.doi.org/10.1016/S0140-6736(09)60318-4]

[5]   Calle EE, Thun MJ, Petrelli JM, Rodriguez C, Heath CW Jr. Body-mass index and mortality in a prospective cohort of U.S. adults. N Engl J Med 1999; 341: 1097-105.
[http://dx.doi.org/10.1056/NEJM199910073411501]

[6]   Pischon T, Boeing H, Hoffmann K, *et al.* General and abdominal adiposity and risk of death in Europe. N Engl J Med 2008; 359: 2105-20.
[http://dx.doi.org/10.1056/NEJMoa0801891]

[7]   Manson JE, Willett WC, Stampfer MJ, *et al.* Body weight and mortality among women. N Engl J Med 1995; 333: 677-85.
[http://dx.doi.org/10.1056/NEJM199509143331101]

[8]   WHO. Obesity and overweight 2015. Available at: http://www.who.int/mediacentre/factsheets/fs311/en/

[9]   Sturm R. Increases in morbid obesity in the USA: 2000–2005. Public Health 2007; 121: 492-6.
[http://dx.doi.org/10.1016/j.puhe.2007.01.006]

[10]   Peeters A, Barendregt JJ, Willekens F, Mackenbach JP, Al Mamun A, Bonneux L. Obesity in adulthood and its consequences for life expectancy: a life-table analysis. Ann Intern Med 2003; 138: 24-32.
[http://dx.doi.org/10.7326/0003-4819-138-1-200301070-00008]

[11]   Barness LA, Opitz JM, Gilbert-Barness E. Obesity: genetic, molecular, and environmental aspects. Am J Med Genet 2007; 143A: 3016-34.
[http://dx.doi.org/10.1002/ajmg.a.32035]

[12]   Joo JK, Lee KS. Pharmacotherapy for obesity. J Menopausal Med 2014; 20: 90-6.
[http://dx.doi.org/10.6118/jmm.2014.20.3.90]

[13]   Akbas F, Gasteyger C, Sjodin A, Astrup A, Larsen TM. A critical review of the cannabinoid receptor as a drug target for obesity management. Obes Rev 2009; 10: 58-67.
[http://dx.doi.org/10.1111/j.1467-789X.2008.00520.x]

[14]   Bray GA, Greenway FL. Current and Potential Drugs for Treatment of Obesity. Endocr Rev 1999; 20: 805-75.
[http://dx.doi.org/10.1210/edrv.20.6.0383]

[15]   de Luis DA, Gonzalez Sagrado M, Conde R, Aller R, Izaola O. Decreased basal levels of glucagon-like peptide-1 after weight loss in obese subjects. Ann Nutr Metab 2007; 51: 134-8.
[http://dx.doi.org/10.1159/000103273]

[16]   Keating GM, Jarvis B. Orlistat: in the prevention and treatment of type 2 diabetes mellitus. Drugs 2001; 61: 2107-19.
[http://dx.doi.org/10.2165/00003495-200161140-00011]

[17]   Torgerson JS, Hauptman J, Boldrin MN, Sjostrom L. XENical in the prevention of diabetes in obese subjects (XENDOS) study: a randomized study of orlistat as an adjunct to lifestyle changes for the prevention of type 2 diabetes in obese patients. Diabetes Care 2004; 27: 155-61.
[http://dx.doi.org/10.2337/diacare.27.1.155]

[18]   Siebenhofer A, Horvath K, Jeitler K, *et al.* Long-term effects of weight-reducing drugs in hypertensive patients. Cochrane Database Syst Rev 2009; Cd007654.

[19]   Aronne LJ, Powell AG, Apovian CM. Emerging pharmacotherapy for obesity. Expert Opin Emerg Drugs 2011; 16: 587-96.
[http://dx.doi.org/10.1517/14728214.2011.609168]

[20]   Moes AJ. Floating delivery and other potential gastric retaining systems Current status on targeted drug delivery to the gastrointestinal tract. Capsugel Library 1993; pp. 97-112.

[21]   Deshpande AA, Rhodes CT, Shah NH, Malick AW. Controlled-Release Drug Delivery Systems for Prolonged Gastric Residence: An Overview. Drug Dev Ind Pharm 1996; 22: 531-9.

[http://dx.doi.org/10.3109/03639049609108355]

[22]   Singh BN, Kim KH. Floating drug delivery systems: an approach to oral controlled drug delivery *via* gastric retention. J Control Release 2000; 63: 235-59.
[http://dx.doi.org/10.1016/S0168-3659(99)00204-7]

[23]   Jain SK, Agrawal GP, Jain NK. Evaluation of porous carrier-based floating orlistat microspheres for gastric delivery. AAPS PharmSciTech 2006; 7: 90. b
[http://dx.doi.org/10.1208/pt070490]

[24]   Jain SK, Awasthi AM, Jain NK, Agrawal GP. Calcium silicate based microspheres of repaglinide for gastroretentive floating drug delivery: preparation and in vivo characterization. J Control Release 2005; 107: 300-9.
[http://dx.doi.org/10.1016/j.jconrel.2005.06.007]

[25]   El-Kamel AH, Sokar MS, Al Gamal SS, Naggar VF. Preparation and evaluation of ketoprofen floating oral delivery system. Int J Pharm 2001; 220: 13-21.
[http://dx.doi.org/10.1016/S0378-5173(01)00574-9]

[26]   Jain SK, Agrawal GP, Jain NK. A novel calcium silicate based microspheres of repaglinide: *In vivo* investigations. J Control Release 2006; 113: 111-6. c
[http://dx.doi.org/10.1016/j.jconrel.2006.04.005]

[27]   Bardonnet PL, Faivre V, Pugh WJ, Piffaretti JC, Falson F. Gastroretentive dosage forms: Overview and special case of Helicobacter pylori. J Control Release 2006; 111: 1-18.
[http://dx.doi.org/10.1016/j.jconrel.2005.10.031]

[28]   Shimpi S, Chauhan B, Mahadik KR, Paradkar A. Preparation and evaluation of diltiazem hydrochloride-Gelucire 43/01 floating granules prepared by melt granulation. AAPS PharmSciTech 2004; 5: e43.
[http://dx.doi.org/10.1208/pt050343]

[29]   Jain SK, Agrawal GP, Jain NK. *In vivo* evaluation of porous carrier-based floating granular delivery system of orlistat. PDA J Pharm Sci Technol 2008; 62: 292-9.

[30]   Thanoo BC, Sunny MC, Jayakrishnan A. Oral sustained-release drug delivery systems using polycarbonate microspheres capable of floating on the gastric fluid. J Pharm Pharmacol 1993; 45: 21-4.
[http://dx.doi.org/10.1111/j.2042-7158.1993.tb03672.x]

[31]   Sangwai M, Sardar S, Vavia P. Nanoemulsified orlistat-embedded multi-unit pellet system (MUPS) with improved dissolution and pancreatic lipase inhibition. Pharm Dev Technol 2014; 19: 31-41.
[http://dx.doi.org/10.3109/10837450.2012.751404]

[32]   Desai J, Khatri N, Chauhan S, Seth A. Design, development and optimization of self-microemulsifying drug delivery system of an anti-obesity drug. J Pharm Bioallied Sci 2012; 4: S21-2.
[http://dx.doi.org/10.4103/0975-7406.94124]

[33]   Dolenc A, Govedarica B, Dreu R, Kocbek P, Srcic S, Kristl J. Nanosized particles of orlistat with enhanced in vivo dissolution rate and lipase inhibition. Int J Pharm 2010; 396: 149-55.
[http://dx.doi.org/10.1016/j.ijpharm.2010.06.003]

[34]   Kim D, Park JH, Kweon DJ, Han GD. Bioavailability of nanoemulsified conjugated linoleic acid for an antiobesity effect. Int J Nanomedicine 2013; 8: 451-9.

[35]   Basak SC, Rahman J, Ramalingam M. Design and *in vivo* testing of a floatable gastroretentive tablet of metformin hydrochloride. Pharmazie 2007; 62: 145-8.

[36]   Yuasa H, Takashima Y, Kanaya Y. Studies on the Development of Intragastric Floating and Sustained Release Preparation. I. Application of Calcium Silicate as a Floating Carrier. Chem Pharm Bull (Tokyo) 1996; 44: 1361-6.
[http://dx.doi.org/10.1248/cpb.44.1361]

[37] Jain AK, Jain SK, Yadav A, Agrawal GP. Controlled release calcium silicate based floating granular delivery system of ranitidine hydrochloride. Curr Drug Deliv 2006; 3: 367-72. a
[http://dx.doi.org/10.2174/156720106778559083]

[38] Kawashima Y, Niwa T, Takeuchi H, Hino T, Itoh Y. Hollow microspheres for use as a floating controlled drug delivery system in the stomach. J Pharm Sci 1992; 81: 135-40.
[http://dx.doi.org/10.1002/jps.2600810207]

[39] Martin A. Micromeritics. Physical Pharmacy IV edn. Philadelphia: Lea Febiger 1993; pp. 431-2.

[40] Streubel A, Siepmann J, Bodmeier R. Floating microparticles based on low density foam powder. Int J Pharm 2002; 241: 279-92.
[http://dx.doi.org/10.1016/S0378-5173(02)00241-7]

[41] Desai S, Bolton S. A floating controlled-release drug delivery system: *in vivo-in vivo* evaluation. Pharm Res 1993; 10: 1321-5.
[http://dx.doi.org/10.1023/A:1018921830385]

[42] Khattar D, Ahuja A, Khar RK. Hydrodynamically balanced systems as sustained release dosage forms for propranolol hydrochloride. Pharmazie 1990; 45: 356-8.

[43] Atyabi F, Sharma HL, Mohammad HA, Fell JT. *In vivo* evaluation of a novel gastric retentive formulation based on ion exchange resins. J Control Release 1996; 42: 105-13.
[http://dx.doi.org/10.1016/0168-3659(96)01344-2]

[44] Saha GB. Fundamentals of Nuclear Pharmacy. Radiolabeling of compounds. New York: Springer-Verlag 1979; pp. 86-91.

[45] Jain SK, Agrawal GP, Jain NK. Porous carrier based floating granular delivery system of repaglinide. Drug Dev Ind Pharm 2007; 33: 381-91.
[http://dx.doi.org/10.1080/03639040600920655]

CHAPTER 5

Multi Targeted Strategies Towards Identification of Potential Drug Candidates from Natural Products in the Management of Obesity

Baddireddi Subhadra Lakshmi[*, 1,2] and **Gopal Thiyagarajan**[2]

[1] *Centre for Food Technology, Anna University, Chennai, India*

[2] *Department of Biotechnology, Anna University, Chennai, India*

Abstract: Obesity, a chronic metabolic disorder, is caused by an imbalance between energy intake and expenditure, and has been associated with insulin resistance, Type 2 Diabetes Mellitus (T2DM), hypertension, myocardial infarction, fatty liver disease, stroke, osteoarthritis and certain cancers. Currently, drugs used for the management of obesity like orlistat (lipase inhibitor) and Phentermine (norepinephrine and dopamine releasing agent) have been reported to exhibit adverse side effects.

Recent advancements in the understanding of biological systems have opened up new possibilities towards a multi targeted approach, designed to target more than one biological mechanism that might ultimately be more effective in producing sustained weight loss along with improvement in comorbidities. Multi-targeted drugs have emerged as a new paradigm in the last decade owing to their advantages in the treatment of complex multifactorial diseases such as obesity and T2DM. Most recently, glucagon-like peptide-1 (GLP-1) mimetics and insulin secretagogues have been reported for their anti-obesity activity, due to their property of delaying the rate of gastric emptying and appetite suppression in CNS, thus promoting satiety and weight loss.

Medicinal plants have been established as rich resources for the identification of potential drug candidates. Most of these isolated natural products exhibit multi-targeted action owing to their diverse and complex structure. Numerous natural bioactive molecules including polyphenols, alkaloids, sterols, glycosides, terpenes and saponins have been identified as potential drug candidates for the management of obesity. Cellular and molecular studies have shown that these natural products suppress appetite and reduce food intake, reduce intestinal absorption of fats, attenuate lipid synthesis and accumulation, stimulate lipolysis, promote oxidation of fatty acids and reduce inflammation.

[*] **Corresponding author Baddireddi Subhadra Lakshmi**: Centre for Food Technology, Department of Biotechnology, Anna University, Chennai – 600 025, Tamil Nadu, India; Tel: +91-44-22350772; Fax: +91-44-22350299; E-mail: lakshmibs@annauniv.edu

Atta-ur-Rahman & M. Iqbal Choudhary (Eds.)

This chapter will focus on the molecular targets and mechanisms involved in weight regulation, provide an insight into the isolation of bioactive compounds from medicinal plants, and the multi targeted strategies for the control of obesity.

Keywords: Adiponectin, Adipogenesis, Allosteric PTP1B inhibitor, Antiobesity drugs, Appetite suppressors, AMPK, β-oxidation, C/EBP, Cholecystokinin agonists, DPP4, GLP1, HSL, Leptin, Lipolysis, Multi targeted drugs, Natural products, Neuropeptide Y antagonist, Obesity, Pancreatic lipase, Partial PPARγ agonist, PPARα, Sirtuins, SREBP, Thermogenesis, UCPs.

INTRODUCTION

Obesity, characterized by surplus of fat mass, is increasing owing to increased consumption of calorically rich diet and lack of physical activity. Obesity occurs when the intake of energy surpasses expenditure, triggering an overgrowth of adipocytes. Epidemiologically, excess of visceral fat, as determined by the waist to hip ratio, has been associated with metabolic disorders [1]. According to the World Health Organization (WHO), a person with BMI (body mass index) greater than 25 Kg/m^2 is overweight, a BMI greater than 30 Kg/m^2 is categorized as obese, while a BMI value ≥40 Kg/m^2 is designated as "morbidly obese".

Obesity is a serious public health concern affecting people all around the world. Globally, the epidemic of obesity is growing rapidly with almost 600 million adults characterized to be obese and around 1.9 million adults (> 18 years) observed to be overweight. The reasons for weight gain could be either due to intrinsic or extrinsic factors. The intrinsic factors include genetic predisposition, epigenetic or endocrine disturbances, while extrinsic factors include increased consumption of high energy-dense foods, limited physical activity and a sedentary life style [2, 3].

Metabolic syndrome is characterized by a coexistence of multiple risk factors, with central obesity being a cardinal feature [4]. The pathogenesis of metabolic syndrome is closely related to alterations in lipogenesis, utilization of fatty acids and energy expenditure. Eventually, these changes affect the storage of lipids in ectopic tissues such as intraperitoneal, skeletal and liver depots, leading to the progression of other complications including insulin resistance, diabetes, dyslipidemia, hypertension, stroke, osteoarthritis, gout, gallbladder disease, pulmonary and cardio vascular diseases [5]. A principal contributor in the progression of obesity is hyperinsulinemia, wherein elevated levels of cellular triacylglycerol and alterations in lipid and glucose metabolism are observed [6].

CURRENT TREATMENT STRATEGIES FOR OBESITY

Although diet and exercise are lifestyle modifications often prescribed for the control of obesity, they usually fail to produce sustainable weight loss [7]. Bariatric surgery has been shown to be a more effective way to reduce weight and decrease comorbidities [8]. However, due to surgical risks, bariatric surgery is reserved for persons who are morbidly obese [9].

Besides surgery and lifestyle modification, therapeutic strategies for the control of obesity include decreased absorption of fat from food, and promotion of energy expenditure [10]. Although many antiobesity agents have been identified in the past decade for the management of obesity, many have been withdrawn from the market owing to their side effects, including gastrointestinal, psychiatric and cardiovascular risk [11]. Currently, drugs including Xenical (orlistat), Qsymia (phentermine and topiramate), Belviq (lorcaserin), Contrave (naltrexone and bupropion) and Saxenda (liraglutide) have been approved by the US-FDA (United States Food and Drug Administration) and EMA (European Medical Agency) for long-term management of obesity. Other anti-obesity pharmacotherapies such as Phentermine, Phendimetrazine, Benzphetamine and Didiethylpropion have been approved by FDA and EMA for short-term weight loss programmes. Antiobesity drugs such as Sibutramine (nor-adrenaline and serotonin reuptake inhibitor), Fenfluramine (serotonin reuptake inhibitor), Rimonabant (cannabinoid-1 receptor antagonist) approved by EMA have been withdrawn from the market due to a higher incidence of cardiac events, stroke, pulmonary hypertension and psychiatric disorders [12, 13]. Therefore, there is a need for more efficacious, tolerable drugs with no or reduced side effects for the long-term management of obesity and its related complications [14].

MEDICINAL PLANTS AS A SOURCE FOR NOVEL DRUGS

For thousands of years, medicinal plants have been widely used for the treatment of various simple to complex diseases. In fact, since the beginning of the 19th century, isolation of pure bioactive compounds from natural products has led to the identification of potential drug candidates. Chemical, biochemical and structural diversity of the compounds isolated from natural products make them desirable candidates for the treatment of multifactorial diseases [15].

The first oral antidiabetic drug candidate, isolated from the extracts of French lilac *Galega officinalis* was identified as a guanidine compound (galegine). This biguanidine was used as a model for the synthesis of metformin, a first-line oral antihyperglycemic drug [15]. Other potential drug candidates from natural products are cromolyn, from *Ammi visnaga* used as a bronchodilator and papaverine from *Papaver somniferum*, which has been used as a base for the synthesis of cerapramil, a known antihypertension agent [16]. Artemisinin and its relative compounds have been developed from *Artemisia annua* and are being used for antimalarial therapy in many developing countries [17]. In recent years, Paclitaxel (Taxol) is the most widely used plant derived anticancer drug identified from the leaves of Taxus species including *Taxus brevifolia* [18].

Natural products and their constituents have been used for the treatment and prevention of obesity and its related complications, emphasizing the therapeutic potential of traditional medicine for the treatment of complex disorders [19, 20]. Green tea has been observed to exhibit antiobesity potential owing to its rich antioxidant activity and a higher content of catechin such as epigalloylcatachin (EGC) and epigalloylcatachin gallate (EGCG) [21]. The polyphenolic constituents of Green Tea cause various combinatorial effects including increased lipolytic activity, reduced appetite, attenuated adipocyte differentiation and increased energy expenditure resulting in loss of weight [22, 23]. The Chinese herb ginseng has been reported to markedly reduce weight gain and body fat with enhanced glucose tolerance. *Panax granatum* has been observed to exhibit lipase inhibitory activity, reduction in energy intake and suppression of fat accumulation in adipocytes, suggesting its antiobesity potential. Moreover, the effect of *P. granatum* on suppression of energy consumption was similar to that of sibutramine [24, 25]. The bioactive molecules from *Aegle marmelos* such as esculetin and umbelliferone have been observed to show significant activity *via* decreased storage of fat in the adipocytes, thereby reducing hyperlipidemia [26]. Galangin (*Alpinia galangal*) has been known to exhibit significant improvement in lipid profile, lipid peroxidation and TG accumulation in liver, resulting in reduced body fatness [27].

Berberine extracted from *Cortex phellodendri* and *Cortidis rhizoma* was originally reported for the treatment of infectious diarrhea in humans [28]. Later, it was found to relieve key symptoms of hyperglycemia and hyperlipidemia associated with obesity and diabetes, and was identified as an insulin secretagogue and sensitizer through modulation of AMPK activity [29, 30]. For many years, the extracts of *Momordica charantia* (bitter melon) have been used traditionally for the treatment of obesity, diabetes and its associated symptoms. A wide range of triterpenoids have been isolated from bitter melon which were observed to exhibit potent antiadipogenic and antihyperglycemic activities in both *in vitro* and *in vivo* experimental studies [31]. The isolated pure molecule sitosterol from *Boerhaavia diffusa* was observed to reduce cholesterol levels by decreasing plasma VLDL-cholesterol and LDL-cholesterol. Phytoconstituent p-synephrine from *Citrus aurantium* has been reported to increase energy expenditure and metabolic rate, resulting in weight loss. The bioactive flavonoids from *Nelumbo nucifera* have been observed to exhibit inhibition of pancreatic lipase and adipocyte differentiation, signifying its antiobesity potential [32, 33]. Recently, two major bioactive compounds such as ephedrine and pseudo-ephedrine from *Sida rhomboidea* have been testified to stimulate appetite suppression and induce weight loss [34].

Further, polyphenols such as curcumin, epigallocathechin-3-gallate (EGCG), quercetin and resveratrol have been observed to attenuate weight gain, blood lipid levels, elevated blood pressure, fat storage, HbA1c levels and insulin resistance [35]. Polyphenols such as caffeoyl, dicaffeoyl and feruloyl quinic acids inhibit the activity of pancreatic lipase and maltase, thereby decreasing obesity and its related disorders including hyperglycemia, hyperinsulinemia and the risk of CVD [36].

MECHANISM AND MOLECULAR TARGETS OF OBESITY

An imbalance in the consumption and utilization of energy results in the development of obesity, due to a dysregulated lipid metabolism including lipogenesis and lipolysis [37]. The mechanism of lipogenesis involves synthesis and storage of fatty acids as triglycerides (TG) in the peripheral tissues such as adipocytes, liver and skeletal muscles, while lipolysis involves the process of degradation of the stored TG into free fatty acids and glycerol [38, 39].

In the regulation of lipid metabolism, adipokines such as leptin and adiponectin are involved in the metabolism of fats, and regulation of insulin sensitivity in peripheral tissues. AMPK (AMP activated protein kinase) plays a significant role in the metabolism of lipids and carbohydrates *via* inactivation of ACC (Acetyl-CoA carboxylase) and activation of fatty acid oxidation through an upregulation of peroxisome proliferator activated receptor α (PPARα), carnitine palmitoyltransferase 1(CPT1) and uncoupling proteins (UCPs) [40]. It has been reported that in the obese state, adipocytes secrete adipokines such as monocyte chemoattractant protein 1 (MCP1) and tumor necrosis factor α (TNFα) in response to inflammatory response, resulting in a high degree of lipolysis [41]. The key targets and their mechanism of action in the regulation of lipid metabolism and obesity can be broadly categorized into five groups:

INHIBITION OF LIPID ABSORPTION

Pancreatic Lipase Inhibitors

Lipases (triacylglycerol hydrolase E.C. 3.1.1.3) are enzymes involved in the digestion of fats such as triglycerides (TG) and phospholipids. In humans, there are two different classes of lipases, such as pre-duodenal lipases (lingual and gastric) and extra-duodenal lipases (hepatic, pancreatic, endothelial and lipoprotein). The pancreatic lipases (PL) are chief lipolytic enzymes synthesized and secreted from the pancreas, playing a vital role in the digestion of triglycerides. The digestion of dietary TG is more important for the action of PL in the small intestine. PL catalyzes the hydrolysis of ester bonds of TG (dietary fats and oils) to yield long chain saturated and unsaturated free fatty acids, diacylglycerols, monoglycerols and glycerol as the lipolytic products. These end products are readily absorbed by the body and thought to be responsible for the progression of obesity. Hence, compounds that can inhibit the activity of PL would be a useful drug candidate for the treatment of obesity [42, 43].

Naturally occurring pancreatic lipase inhibitors are orlistat and tetrahydrolipstatin produced from *Streptomyces toxytricini* [44]. Orlistat inhibits the activity of lipase by covalent bond interaction with Serine at the active site of the enzyme [45]. Although, orlistat is one of the US-FDA approved drugs for the treatment of obesity, it exhibits some gastrointestinal related adverse effects such as flatulence and oily stools. Therefore, current research is focusing towards identification of newer PL inhibitors derived from plants or other natural sources which do not cause any side effects [46]. Phytochemicals from traditional medicine provide an excellent opportunity for the discovery of novel therapeutics. A range of extracts derived from plants used in traditional medicine have been known to exhibit lipase inhibitory activity including *Platycodi radix* [47], *Panax japonicus* [48], *Nelumbo nucifera* [49], *Salacia reticulata* [50] as shown in Table **1**.

Table 1. List of plant extracts showing pancreatic lipase inhibitory activity.

Name of the Plant and active concentration (IC50)	References
Juglans mandshurica fruit (2.3 mg/mL)	[42]
Adonis palaestina (937.5 μg/mL), *Anthemis palestina* (107.7 μg/mL), *Chrysanthemum coronarium* L. (286.1 μg/mL), *Convolvulus althaeoides* L. (664.5 μg/mL), *Hypericum triquetrifolium* (236.2 μg/mL), *Malva nicaeensis* (260.7 μg/mL), *Ononis natrix* L. (167 μg/mL), *Origanum syriaca* L. (234 μg/mL), *Paronychia argentea* L. (342.7 μg/mL), *Reseda alba* L. (738 μg/mL) and *Salvia spinosa* L. (156.2 μg/mL)	[51]
Aframomum melegueta (90%) and *Spilanthes acmella* (40%)	[52]
Alpinia zerumbet rhizome (5.00 μg/mL)	[53]
Artocarpus lakoocha fruit (82.49%)	[54]
Baccharis trimera leaf (78%)	[55]
Bergenia crassifolia rhizomes (3.4 μg/mL)	[56]
Cassia angustifolia (0.81 mg/mL)	[57]
Cassia auriculata (6.0 mg/mL)	[58]

(Table 1) cont.....

Name of the Plant and active concentration (IC50)	References
Cassia siamea roots (74.3%), *Chukrasia tabularis* leaves (67.6%), *Ferula asafoetida* resin (72.5%), *Justicia gendarussa* (61.1%), *Lagerstroemia indica* Fruits (61.2%) and *Vigna radiata* roots (64.6%)	[59]
Morinda citrifolia (21.0%), *Centella asiatica* (25.3%) and *Momordica charantia* (25.8%)	[60]
Coscinium fenestratum stems (160 µg/mL)	[61]
Cudrania tricuspidata (9.91 µg/mL)	[62]
Dioscorea nipponica root (10 µg/mL)	[63]
Eleusine indica (31.36%)	[64]
Lepidium sativum L. (1.28 mg/mL)	[65]
Mangifera indica L. leaves (75%)	[66]
Rosmarinus officinalis (7 mg/mL) and *Mentha Spicata* (7.85 mg/mL)	[67]
Passiflora nitida (21.2 µg/mL)	[68]
Rheum palmatum L. (53.8) and *Prunella vulgaris* L. (74.7%)	[69]
Shorea roxburghii bark (31.6 µg/mL)	[70]
Viscum album (33.3 mg/mL) and *Sorbus commixta* leaf (29.6 mg/mL)	[71]
Vitis vinifera L. seeds (30%)	[72]

The phytochemicals exhibiting pancreatic lipase inhibitory activity are mostly polyphenols [66, 73 - 75]. Among the natural PL inhibitors, various types of tea such as black, green and oolong tea have been well studied. Polyphenols including catechin, epigalloylcatachin isolated from tea (leaves extract) have shown significant PL inhibitory activity [76, 77]. These types of polyphenols need galloyl moieties in their chemical structure for efficient PL inhibition [78]. Phenolic compounds from grape seeds such as epigallocatechin-3-gallate, kaempferol and quercetin have been reported to show a strong inhibition of PL activity [79]. Furthermore, tannins, ellagitannin and proanthocyanidins isolated from berries (strawberry, blueberry, arcticberry, raspberry lingonberry and bearberry), *Pisum sativum* (pea plant), *Picea abies* (Norway spruce) and *Plantago lanceolata* have been observed to exhibit significant inhibition of PL activity [80, 81]. Table **2** lists the active constituents from plants exhibiting pancreatic lipase inhibition.

Table 2. List of active phytochemicals which exhibit pancreatic lipase inhibition.

Name of the Plant	Active Constituents (IC50)	References
Accanthopanax sessiliflorus	Sessiloside and chiisanoside (0.36 and 0.75 mg/ml)	[82]

(Table 2) cont.....

Name of the Plant	Active Constituents (IC50)	References
Camellia sinensis	Theaflavins, theaflavin 3-O-gallate, theaflavin 30-O-gallate, theaflavin 3,30-O-gallate, epigallocatechin gallate, epicatechin gallate, catechins, 2 quercetin glycosides, quinic acid, gallic acid and caffeine	[83, 79]
Coffea canephora	Caffeine, chlorogenic acid, neochlorogenic and feruloylquinic acids	[36]
Cynometra cauliflora	Kaempferol 3-*O*-rhamnoside (186.5%)	[84]
Dioscorea nipponica	Dioscin (20 µg/ml), diosgenin (28 µg/ml), prosapogenin C (42.2 µg/ml), gracillin (28.9 µg/ml)	[63]
Gardenia jasminoids	Crocin (28.63 µmol)	[71]
Panax japonicus	Chikusetsusaponins (125–500 µg/ml)	[48]
Salvia officinalis L.	Carnosic acid (12 µg/ml) and oleanolic acid (83µg/ml)	[85]
Scabiosa tschiliensis	Prosapogenin 1B (0.12 mg/ml)	[69]
Thea sinensis (oolong tea)	(-)-epigallocatechin 3,5-di-O-gallate (0.098 µM), assamicain A (0.120 µM), theasinensin D (0.098 µM), oolongtheanin 30-O-gallate (0.068 µM), theaflavin (0.106 µM)	[78]

SUPPRESSION OF APPETITE

Appetite suppression has been implicated as a first line therapeutic strategy in the management of obesity [86]. A decrease in body weight through appetite suppression is regulated through neurohormonal mechanisms in the central nervous system (CNS). Increasing evidence suggests that several neurotransmitters such as histamine, dopamine, serotonin and activities of their respective receptors are closely correlated with regulation of satiety and appetite [87]. These receptors collectively enable researchers to identify targets for the control of obesity *via* a reduced intake of energy [88]. The gastrointestinal tract plays an essential role in the secretion of various appetite and satiety signaling molecules [89]. The Arcuate nucleus in the hypothalamus is a crucial site in the brain involved in the regulation of appetite. Only a few gut hormones and neuropeptides have been studied extensively for their effective role on appetite and energy expenditure. The gut hormones and enzymes that affect food intake are pancreatic polypeptide (PP), peptide YY_{3-36} (PYY), glucagon like peptide 1 (GLP1), amylin, ghrelin, cholecystokinin (CCK) and dipeptidyl peptidase 4 (DPP4) [89, 90].

Most of the gut hormones are anorexigenic and promote satiation and satiety except ghrelin, which is actively involved in the stimulation of appetite [91]. Neuropeptide Y (NPY) is the neuropeptide secreted from CNS involved in the stimulation of appetite. Further, leptin, an adipocyte related hormone, is observed to regulate appetite in a CNS dependent manner. Hence, identification of potential drug compounds that can stimulate or inhibit secretion of these peptides at the cellular level could be an attractive strategy.

Recently, research on gut hormones, particularly GLP1 and DPP4 is growing rapidly owing to their satiety-related weight lowering effect in humans [92]. In a placebo controlled clinical trial, administration of Liraglutide (GLP1 agonist) to diabetic patients was observed to reduce weight by 7-8% and is a target for development of antiobesity drugs [93].

Glucagon Like Peptide 1 Analogues and Dipeptidyl Peptidase 4 Inhibitors

Glucagon like peptide 1 (GLP1), a gut hormone, has been recently identified as a novel and promising target for the development of antiobesity drugs. GLP1 is normally synthesized and secreted from the gastrointestinal L cells. After subsequent selective cleavage of GLP1, two active amide fragments are obtained as GLP 17–37 and GLP 17–36. Among them, the fragment GLP 17-36 is found to be a major circulating form after ingestion of a meal. GLP1 receptors are ubiquitously expressed in the central nervous system (CNS) and peripheral tissues, and are inactivated by another gut peptide DPP4 (dipeptidyl peptidase 4), limiting the half-life of circulatory GLP1 to 1-2 min [89]. Binding of this peptide to the GLP1 receptors present in the stomach results in satiation (fullness of stomach) and possibly termination of meal. Treatment with GLP1 and its analogues showed a dose dependent decrease in food intake in laboratory animals as well as in lean and obese human subjects [94]. Hence, two major strategies have been implicated to extend the short half-life of GLP1. The first is production of more efficient and stable GLP1 analogues, and the other is inhibition of the enzymatic activity of DPP4. To date, stabilization of GLP1 have been observed to exhibit better results in weight management. Discovery of Exendin 4, a GLP1 analogue, from the venom of a Gila monster (lizard), has been a great breakthrough, based on which, Eli Lilly with Amylin Pharmaceuticals have developed a trade mark drug Byetta® which is in use as an insulin secretogogue. Reports have shown that, although administration of Exendin improved glycemic control with a decrease in body weight, some side effects including nausea and difficulties in subcutaneous injection [95, 96] were observed.

Table **3** lists the GLP1 analogues and DPP4 inhibitors identified from plants. Some of the notable compounds include the triterpenoid saponins such as ginsenoids Rb1, Rb2, Re and Rb3 and Compound K which showed efficient GLP1 secretion. Compound K, and ginsenoid Rb2 from *Panax ginseng* have been reported to secrete GLP1 in human enteroendocrine NCI-4716 cells [97, 98], while the ginsenoid Rb1 was observed to enhance the secretion of GLP1 and plasma insulin with a concomitant decrease in food intake, body weight and fat mass and fasting blood glucose in HFD induced obese rats. Additionally, ginsenoid Re have been shown to secrete GLP1 with reduced blood glucose level in *ob/ob* mice [99]. Similarly, ginsenoid Rg3 (*Panax ginseng*) was found to increase the secretion of GLP1 in rodent β cell line with a corresponding decrease in blood glucose level in ICR mice [100]. Procyanidin from the seeds of *Vitis vinifera* have been reported to inhibit DPP4 gene expression in intestinal human cells (caco2) as well as diet induced obese rats [101].

Table 3. List of GLP1 analogues and DPP4 inhibitors from plant sources.

Name of the Plants	Active Constituents	Biological and *in vitro* Activity	References
Anemarrhena asphodeloides	Aqueous extract	Ameliorates GLP1 secretion in human L cell line.	[105]
Berberis aristata	Bark extract	Enzymatically inhibits DPP4 activity.	[107]
Blupleurum falcatum	Hexane extract	Increases GLP1 secretion in human L cell line and decreases blood glucose in *db/db* mice.	[106]
Citrus aurantium	Hexane extract	Enhances GLP1 levels in human L cell line.	[104]
Gentiana scabra	Loginic acid (Root extract)	Increases G-protein coupled GLP1 activity, increases insulin secretion and attenuates hyperglycemia in *db/db* mice.	[102]
Hoodia gordonii	Gordonoside F	Increases plasma GLP1 level and decreases food intake *via* cannabinoid receptor mediated manner and increases glucose dependent insulin secretion in isolated rat islets and C57BL/6 mice.	[103]
Mangifera indica	Methanol extract	Inhibits DPP4 activity.	[109]
Momordica charantia	Fruit extract	Inhibits DPP4 activity.	[108]
Ocimum sanctum	Leaves extract	Inhibits DPP4 activity.	[108]
Panax ginseng	Compound K	Secretes GLP1 in human enteroendocrine NCI-4716 cells.	[98]
Panax ginseng	Ginsenoid Rb2	Secretes GLP1 in human enteroendocrine NCI-4716 cells.	[97]
Panax ginseng	Ginsenoid Re	Secretes GLP1, reduces blood glucose in *ob/ob* mice.	[99]
Panax ginseng	Ginsenoid Rg3	Secretes GLP1 in rodent β cell line and decreases blood glucose in ICR mice.	[100]
Vitis vinifera	Procyanidin (Seed)	Inhibits activity of DPP4 gene expression in intestinal human cells (caco2) and diet induced obese rats.	[101]

Administration of root extracts of *Gentiana scabra* enriched with loginic acid was observed to increase the G-protein dependent GLP1 and insulin secretion, resulting in attenuation of hyperglycemia in *db/db* mice [102]. In another study, mice supplemented with gordonoside F from *Hoodia gordonii* was found to increase cannabinoid receptor mediated GLP1 secretion with concurrent decrease in food intake, enhancing glucose dependent insulin secretion in isolated rat islets and C57B/6 mice [103]. *Citrus aurantium* (Hexane extract), *Blupleurum falcatum* (Hexane extract) and *Anemarrhena asphodeloides* (Ethylacetate extract) have been reported to increase GLP1 secretion in human L cell line and decrease blood glucose level in *db/db* mice [104 - 106].

Inhibition in the enzymatic activity of DPP4 was found to increase the circulating activity of GLP1. Thus, various extracts of *Berberis aristata* (Bark), *Mangifera indica* (methanolic extract) *Momordica charantia* (Fruit) and *Ocimum sanctum* (Leaves) were assessed for their enzymatic inhibitory activity of DPP4, which showed a dose dependent DPP4 inhibition [107 - 109]. Various *in vitro* and animal experimental studies have shown that DPP4 inhibitory and GLP1 stimulatory activity of bioactive extracts and constituents could be an alternative for the control of weight gain and obesity.

Cholecystokinin Agonists

Cholesystokinin (CCK) is synthesized and secreted from I-cells in the gastrointestinal lining of small intestine. CCK is produced through selective post-translational mediated breakdown of the pre pro-CCK polypeptide, followed by proteolytic treatment to yield a varying combination of active polypeptides. CCKs vary with the number of amino acids present in the configuration such as CCK8, CCK22, CCK33 and CCK58 [93, 110]. After ingestion of nutrients, circulating levels of CCK begin to rise at 15 min, attaining a peak at 25 min and remain elevated for about 3h. At present, two active G protein coupled CCK receptors such as CCK1 and CCK2 have been identified. CCK1 receptors are mainly found in the gastrointestinal tract, vagus nerve and myenteric plexus, whereas CCK2 receptors are widely present in the brain. Studies confirmed that CCK triggered satiation is chiefly dependent on the CCK1 receptors [89]. The stimulatory effect of CCK has been observed to counteract the expression of ghrelin [111]. Experimental rats treated with CCK peptide were observed to exhibit significant reduction in their appetite. The appetite inhibitory effect of CCK was also observed in obese rats [112]. Although the administration of CCK peptide has shown promising effect on the reduction of food intake, the possibility of CCK as an antiobesity drug, has not yet been proven.

Limited data is available on the plant products that have CCK antagonizing property. Administration of fatty acids and oils (3 g), isolated from *Pinus koraiensis* (pine nut), to obese female patients were reported to enhance 60% secretion of CCK8 (satiety hormone) and a reduction in diet intake [113, 114].

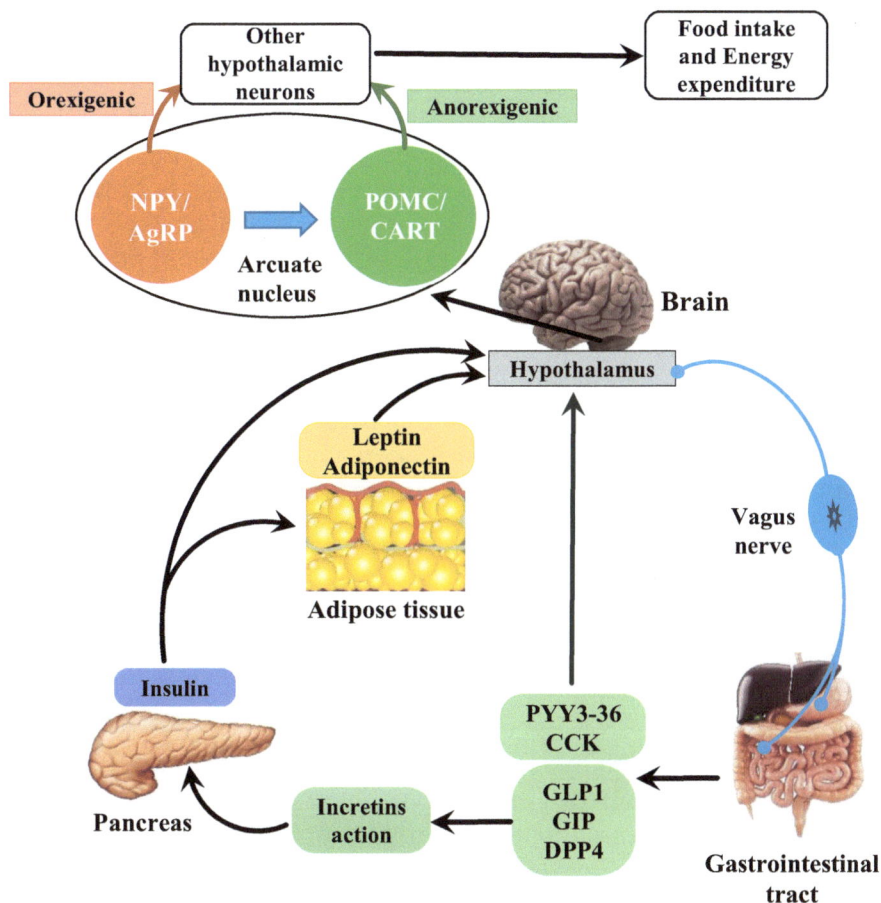

Fig. (1). Schematic representation of gut and neuro peptide signalling in the regulation of appetite.

Neuropeptide Y Antagonist

Regulation of diet and body weight are counterbalanced in the central nervous system [115]. Various stimuli from satiety hormones and nutrient signaling are collectively sensed and incorporated at the arcuate nucleus of hypothalamus in the CNS *via* vagal nerves and brainstem. As illustrated in the Fig. (**1**), appetite inducing (orexigenic) neuropeptide Y (NPY) and agouti related proteins (AgRP) activating neurons counterbalance the regulation of anorexigenic pro-opiomelanocortin (POMC) and cocaine-amphetamine regulated transcript (CART) expressing neurons. Moreover, neuronal signal at Y1 and Y5 receptors involve the activation of orexigenic (appetite stimulant) effects of NPY. Signaling at neuronal Y2 and Y4 receptor activates an anorexic (satiation) effect owing to their presynaptic inhibition of NPY peptide release. Therefore, small molecules or agents that show antagonism towards the Y1 and Y5 receptors could be explored as a potential therapeutic utility in the management of obesity [96, 116].

Some natural appetite suppressants have been reported, which reduce the expression of hypothalamic neuropeptide Y (NPY), and regulate the secretion of leptin from adipocytes [117]. Administration of crude saponin, isolated from Korean ginseng, to HFD fed obese rats was observed to reduce the levels of NPY and leptin [118]. Chakasaponin II from the flower bud of *Camellia sinensis* L., decreased mRNA levels of neuropeptide Y (NPY) in experimental animals [119].

Leptin

Leptin, an adipose tissue secreted hormone, has been found to be involved in both the short and long-term regulation of energy balance [120]. Obese mice that were administered leptin were found to exhibit decreased food intake and increased energy expenditure with a 30% reduction in weight [121]. Moreover, an inborn deficiency of leptin in humans was observed to result in early-onset obesity, which responded to leptin therapy [122]. Circulating levels of leptin have been directly correlated with both the state of feeding and degree of adiposity. Additionally, obese patients have been reported to exhibit elevated levels of circulating leptin, suggesting the concept of leptin resistance [123].

Leptin receptors are members of glycoprotein 130 (gp130) of cytokine receptors and are widely expressed in the hypothalamus [124]. Hypothalamic neurons such as NPY/AgRP and POMC/CART are reported to express leptin receptors. Activation of leptin receptors trigger the activation of Janus kinase 2 (JAK2), which, in turn, phosphorylates signal transducer and activator of transcription 3 (STAT3), resulting in increased expression of pro-opiomelanocortin (POMC), and inhibition of AgRP [125, 126]. Additionally, stimulated JAK2 phosphorylates insulin receptor substrate (IRS), resulting in activation of phosphoinositide 3 kinase (PI3K), which subsequently increases the expression of POMC, while suppressing NPY and AgRP. Further, AMP activated protein kinase (AMPK), an energy sensor, is activated at low cellular ATP levels, which in turn induces appetite and feeding behavior. Activation of the leptin receptor inhibits the expression of AMPK at multiple sites of the hypothalamus [127]. Leptin-mediated regulation of appetite has been associated with the ARC signalling (Fig. **1**). Leptin downregulates the neuronal expression of NPY/AgRP, thereby suppressing the expression of neuropeptides, whereas leptin activates POMC expression and upregulates the expression of POMC/CART signaling in the ARC of hypothalamus [3]. Although the role of leptin in the regulation of appetite has been widely known, there are reports of some people with obesity exhibiting leptin receptor resistance [128].

Many natural appetite suppressants have been identified from food supplements for the control of appetite. For example, a south African Plant *Hoodia gordonii* has been demonstrated as a natural appetite suppressant [129]. The extract of *H. gordonii* was found to increase the neuronal ATP content at the hypothalamus of rat brain, resulting in decreased food intake [130]. Studies showed that EGCG isolated from green tea was observed to strongly inhibit fatty acid synthase (FAS), which is involved in the conversion of fatty acids to acetyl-CoA and malonyl-CoA. An inhibition of FAS in mice has been reported to decrease feeding behavior and reduce body weight [131]. An Indian edible cactus, *Caralluma fimbriata*, in a clinical study, was observed to exhibit a reduction in the hip to waist ratio, appetite and body weight, suggesting its potential as an antiobesity drug [132]. Table **4** shows the list of compounds from Plants which are used as Appetite Suppressors and their metabolic effect.

Table 4. List of natural plant products modulating appetite and satiation.

Name of the Plants	Active Compounds	Metabolic Effects	References
Camellia sinensis (leaf)	(-)-Epigallocathechin gallate (EGCG)	Reduces food intake *via* inhibiting fatty acid synthase (FAS), decreases acetyl- CoA and malonyl CoA. 82 mg/kg in Sprague Dawley rats (7 days) decreases 53% of body weight; 81 mg/kg in lean Zucker rats (8 days) decreases 32% of body weight; 2 mg/kg in obese Zucker rats (4 days) decreases 11% of body weight.	[133 - 136]
Camellia sinensis L.	Chakasaponin II	Suppresses expression of gene neuropeptide Y (NPY) and stimulates the release of appetite suppressor, serotonin (5-HT) in the hypothalamus of the mice.	[119]
Caralluma fimbriata (cactus)	Pregnane glycosides (Crude ethanolic extract)	1 g/day in overweight adult Indian men and women (60 days) decreased 2.5% of body weight.	[132]
Coix lachrymajobi var. mayeun (seed)	Crude aqueous extract	500 mg/kg in Sprague Dawley rats with HFD (4 weeks) decreases 36% of body weight.	[137]
Garcina cambogia	(-)-Hydroxycitric acid (HCA)	Stimulates the release of appetite suppressor, serotonin (5-HT). 154 nmol HCA/kg in Zucker obese rats (92 days) decreases 8% of body weight.	[138, 139]

(Table 4) cont.....

Name of the Plants	Active Compounds	Metabolic Effects	References
Hoodia gordonii and *Hoodia pilifera*	Steroidal glycoside	Increases intracellular ATP content in the hypothalamic neurons, and administration of intra-cerebroventricular injection (24 h) results in 40–60% reduction in food intake.	[129, 130, 140, 141]
Panax ginseng (root)	saponins	Suppresses expression of gene neuropeptide Y (NPY) and stimulates appetite suppressant serotonin (5-HT). 200 mg/kg in Sprague Dawley rats with HFD (3 weeks) decreases 37% of body weight.	[118]
Phaseolus vulgaris and *Robinia pseudoaccacia*	Lectins	100 mg/kg of lectin in Harlan-Wister rats (16 h) decreases 8-fold of food intake	[142]
Pinus koraiensis (pine nut)	Fatty acid and oils	3 g in obese women (4 h) 60% increase in cholecystokinin-8 (CCK) (satiety hormone) secretion	[113, 114]

Protein Tyrosine Phosphatase 1B Inhibitors

PTP1B is a negative regulator of the insulin and leptin signaling and is a key target extensively studied for its role in diabetes and obesity. Experimental methods have strongly implicated PTP1B as an essential phosphatase, in the modulation of insulin and leptin signaling cascade [20]. PTP1B is the first PTP isolated and purified from human placenta [143], and is encoded by the gene *ptpn1* which ubiquitously expresses a 50 kDa enzyme mainly bound to the endoplasmic reticulum through the proline-rich C-terminal segment [144].

In the insulin signaling pathway, binding of insulin stimulates autophosphorylation of IRβ and phosphorylation of IRS1/2 which further activates Akt and PI3K, leading to an increase in the translocation of Glut4, and transportation of extracellular glucose. PTP1B, is well known to inactivate PTK such as IRβ and IRS1/2 *via* dephosphorylation of the phosphorylated IRβ. Further, it inhibits insulin-stimulated recruitment and phosphorylation of the p85 of PI3K, and Glut4 translocation thereby negatively regulating the insulin signaling cascade [145]. PTP1B has also been postulated as a down regulator of leptin signaling *via* ob-receptor (OBR) mediated JAK-STAT mechanism. Upon binding of leptin to its leptin receptor, Janus kinases (JAK 1/2), two cytosolic PTKs, phosphorylate the signal transducer and activator of transcription (STAT). Several *in vitro* and *in vivo* studies have demonstrated that an over expression of PTP1B results in inhibition of JAK2 and STAT3 phosphorylation, and, attenuates the leptin mediated STAT signal transmission [146]. Fig. (**2**) shows the key events involved in the insulin and leptin signaling.

Moreover, in obesity and diabetes, an elevated level of leptin and leptin resistance has been associated with an upregulation of PTP1B *via* dephosphorylation of JAK2 [147]. However, an improved insulin sensitivity observed in PTP1B null mice fed on high fat diet could not be completely correlated with the reduction in weight gain. An over expression of PTP1B in mice hypothalamic cells resulted in a down regulation of JAK2 and STAT3 phosphorylation and attenuated leptin mediated signaling. Neuronal PTP1B null mice improved leptin stimulated hypothalamus signaling and were observed to decrease feeding, reduce weight, adiposity and increase energy expenditure, suggesting that PTP1B could be a crucial target for development of antiobesity drugs [148].

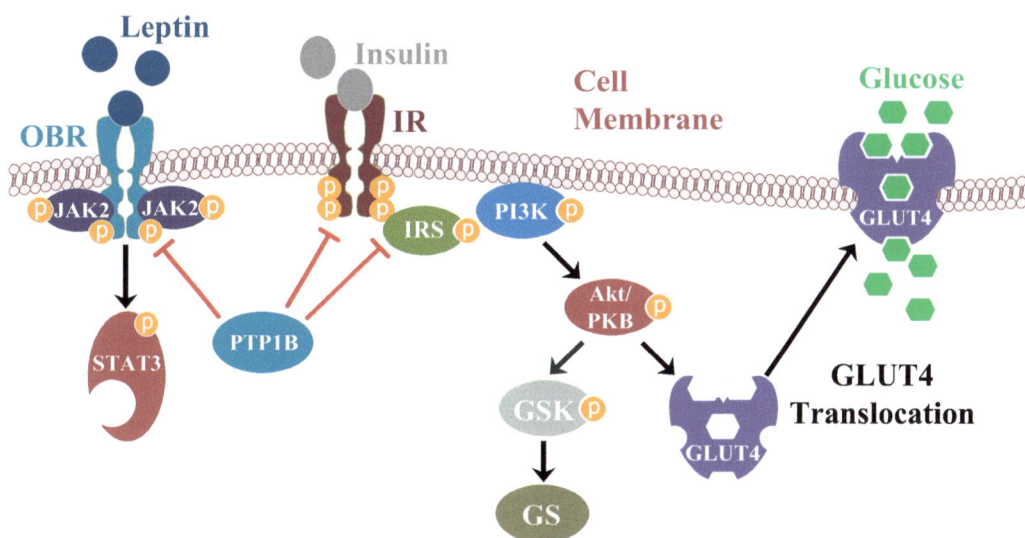

Fig. (2). Negative regulation of PTP1B in insulin and leptin signaling pathway.

Among the nearly 300 PTP1B inhibitors that have been identified and isolated from natural sources so far, majority of them belong to the phenolics and terpene group of compounds [149]. Phenolics such as lignans, coumarins and terpenes, such as diterpenes, sesquiterpenes, triterpenes, steroids and triterpenoid glucosides, along with the medicinal plants are summarized in Table **5**, with their respective inhibitory concentration (IC50) values assessed through *in vitro* recombinant human PTP1B inhibition.

Table 5. List of plants showing *in vitro* PTP1B inhibitory activity.

Name of the Plant	PTP1B Inhibitors and Biological Activity	References
Artemisia minor	Caffeic acid (3.06 μM)	[150]
Astilbe koreana	3-Oxoolean-12-en-27-oic acid (6.8 μM), 3b-Hydroxyolean-12-e--27-oic acid (5.2 μM),	[151]
Berberis sp.	Berberine mimics insulin action, enhances glucose uptake in L6 skeletal muscle and 3T3L1 adipocytes, and ameliorates glucose tolerance in *db/db* mice.	[152]
Broussonetia Papyrifa	Broussochalcone (21.5 μM)	[153]
Cichorium intybus (leaves)	Chlorogenic acid (3.82 μg/mL) inhibits PTP1B activity, Tannins (methanol extract) enhances glucose uptake with inhibition of adipogenesis, caffeoyl derivatives inhibits adipogenesis and regains insulin sensitivity in 3T3L1 adipocytes and HFD, STZ-induced rats.	[154, 155]
Cornus officinalis	Ursolic acid (3.08 μM)	[156]
Costus pictus	Methyl tetracosanate (1ng/mL)	[157]
Crocus sativus L. (flower)	Oral administration of safranal (20 mg/kg BW) improved impaired glucose tolerance in C2C12 myotubes and diabetic *KK-Ay* mice.	[158]
Cudrania tricuspidata	Cudratricusxanthone N (2.0±0.4 μM) and Cudraflavanone D (5.7±1.5 μM), non-competitive inhibitors	[159]
Curcuma longa (rhizome)	Curcumin reduces serum insulin and leptin levels minimizes increased synthesis of TG and VLDL and reduces hepatic mediated overexpression of PTP1B activity.	[160]
Cyclocarya paliurus	Myricetin-3-*O*-β-D-glucuronide (9.47±3.31 μg/mL) and 4-Di-*O*-β-D-glucopyranoside (10.50±2.67 μM)	[161]
Erythrina Mildbraedii	Abyssinone-VI-4-O-methyl ether (14.8 μM)	[162]
Orthosiphon aristatus	Betulinic acid suppresses hypothalamic expression of protein tyrosine phosphatase 1B (PTP1B) and improves antiobesity effect of leptin in obese rats fed with HFD	[163]
Paeonia lactiflora (roots)	1,2,3,4,6-Penta-O-galloyl-D-glucopyranose shows *in vitro* inhibition of PTP1B activity and improves insulin sensitivity in hepatoma cells (HCC-1.2).	[164]
Papaver somniferum L.	Papaverine inhibits *in vitro* PTP1B enzymatic activity and reduces fasting blood glucose in Balb/c mice.	[165]
Phoradendron reichenbachianum	Moronic acid (13.2 μM), Morolic acid (9.1 μM), Oleanolic acid (9.5 μM) and Ursolic acid (2.3 μM)	[166, 167]
Pongamia pinnata (fruit)	Pongamol and karanjin shows antihyperglycemic potential of *P. pinnata* in STZ-induced diabetic rats and diabetic *db/db* mice	[168, 169]
Psoralea corylifolia	Psoralidin (9.4±0.5 μM), non-competitive PTP1B inhibitor	[170]
Rhododendron brachycarpum	Rhododendric acid (6.3 μM) and Ursolic acid (3.1 μM)	[171]

(Table 5) cont.....

Name of the Plant	PTP1B Inhibitors and Biological Activity	References
Sambucus adnata	Ursolic acid (4.1 µM)	[172]
Sorbus commixta	Lupeol (5.6 µM) and Lupenone (13.7 µM), non-competitive inhibitor	[173]
Symplocos paniculata	Corosolic acid (7.2 µM) and Ursolic acid (3.8 µM)	[151]
Syzygium cumini (seed)	Vitalboside A enhances insulin sensitivity *via* upregulating PI3K dependent glucose uptake in myocytes and adipocytes, inhibits formation of lipid accumulation in 3T3L1 adipocytes.	[174]
Weigela subsessilis	Ilekudinols A (29.1±2.8 µM) and ilekudinols B (5.3±0.5 µM), non-competitive PTP1B inhibitor	[175]

Although several natural PTP1B inhibitors have shown characteristic activities, currently there are no clinically approved PTP1B inhibitors available for the treatment or control of obesity and diabetes. Identification of more pharmacologically active PTP1B inhibitors are facing two major challenges, including higher charge at the catalytic site of PTP1B and structural homogeneity with other PTPs, resulting in less selectivity. Therefore, identification of a safe, specific, selective and bioavailable PTP1B inhibitor has been a challenging issue [20].

A few selective PTP1B inhibitors with satisfactory pharmacological efficacy have been documented. TTP8, a synthetic PTP1B inhibitor from TransTech Pharma Inc. has entered into Phase II clinical trials [176]. Trodusquemine (MSI-1436), from Ohr Pharmaceutical Inc. is another drug in Phase I clinical testing. Trodusquemine, a cholesterol derived spermine metabolite was initially isolated from the liver of dogfish shark and later reported as a potent insulin sensitizer and weight gain attenuator [177].

Structurally, the active site of PTP1B contains a PTP loop and WPD loop. The PTP loop encompasses His 214 – Arg 221 while the WPD loop (Trp 179, Pro 180, Asp 181) is located just above the active site, closing over the substrate binding pocket. In the inactive form of PTP1B, the WPD loop establishes an open conformation, whereas it forms a cover over the active site Cys 215 upon binding of the substrate resulting in closed conformation. Additionally, the role of WPD loop in PTP1B has been well studied, and the closure of WPD loop has been found to be a significant event in the catalytic inhibition of PTP1B activity [149]. Wiesmann *et al.* (2004) have identified a unique adjacent site situated near the active site of PTP1B known as allosteric site. The allosteric site is located nearly 20 Å away from the catalytic site (Cys215) of the active PTP loop (His214–Arg221) [178]. Unlike the positively charged active site of PTP1B, the allosteric site is found to be unique and selectively present in PTP1B. This substantially less polar site is not well conserved among other PTPs [179]. Inhibition of PTP1B at the allosteric site is now attracting attention as an alternative target for obesity and diabetes. Interestingly, compound 2, a synthetic allosteric inhibitor showed potent inhibition of PTP1B with limited selectivity than other PTPs [178].

Chlorogenic acid and cichoric acid isolated from *Cichorium intybus* (leaves) have been observed as non-competitive inhibitors of PTP1B. *In silico* analysis using molecular docking and simulation revealed the CGA and CHA to be novel PTP1B inhibitors and were observed to inhibit PTP1B at the allosteric site [154, 180]. Further, key structural characteristics of triterpenes towards their role in PTP1B inhibition have been identified. The OH moiety at C-3 and COOH moiety at C-27 or C-28 positions of the triterpenoids are found to be crucial elements of oleanane type of terpenes in terms of their inhibitory activity [151, 181]. The ursane type of triterpenoids isolated from *Rhododendron brachycarpum* (leaves) have also been observed to possess similar structural elements enabling hydrogen bond interactions with the catalytic site of PTP1B. Recently, Vitalboside A from *Syzygium cumini* (seed) has been reported as an allosteric inhibitor of PTP1B and observed to increase insulin sensitivity and inhibit storage of lipid in adipocytes [174]. Lupane type triterpenes, such as Lupeol and Betulinic acid were found to possess enzymatic and neuronal inhibitory activity of PTP1B and have been identified as novel allosteric inhibitors by molecular docking and dynamic simulation studies [182]. Therefore, identification of rationally selective and potent natural PTP1B inhibitors at the allosteric site could be a promising approach for the management of obesity.

INHIBITION OF ADIPOGENESIS

Obesity is characterized by an increased adipose mass of both the number of adipocytes (hyperplasia) and adipocyte size (hypertrophy), involving controlled process of adipocyte determination and differentiation. Adipogenesis is a well-orchestrated cascade that requires expression of many transcriptional genes including the CCAAT/enhancer-binding protein (C/EBP) gene family and peroxisome proliferator activated receptor γ (PPARγ) [183]. Among the C/EBP family of genes, CEBP β and δ along with PPARγ are expressed rapidly in response to signaling, during initiation of adipogenesis. In addition, insulin responsive lipogenic gene, the steroid regulatory element binding protein (SREBP1c) is also activated in the process of adipogenesis [183]. PPARs are expressed as two isoforms, PPARγ1 and PPARγ2. The expression of PPARγ1 is observed in liver, muscle, colon and macrophage, whereas, PPARγ2 is exclusively expressed in adipocytes [184]. During the terminal stage of differentiation, C/EBPα and PPARγ2 are coordinately expressed along with

SREBP1c to generate mature adipocytes. Therefore, it is clear that PPARγ2 and C/EBPα are the major transcription factors in the process of adipogenesis, functioning synergistically in developing differentiated and insulin responsive mature adipocytes [185] (Fig. **3**).

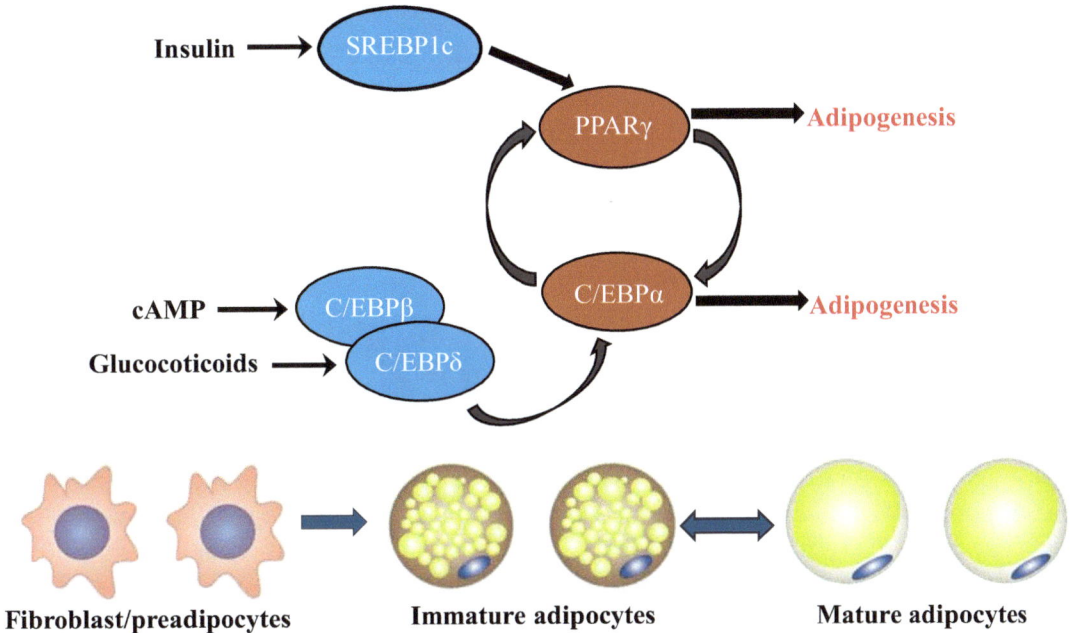

Fig. (3). Regulation of Adipogenesis.

Peroxisome Proliferator Activated Receptor γ (PPARγ)

PPARγ has been reported as a master modulator of adipogenesis, fluid homeostasis and inflammation [186]. PPARγ-mediated genes are differently controlled by ligands or agonists, resulting in phosphorylation and activation of the ligand binding domain (LBD) of PPARγ [187]. In the absence of ligand, the PPARγ/RXR heterodimer forms complex with the multifaceted corepressor protein such as nuclear receptor corepressor 1 (NCoR) and the silencing mediator of retinoic acid and thyroid receptor (SMRT). This complex blocks the transcriptional activation of PPARγ, and maintains minimal levels of PPARγ expression. Upon binding of the agonist, dissociation of corepressors from the PPAR/RXR complex leads to the recruitment and activation of coactivators such as PPARγ coactivator 1α (PGC1α), CREB binding protein (CBP), SRC1 (steroid receptor coactivator 1) and Mediator 1 (MED1) including PBP/TRAP220/DRIP205. Therefore, differential activation of these coactivators by PPARγ is crucial in the regulation of various transcriptional machinery [188].

SREBP1c and PPARγ are critical players in adipocytic and hepatic lipid metabolism and homeostasis [189]. During overweight conditions, SREBP1c predominantly upregulates lipogenic genes such as acetyl-CoA carboxylase (ACC) and fatty acid synthase (FAS), and decreases the expression of acetyl-CoA oxidase and PPARα. Moreover, activation of Akt significantly upregulates the expression of hepatic SREBP1c, and the subsequent accumulation of lipid in liver [190, 191]. In the liver, SREBP1c is regulated by PPARα, a peroxisomal catabolic protein. During insulin resistant obese conditions, insufficient insulin fails to repress hepatic glucose production, causing hyperglycemia. Similarly, unregulated lipid metabolism results in a downregulation of PPARα, thereby leading to the development of hyperlipidemia and liver steatosis [189]. Hence, agents that suppress overexpression of PPARγ, SREBP1c, C/EBPα, ACC and FAS in the adipose tissue as well as liver could decrease the degree of TG accumulation in obese patients [192].

Numerous natural products and their active molecules have been documented for their adipogenic inhibitory activity (Table **6**). *In vivo* experiments using HFD induced obese animals *and Hibiscus sabdariffa* L. and *Camellia sinensis* L. (green tea) extracts have shown negative regulatory effect of these plants on adipogenesis [21]. Further investigation of these extracts using 3T3L1 adipocytes and experimental animals have shown an inhibition at the early stage of adipocyte differentiation by modulation of the activity of PPARγ, CEBPα, SREBP1c and phosphorylation of AMPK, P13K and MAPK, with a reduction in lipid and total TG [22, 193]. Further, green tea has also been observed to exhibit a decrease in oxidative stress and inflammatory conditions *via* downregulation of the expression of cytokines such as IL1β, TNFα and catalase, resulting in reduced lipid peroxidation in HFD C57Bl/6NH mice [21].

Leaf extracts of *Anredera cordifolia, Aster pseudoglehni* L., *Camellia japonica* L. and *Cirsium brevicaule* have been observed to suppress accumulation of fat *via* downregulation of PPARγ, CEBPα and SREBP1c in HFD fed obese mice [194 - 197]. Crude extracts of *Dimocarpus longans* reduce hepatic lipid storage through PPARγ mediated gene regulation of SREBP1c and FAS activities in high caloric diet induced SD rats [198]. Luteolin (*L. japoinica*) and *Rosmarinus officinalis* L. leaf extracts have been reported to inhibit the inflammatory cytokines MCP1, TNFα and IL6 and modulate the expression of PPARγ2, GLUT4, adiponectin and leptin in 3T3L1 adipocytes and lean (*Le, fa/+*) and obese (*Ob, fa/fa*) female Zucker rats, resulting in decreased serum TG, cholesterol and other lipid levels [199, 200].

Catechin and quercetin attenuate inflammation through decreasing PPARγ, MAPKs and p38, thereby increasing the circulating levels of adiponectin in

3T3L1 cells and high fructose induced rats [201]. Further, the presence of catechin in green tea has been observed to stimulate hepatic lipolysis and modulate lipid metabolism, suggesting an antiadipogenic potential of green tea [202]. Recently, isolated pure compounds such as halfordinol, esculetin and umbelliferone from *Aegle marmelos* L., Platyphyllonol-5-O-β-D-xylopyranoside from *Alnus hirsute*, Mangiferin and hesperidin from *Cyclopia maculata*, Acetylshikonin from *Lithospermum erythrorhizon*, Isorhamnetin 3-O-β-D-gluco-pyranoside from *Salicornia herbacea* L. and 6-Gingerol from *Zingiber zerumbet* L. were found to suppress adipogenesis through downregulating expression of PPARγ, CEBP1α and SREBP1 and upregulating pAMPK in differentiated 3T3L1 preadipocytes and HFD fed obese animals [26, 197, 203 - 205]. The triterpenoids isolated from *Momordica charantia* have been observed to decrease the differentiation of preadipocytes *via* modulating the G2/M cell cycle and inhibiting lipid accumulation with increase in secretion of adiponectin in 3T3L1 adipocytes [206].

Adiponectin

Despite regulation of lipid metabolism, adipose tissue is observed to secrete numerous adipokines and cytokines such as adiponectin, resistin, visfatin, retinol-binding protein 4 (RBP4), apelin, vaspin and cytokines including TNFα and IL1β [207]. Adipokines are involved in the induction of low-grade inflammation in patients with insulin resistance and obesity. Among the adipocyte derived molecules, adiponectin and leptin enhance insulin action, while IL1β, TNFα and resistin impair insulin action. Adiponectin plays an important function in diabetes, CVD and metabolic syndrome [208]. Subjects with insulin resistance and obesity have lower adiponectin levels. Several factors including proinflammatory cytokines, TNFα and catecholamines are involved in the downregulation of the circulating levels of adiponectin in adipocytes [209]. However, during weight loss or treatment with thiazolidinediones (PPARγ), the serum levels of adiponectin increase with improved insulin sensitivity [210]. Adiponectin and leptin are two important adipokines involved in energy metabolism, making them key research areas for obesity and diabetes.

Studies have identified a fat secretory hormone, adiponectin or ACRP30 (adipocyte complementary related protein-30kDa), with antidiabetic and antiobesity potential [211]. The expression of adiponectin was originally observed during the process of adipogenesis and is regulated *via* two receptors: AdipoR1 which is mostly expressed in skeletal muscle, and, AdipoR2 which is exclusively present in the liver. Binding of adiponectin with AdipoR1 or AdipoR2 results in the activation of adenosine monophosphate kinase (AMPK), and PPARγ. Activated AMPK enhances insulin sensitivity in muscle and adipose tissues and suppresses hepatic *de no* lipogenesis and gluconeogenesis while promoting fatty acid oxidation in the liver [212] (Fig. **4**).

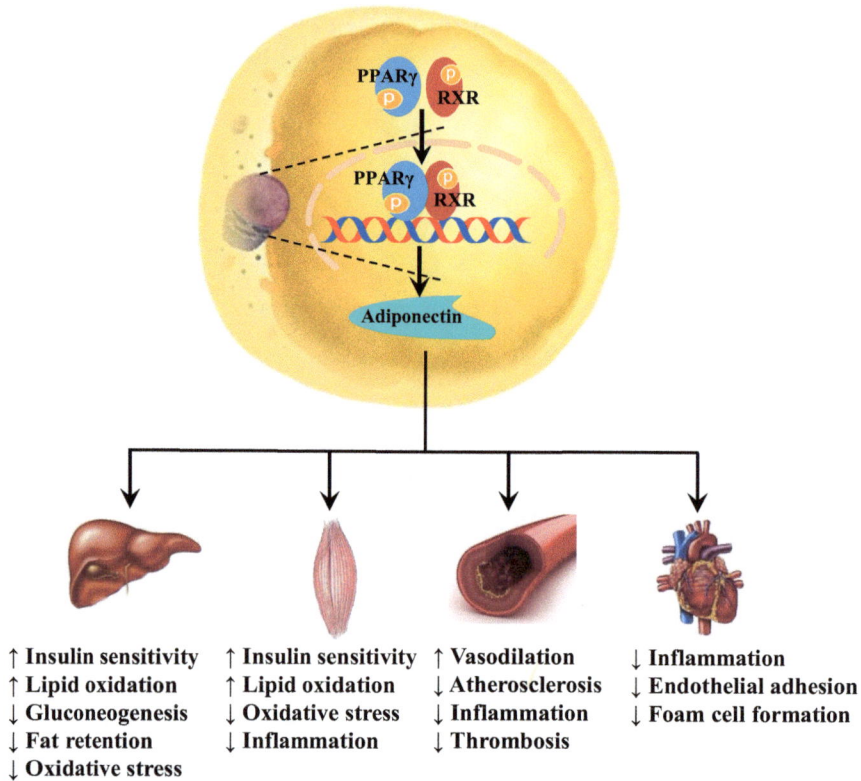

Fig. (4). Effect of adiponectin on regulation of peripheral lipid and carbohydrate metabolism, oxidative stress and inflammation.

Administration of adiponectin has been observed to increase fatty acid oxidation in muscle and liver with decreased hepatic glucose production. The level of serum adiponectin was seen to be lesser in unhealthy obese subjects, whereas it was found to increase during weight loss [210]. Additionally, Bauche *et al.* (2007) have reported that an overexpression of adiponectin was sufficient to ameliorate insulin sensitivity in HFD obese mice [213]. Recently, AdipoRon, an orally active small molecule has been identified and reported as an adiponectin receptor agonist. Oral administration of AdipoRon was found to exhibit improved insulin sensitivity with normal glucose tolerance in mice. In addition, binding of this small molecule to adiponectin receptors was observed to significantly ameliorate diabetes and increase the life expectancy of obese mice [214]. Therefore, molecules exhibiting agonism to adiponectin receptor would be a promising target for the therapeutic intervention of T2DM, insulin resistance and obesity.

Plants and their compounds have been found to exhibit beneficial effects towards secretion of adiponectin. Hypoadiponectenemia, a serious pathological condition, is often seen in obesity, insulin resistance and diabetes. Ethanolic extract from *Coprinus comatus* and *Morus alba* L. (leaves) have been observed to increase circulatory levels of adiponectin, and, inhibit fat accumulation through decreasing the level of PPARγ, CEBPα, LPL and aP2 in 3T3L1 adipocytes. These extracts reduced body weight *via* downregulation of PPARγ and Akt in HFD fed rats [215, 216]. *Tecomella undulata* (Bark extract) has also been observed to regulate adiponectin secretion along with sirtuins 1 (SIRT1), by reducing adipogenesis and its related adipocyte markers including PPARγ, C/EBP, E2F1 and LPL levels in diet induced obese mice [217]. The root extracts of *Adenophora triphylla* have also been observed to increase circulating levels of adiponectin through activating AMPK and PPARα, and inhibiting HMG-CoA reductase gene expression in HFD fed C57BL/6 mice [218]. Table **6** shows the antiadipogenic potential of plant compounds.

Recent studies have shown that bioactive molecules such as catechin and quercetin increase the level of adiponectin by attenuating adipogenesis and inflammatory factors such as PPARγ, JNK and p38 in 3T3L1 adipocytes, and high fructose induced experimental rats [201]. Moreover, sulforaphane from medicinal plants has been reported to suppress lipogenesis in HFD fed mice *via* upregulating the expression of adiponectin, AMPKα and ACC activities, and reducing the levels of PPARγ and CEBPα [219]. Luteolin (*L. japoinica*) has been observed to increase the action of insulin *via* stimulating PPARγ2, adiponectin and leptin, while decreasing inflammatory cytokines such as MCP1, TNFα and IL6 in 3T3L1 adipocytes [199].

Table 6. List of natural inhibitors of adipocyte differentiation.

Name of the Plants	Active Extract and Molecules	Biological Activity	References
Aegle marmelos L.	Halfordinol, esculetin and umbelliferone	Decreases adipocyte lipid storage, ameliorates hyperlipidemia in HFD male SD rat.	[26]
Allium fistulosum L.	Root extract	Reduces body weight, adipose tissue weight and adipocyte size through down regulation of lipogenesis in HFD mice	[220]

(Table 6) cont.....

Name of the Plants	Active Extract and Molecules	Biological Activity	References
Alnus hirsute	Platyphyllonol-5-O-β-D-xylopyranoside	Attenuates adipocyte differentiation *via* modulation of lipogenic induction factors such as PPARγ and C/EBPα in differentiating 3T3L1 adipocytes.	[197]
Angelica keiskei	Ashitaba extract	Inhibits lipid accumulation in 3T3L1 and HepG2 cells; reduces weight *via* AMPK and downregulates PPARγ, SREBP1c, CEBPα, and FAS.	[221]
Anredera cordifolia	Leaves extract	Suppresses lipid accumulation and downregulates PPARγ, CEBPα, SREBP1c, increases Phosphorylation of AMPK HFD mice.	[196]
Aster pseudoglehni L.	Leaves Extract	Suppresses expression of adipogenesis related genes including PPARγ, C/EBPα, and SREBP1c in HFD mice.	[222]
Berberis aristata	Berberine	Reduces body weight and causes significant improvement in glucose tolerance in *db/db* mice (ip. 5 mg/kg body weight) and reduced lipid accumulation in 3T3L1 adipocytes.	[223]
Camellia japonica L.	Leaves extract	Modulates synthesis of lipid *via* reduction in SREBP-1c levels, regulates hepatic TG synthesis in HFD fed SD rats.	[194]
Camellia sinensis L.	Epigallocatechin-3-gallate (EGCG)	Decreases adipogenic genes such as PPARγ, C/EBPα, SREBP-1c, adipocyte FABP4, LPL and FAS in experimental animals.	[21, 22]
Camellia sinensis L. and *Euonymus alatus*	Catechin and quercetin	Attenuates lipid inflammation through decreasing PPARγ, (MAPKs) JNK and p38; increases adiponectin in 3T3L1 cells and high fructose induced rats.	[201, 224, 225]
Cirsium brevicaule	Leaves extract	Inhibits activation of FAS and suppresses lipid accumulation, affecting adipogenic markers such as SREBP1c, C/EBPα and PPARγ in HFD fed mice.	[195]

(Table 6) cont.....

Name of the Plants	Active Extract and Molecules	Biological Activity	References
Coprinus comatus	Ethanolic extract	Decrease in lipid accumulation *via* decreasing level of PPARγ and CEBPα, LPL and aP2, increases adiponectin and pAkt in 3T3L1 adipocyte (150 mg/mL); reduces the body weight *via* downregulating PPARγ and Akt in HFD fed rats.	[216]
Cyclopia maculata	Mangiferin and hesperidin	Inhibits intracellular TG and fat accumulation *via* decreasing PPAR2 expression in differentiating 3T3L1 adipocytes.	[203]
Dimocarpus longans	Crude extract	Reduces dietary fat absorption, and normalizes hepatic mediated PPARγ gene regulation through suppression of pancreatic activity and SREBP1c and FAS gene expression in high caloric diet induced SD rats.	[198]
Dioscoreae tokoronis	Root extract	Decreases total TG, total plasma cholesterol and low-density lipoprotein-cholesterol (VLDL) and inhibits expression of SREBP1 as well as FAS in adipocytes and hepatocytes of HFD fed mice.	[226]
Hibiscus sabdariffa L.	Leaf extract	Attenuate progress of liver steatosis *via* downregulating expression of SREBP1c and PPARγ, reduces mRNA level of inflammatory factors such as IL1, TNFα mRNA and lipid peroxidation and increases catalase mRNA in HFD C57Bl/6NHsd mice.	[227]
L. japoinica	Luteolin	Increases insulin action, decreases inflammatory cytokines (MCP1, TNFα and IL6) and induces expression of PPARγ2 and GLUT4, adiponectin and leptin in in 3T3L1 adipocytes.	[199]
Lithospermum erythrorhizon	Acetylshikonin	Suppresses adipocyte differentiation and adipogenic transcription factor in HFD mice.	[228]

(Table 6) cont.....

Name of the Plants	Active Extract and Molecules	Biological Activity	References
Momordica charantia	Triterpenoid extract	Secretes GLP1, decreases food intake, body weight and fat mass, reduces preadipocyte differentiation through G2/M cell cycle arrest; inhibits lipid accumulation and increases adiponectin level in 3T3L1 adipocyte.	[206]
Morus alba L.	Mulberry leaves extract	Increases lipid accumulation *via* expression of CEBPα and PPARγ, increases adiponectin secretion in 3T3L1 adipocytes.	[215]
Nelumbo nucifera	Whole plant extract	Inhibits differentiation of adipocytes and activity of pancreatic lipase, decreases lipid accumulation *via* attenuation of PPARγ, GLUT4, and leptin expression in cultured human adipocytes and in the hepatocytes of HFD fed C57Bl/6 mice.	[32, 33]
Petasites japonicus	Flower buds extract	Blocks lipid storage *via* attenuation of adipogenic transcription factors such as PPARγ2, CEBPα and SREBP1c HFD mice.	[229]
Pinus koraiensis	Leaves extract	Suppresses fat accumulation and intracellular TG storage through downregulation of lipogenic factors including PPARγ and CEBPα in the differentiated 3T3-L1 adipocytes, attenuates expression of FABP and GPDH in HFD male rats.	[228]
Polygonum aviculare L.	Crude extract	Reduces the elevated mRNA expression of SREBP1c, PPARγ, FAS and aP2 in adipocytes of obese mice.	[230]
Radix astragali	Cycloastragenol	Suppresses accumulation of lipid droplet in 3T3L1 and HepG2 cells.	[231]

(Table 6) cont.....

Name of the Plants	Active Extract and Molecules	Biological Activity	References
Rosmarinus officinalis L.	Leaves	Decreases circulating level of TNFα, IL1β and leptin while upregulating levels of adiponectin. The extract stimulates gene expression of PGC1α and diminishes serum TG, total cholesterol and insulin levels in lean (*Le, fa/+*) and obese (*Ob, fa/fa*) female Zucker rats.	[200]
Salicornia herbacea L.	Isorhamnetin 3-O-β-D-glucopyranoside	Suppresses adipogenesis and downregulates expression of PPARγ, CEBP1α and SREBP1 through upregulation of pAMPK in differentiated 3T3L1 preadiocytes.	[205]
Schisandra chinensis	Peel extract	Suppresses transcriptional expression of genes such as C/EBPβ, C/EBPα, PPARγ and blocks late phase adipogenesis marker aP2 during differentiation of 3T3L1 and downregulates activity of Akt and GSK3β, reduces progression of adipogenesis in diet induced obese mice.	[232]
Tecomella undulata	Bark extract	Regulates adipogenesis by reducing adipocytes markers such as PPARγ, C/EBP, E2F1, leptin and LPL levels, increases the activation of SIRT1 and adiponectin in differentiated adipocytes and exhibits betterment in lipid and glucose levels in diet induced obese mice.	[217]
Vaccinium corymbosum L.	Peel extract	Inhibits lipid accumulation *via* diminishing expression of PPARγ, C/EBPβ and C/EBPα genes during progression of adipocytes, also reduces expression of genes including aP2 and FAS in HFD induced obese mice.	[233]

(Table 6) cont.....

Name of the Plants	Active Extract and Molecules	Biological Activity	References
Zanthoxylum bungeanum	Fruit	Modulates body weight loss in WAT and decreases serum lipid profile such as TG and cholesterol levels, reduces accumulation of fat *via* downregulation of lipogenic genes and proteins including PPARγ, C/EBPα, SREBP1c and FAS in the hepatic tissue of obese C57Bl/6 mice	[234]
Zingiber zerumbet L.	6-Gingerol	inhibits adipogenesis, decreases PPARγ, CEBPα, Akt, GSK3β, fatty acid synthase (FAS) and adipocyte-specific fatty acid binding protein (aP2) in 3T3L1 cells.	[235]

Partial PPARγ Agonists

In T2DM, administration of PPARγ activators such as the thiazolidinediones (rosiglitazone and pioglitazone) showed significant improvement in insulin sensitivity, with a concomitant reduction in blood glucose concentrations, reflecting the essential role of PPARγ in the regulation of glucose and lipid metabolism [236]. Although, agonism of PPARγ is a good target for the control of diabetes, its usage is limited, since it causes many adverse effects including adipogenesis, edema and certain types of cancer [237]. Therefore, researchers are focusing on development of novel partial PPARγ agonists or selective PPARγ modulators (SPPARMs) with improved insulin sensitivity and lower complications [238] (Fig. **5**).

The ligands, functioning as partial agonists to PPARγ, exhibit diverse binding modes than the full classical PPARγ agonists (TZDs) [239]. The mechanism of activation of PPARγ by TZDs is dependent on the interaction of molecular switch present at the α-H12. Upon binding of PPARγ ligands, the α-H12 helix forms bond with the ligand activated domain, AF-2 and closes the ligand binding region. This active form enables binding with several coactivator factors involved in the various cellular transcription pathways [240]. Binding of PPARγ ligand, such as TZDs to the PPARγ protein, results in a "U" or "Y" conformation, which comprises of a polar head and a hydrophobic tail. This polar head group forms hydrogen bonds and a net charge with the TYR473, HIS449, HIS323 and SER289 of PPARγ. Formation of this net charge is essential for the conformational change of α-H12 helix and complete activation of PPARγ [241]. Unlike full PPARγ agonists, the partial agonists are observed to activate PPARγ by an α-H12 helix independent machinery [242]. The partial PPARγ agonist causes reduction in α-H12 helix stabilization, which in turn, decreases the recruitment and transcriptional activity of coactivators [243]. Therefore, crucial interactions at the ligand binding domain (LBD) of partial agonists are mostly different from the full agonists [239].

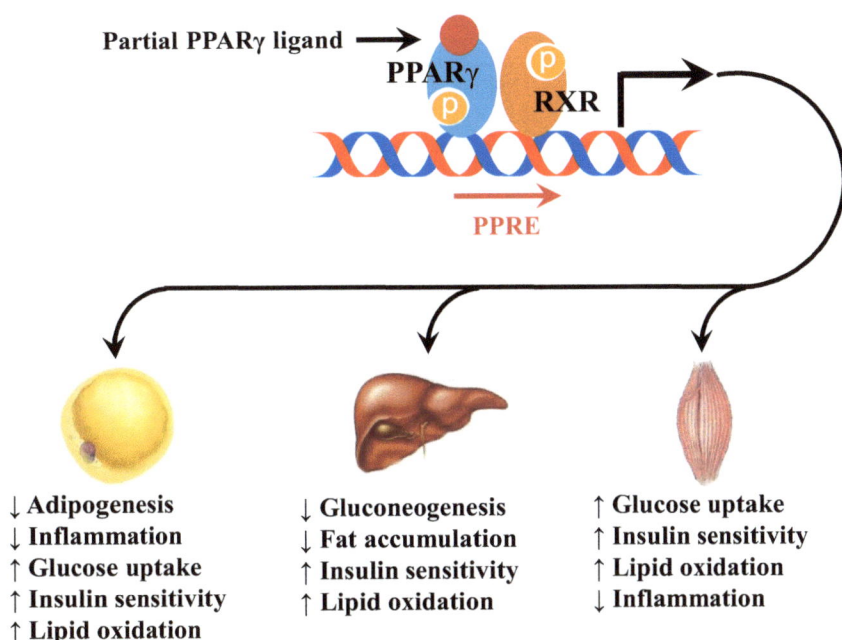

Fig. (5). Beneficial effect of partial PPARγ agonist in the regulation of biological processes.

Table **7** summarizes the SPPARMs that have been identified which are known to exhibit novel partial agonistic activity through PPARγ-mediated reporter gene assays. These compounds, such as amorphastilbol, biochanin A, genistein, resveratrol, sargaquinoic acid and sargahydroquinoic acid were found to have dual agonistic PPAR activity (PPARα and PPARγ). Among these SPPARMs, amorphastilbol (*Robinia pseudoacacia*), amorfrutin B (*Amorpha fruticosa* L.), amorfrutin 1 (*Glycyrrhiza foetida* L.) and honokiol (*Magnolia officinalis*) were found to reduce weight in high fat diet (HFD) fed obese mice. Interestingly, these molecules also showed potent insulin sensitizing activity, and did not cause thiazolidinedione-dependent adverse effects such as hepatomegaly, hepato-toxicity, fluid retention and osteoblastogenesis [244 - 247]. Other natural products including magnolol and resveratrol were observed to decrease fasting blood glucose, and improve metabolic related abnormalities in animal models with diabetes. In addition, amorfrutin 1 is the only natural PPARγ modulator reported to suppress phosphorylation of Ser273, which is most essential for functional activity of partial PPARγ inhibition [247]. Therefore, identification of novel partial PPARγ agonists from natural resources would be useful for the control of obesity and its related diseases such as dyslipidemia.

Table 7. Plants showing partial PPARγ agonistic activity.

Partial PPARγ Agonist	Plant's Name	Biological Activity	References
Amorfrutin 1	*Glycyrrhiza foetida* L	Partial agonist (EC50=0.46 µM) and selectively activates gene expression of PPARγ in human adipocytes, enhances insulin sensitivity *via* attenuating inflammatory factors without changes in fat storage, reduces rosiglitazone mediated undesirable side effects including hepatotoxicity in HFD and db/db mice	[247]
Amorfrutin 2	*Glycyrrhiza foetida* L.	Shows partial agonism to PPARγ (EC50=1.2 µM) with maximal efficacy 70% lower than rosiglitazone	[247]
Amorfrutin B	*Amorpha fruticosa* L.	Partial agonist with EC50 of 0.073 µM and shows 4-fold lower efficacy than rosiglitazone, modulates PPARγ associated gene expressions in human adipocytes and insulin resistant obese mice, exhibits hepato-protective potential and ameliorates insulin resistance, glucose intolerance and blood lipid parameters, reduces side effects including body weight gain, fluid retention and osteoblastogenesis.	[246]
Amorphastilbol	*Robinia pseudoacacia*	As dual PPAR agonist, shows 83% activation of human PPARγ (EC50 = 5 µM) and liver specific PPARα activation, reduces impairment of glucose and lipid metabolism in *db/db* mice without unwanted side effects, such as hepatomegaly and weight gain.	[244, 245]
Biochanin A	*Origanum vulgare* L.	As partial agonist (EC50 = 39.5 µM), shows a 3-fold lower efficacy than pioglitazone, and, stimulates adipogenesis in 3T3-L1 adipocytes (1-5 µM) along with inhibition of adhesion of monocyte in the activation of TNFα in HUVEC (1 µM).	[248]
(−)-Catechin	*Camellia sinensis* L.	PPARγ agonist (IC50 = 9.9 µM), regulates expression of PPARγ linked genes and triggers adipocyte differentiation in human bone marrow mesenchymal stem cells.	[225]
Deoxyelephantopin	*Elephantopus scaber* L.	Partial agonist (1–20 µM). Induces the transcriptional activity of PPARγ.	[249]

(Table 7) cont.....

Partial PPARγ Agonist	Plant's Name	Biological Activity	References
Falcarindiol	*Notopterygium incisum*	As partial agonist (1–30 μM), it stimulates adipogenesis and glucose transport in 3T3L1 adipocytes.	[250]
Genistein	*Glycine max* L.	Dual PPARγ agonist. As partial PPARγ agonist (EC50 at 18.7 μM) shows 4-fold lower activity than pioglitazone, enhances adipogenesis in 3T3L1 adipocytes (1-30 μM) *via* activating PPARγ promoter activity and inhibits monocyte adhesion associated TNFα activity in HUVEC and stimulates activity of PPARα.	[248, 251, 252]
Honokiol	*Magnolia officinalis*	Dual agonist of PPARγ and RXRα, partial PPARγ agonist (EC50 = 3.9 μM), induces glucose uptake and inhibits adipogenesis in 3T3L1 cells (1–10 mM), reduces blood glucose levels in Type 2 diabetic *KKAy* mice, without body weight gain.	[253]
2-Hydroxychalcone	*Trifolium pratense*	Shows partial agonism to PPARγ with EC50 at 3.8 μM (maximal efficacy about 3-fold lower than rosiglitazone)	[252, 254]
6-Hydroxydaidzein and 6-Hydroxy- *O*-desmethylangolensin	*Pueraria thomsonii*	Partial agonist with IC50 at 3.3 μM and EC50 at 27.7 μM	[255]
Kaempferol	*Euonymus alatus*	PPARγ (IC50 at 23.1 μM), stimulates insulin mediated glucose uptake with inhibition of adipogenesis in 3T3L1 adipocytes (5–50 μM).	[224]
Luteolin	*Scoparia dulcis*	As partial PPARγ agonist (EC50 at 15.6 μM), it shows 3-fold lower activity than rosiglitazone and suppresses adipogenesis, functions as a full PPARγ agonist with GLUT4 expression in 3T3L1 adipocytes and modulates IL8 secretion in human corneal epithelial cells.	[256]
Magnolol	*Magnolia officinalis*	Dual agonism to PPARγ and RXRα, as partial agonist (EC50 at 1.6 μM), induces the recruitment and activation of TRAP220/DRIP2 and stimulates glucose uptake and adipogenesis in 3T3L1 adipocytes (10 μM), reduces plasma insulin and fasting blood glucose levels, improves diabetic nephropathy in diabetic Goto-Kakizaki rats.	[257 - 259]
Quercetin	*Euonymus alatus*	Partial agonist with IC50 at 26.0 μM, induces the insulin stimulated glucose uptake without upregulation of adipogenesis and suppresses rosiglitazone dependent differentiation of 3T3L1 cells (5–50 μM).	[224]

(Table 7) cont.....

Partial PPARγ Agonist	Plant's Name	Biological Activity	References
Resveratrol	*Vitis vinifera L.*	As partial PPARγ agonist (IC50 at 27.4 µM), regulates metabolism of glucose and lipid and inflammatory factors through interacting with PPARγ in many *in vitro* and *in vivo* models and enhances insulin sensitivity in T2DM patients, also functions as PPARα agonist.	[260 - 262]
Sargaquinoic acid and Sargahydroquinoic acid	*Sargassum yezoense*	Both function as partial agonists (1–30 µM), enhance adipogenesis in 3T3L1 adipocytes though enhancing expression of genes involved in adipocyte phenotype and activate PPARα (1–30 µM).	[263]
Vitalboside A	*Syzygium cumini*	Partial agonist (1–10 µg/mL), improves insulin sensitizing effect through increasing PI3K dependent glucose uptake, suppresses accumulation of lipid with enhancement in adiponectin secretion.	[174]

ENERGY EXPENDITURE

Thermogenesis

Body fat is regarded as an obligatory energy storage form to be used during fasting, rigorous physical exercise, cold and survival. Chronic intake of high calorie food and decreased energy expenditure are two components which lead to storage of excess fat in adipocytes, causing obesity. Brown adipose tissuc (BAT) in mammals is considered as a site for adaptive non-shivering thermogenesis *via* dissipating excess energy as heat [264]. Unlike white adipose tissue, BAT has a high degree of sympathetic innervation and mitochondria mediated thermogenic component, uncoupling protein 1 (UCP1). UCP 1 is a responsible factor for dissipating energy by oxidation of fatty acids *via* oxidative phosphorylation. The role of BAT in small animals has been well demonstrated as a chief organ of sympathomimetic activated thermogenesis during cold exposure, thereby regulating body fat and energy expenditure [265]. The sense of coldness is recognized through temperature sensors including transient receptor potential (TRP) channels, which transmit difference in surrounding environment including pain, touch, taste, osmolarity and temperature. Thus, cold mediated activation of TRP proteins on sensory neurons are transmitted to the brain, wherein it increases activation of sympathetic nerves reaching BAT. Neurotransmitters including norepinephrine from sympathetic nerve endings trigger UCP1 dependent thermogenesis and fatty acid oxidation in brown adipocytes [266]. Therefore, identification of compounds that stimulate upregulation of UCP1 mediated thermogenesis would be a beneficial approach for development of new therapeutics for the control of obesity.

Extracts of *Solanum tuberosum* have been observed to activate the expression of UCP1 in brown adipocytes and liver, resulting in decreased weight. Many natural extracts and compounds such as catechins (tea), capsaicin (chilli), piperine (pepper) and gingerols, shogaol, and 6-paradol from ginger have been observed to reduce body fat through increased energy expenditure. Table **8** lists the compounds which are thermogenic activators for energy expenditure. Administration of pungent capsaicin (chilli peppers) to experimental animals showed an increase in BAT thermogenesis through activation of TRPV1 (in tongue), hot sensor of TRP family proteins, while capsinoids, the non-pungent type of red pepper activates TRPV1 *via* sensory neurons situated in the gastric and intestinal mucosa [267]. Oral administration of capsinoids in human subjects activates BAT thermogenesis through stimulation of cold sensor, thereby reducing body fatness [268]. Although sensory neuron TRPV1 stimulators possess higher BAT thermogenesis to that of cold exposure, it is considered that TRPV1 is not a cold but hot sensor, which is activated at higher temperature of 43 °C. In contrast, TRPM8 and TRPA1 are two cold sensors activated at a temperature of 20 °C. Natural compound menthol (Mint), stimulates cold activated regulation of BAT thermogenesis *via* TRPM8 dependent manner, resulting in decreased weight in HFD animals [269]. Furthermore, ally- and benzyl-isothiocyanates, cinnamaldehyde and epigallocatechingallate were found to stimulate TRPA1 neuronal sensor dependent activation of thermogenesis in brown adipocytes [270, 271].

Table 8. List of thermogenic regulators involved in energy expenditure.

Name of the Plant	Thermogenic Inducers	Biological Activity	References
Brassica geniculata (Mustard) and *Eutrema japonicum* (Wasabi)	Ally- and benzyl-isothiocyanates	Activates BAT thermogenesis *via* TRPA1 receptor	[270]
Camellia sinensis (Green tea)	Epigallocatechin gallate	Thermogenic and antiobesity *via* activation of TRPA1	[271]
Capsicum annuum (Chili peppers)	Capsaicin (pungent)	Activates UCP1 *via* TRPV1 receptor in the tongue, thermogenesis, and reduces body fatness in animals and human subjects	[267]
Capsicum annuum (Red pepper, non-pungent type)	Capsinoids	Activates UCP1 *via* TRPV1 receptor in the gastric and intestinal mucosa, thermogenesis and reduces body fatness in human subjects	[268, 272]

(Table 8) cont.....

Name of the Plant	Thermogenic Inducers	Biological Activity	References
Cinnamomum verum (Cinnamon)	Cinnamaldehyde (bark of cassia)	Stimulates thermogenesis *via* TRPA1 receptor	[270]
Mentha arvensis (Mint)	Menthol	Stimulates BAT thermogenesis *via* cold receptor TRPM8 in diet induced obese animals	[269]
Piper nigrum (Black and white pepper)	Piperine	Activates BAT thermogenesis *via* TRPV1 and reduces body fat	[272]
Zingiber officinale (Ginger)	Gingerols, Shogaol, and 6-paradol	Activates BAT thermogenesis *via* TRPV1 and reduces body fat	[264]

MODULATION OF LIPID METABOLISM

Development of pharmacological targets for the management of obesity demands an understanding of the delineation factors involved in dietary fat storage, lipolysis and oxidation. The preliminary approach in lipolysis is hydrolysis of triglycerides (TG) into glycerol and free fatty acids. Another approach is oxidation of fatty acids synthesized in adipocytes, liver and muscles [273]. However, an increased degree of lipolysis would contribute to a high amount of circulatory free fatty acids, leading to development of dyslipidemia, a major complication of metabolic syndrome [273]. Moreover, in adipocytes, fatty acids for TG synthesis are derived from circulating lipoproteins including chylomicrons and very low density lipoproteins (VLDL). The enzyme lipoprotein lipase (LPL) catalyzes hydrolysis of these lipoproteins to yield free fatty acids and glycerol. This hydrolytic activity of LPL is controlled by the transcription factor PPARγ [274].

Lipolysis

Adipose tissue is the main energy depot in mammals. Under normal conditions, adipocytes synthesize and store excess energy as TG in fat droplets. During insulin resistance, fasting state and physical exercise, the adipose tissue breaks down and transports the non-esterified fatty acids (NEFAs) to peripheral tissues, where NEFAs are oxidized or stored as energy *via* lipolysis [275]. As illustrated in the Fig. (**6**), the process of lipolysis is stimulated by noradrenaline released from sympathetic nerves *via* β3-adrenoceptors. Binding of noradrenaline leads to the activation of adenylyl cyclase (AC) *via* Gs protein coupled β3-adrenoceptors, which results in cyclic adenosine monophosphate (cAMP) dependent stimulation of protein kinase A (PKA). Similarly, another neurotransmitter, NYY, released from sympathetic nerves inhibits the mechanism of lipolysis by inhibition of Gi protein coupled receptors. Thus, in adipocytes, endocrine factors including natriuretic peptides, adrenaline and insulin are key regulators of lipolysis [276].

Protein kinase A (PKA) promotes the phosphorylation of target protein such as hormone sensitive lipase (HSL) and perilipin 1 (PLN). Perilipin 1 stimulates hydrolysis of TG *via* sequential phosphorylation and activation of key enzymes such as adipose triglyceride lipase (ATGL) and hormone-sensitive lipase (HSL) and monoglyceride lipase (MGL) [276]. During the state of high plasma insulin, lipolysis is suppressed by activation of phosphodiesterase, which catalyzes the conversion of active cAMP into inactive 5'-AMP, leading to decreased PKA dependent activation of HSL. ATGL, HSL and MGL are three key enzymes essential for complete hydrolysis of TG into diacylglycerol (DG), monoacylglycerol (MG) and free fatty acids (FFAs). In addition, CGI58 (coactivator comparative gene identification 58) is reported to be required for full activation of ATGL [277, 278].

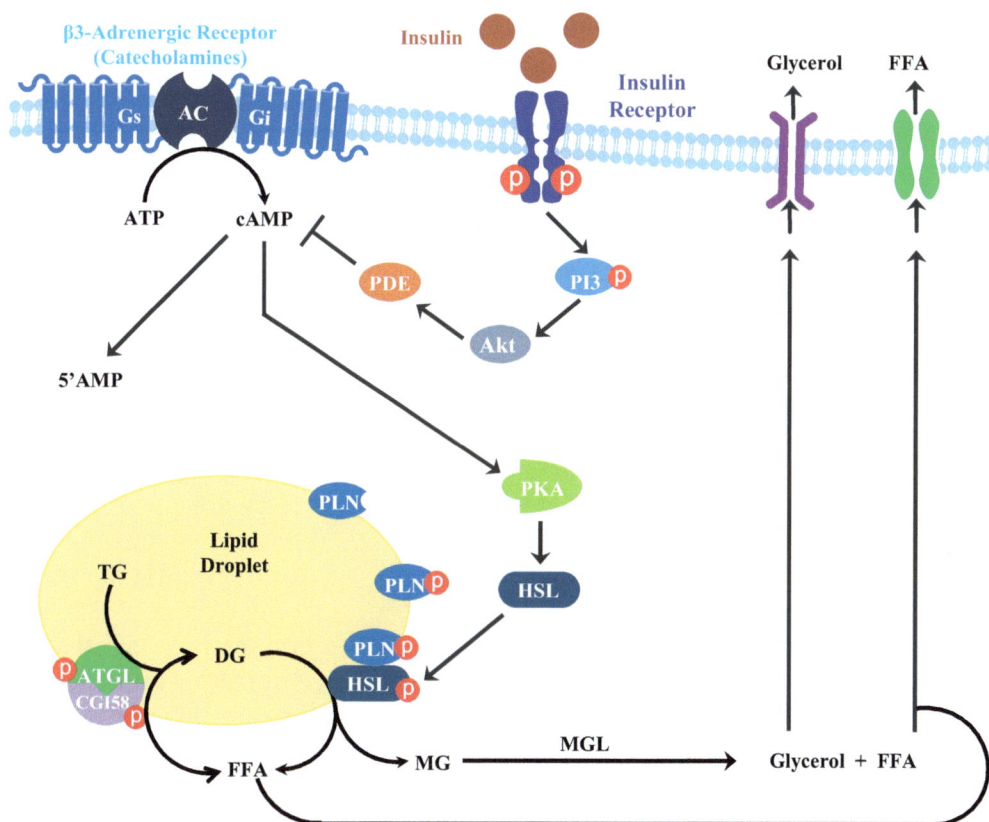

Fig. (6). Mechanism of lipolysis.

Various flavonoids present in the *Nelumbo nucifera* (leaves) have been reported to activate the β-adrenergic receptor. The dietary supplementation of *Nelumbo nucifera* leaf extract has been observed to suppress body weight gain in A/J mice fed with HFD [279]. Table **9** shows the list of natural plants involved in lipolysis. The Root extracts of *Panax ginseng* have been reported to enhance lipolysis through increasing activity of PPARα, AMPK and PKA-dependent upregulation of HSL in hepatocytes, skeletal myocytes and HFD fed obese mice [24, 25]. Studies on *Brassica rapa* L. (Root) extracts showed increasing levels of lipolysis-associated genes including β3-adrenergic receptor, ATGL, HSL and UCP in adipocytes of experimental animals and 3T3L1 cells [280]. Treatment with *Cyamopsis tetragonoloba* L. bean extract to the HFD fed Wister rats was observed to decrease adipose TG level with increased HSL activity [281]. *Allium nigrum* extract was shown to activate lipolysis *via* increasing activity of Sirt1, ATGL, HSL and perilipin while decreasing the level of CD36 in 3T3L1 adipocytes and HFD induced diabetic mice [282]. Curcumin, the active constituent of *Curcuma longa* L., was found to modulate activity of lipolytic genes including ATGL and perilipin *via* increased activation of AMPK in adipocytes. Furthermore, curcumin was reported to suppress the expression of inflammatory cytokines including MCP1 and NFκB in 3T3L1 adipocytes, thereby reducing inflammation mediated lipolysis [283, 284].

β-Oxidation

Although a counterbalance in the process of lipogenesis and lipolysis is important in the regulation of body weight, the mechanism of lipid oxidation is also considered in the management of weight reduction strategy. Oxidation of fatty acids is the main process, wherein fatty acids released *via* lipolysis are oxidized in the peripheral organs such as liver and skeletal muscle, serving as a major source of energy [37]. Furthermore, a marked dysregulation of fatty acid oxidation was observed in the progression of morbid obesity [285]. The mechanism of β-oxidation is tightly regulated within the matrix of mitochondria. Carnitine palmitoyltransferase 1 (CPT1) is the main regulatory enzyme of mitochondrial β-oxidation (Fig. **7**). CPT1 catalyzes the key step in the conversion of fatty acyl-CoA into fatty acyl-carnitine, which is then transported into the mitochondrial matrix [286]. Acyl-CoA oxidase (ACO) is another key peroxisomal enzyme, actively involved in the oxidation of fatty acid [287]. Further, fatty acid oxidation involves stepwise activation of four enzymes namely acyl-CoA dehydrogenase, enoyl-CoA hydratase, 3-hydroxyacyl-CoA dehydrogenase and 3-ketoacyl-CoA thiolase [288].

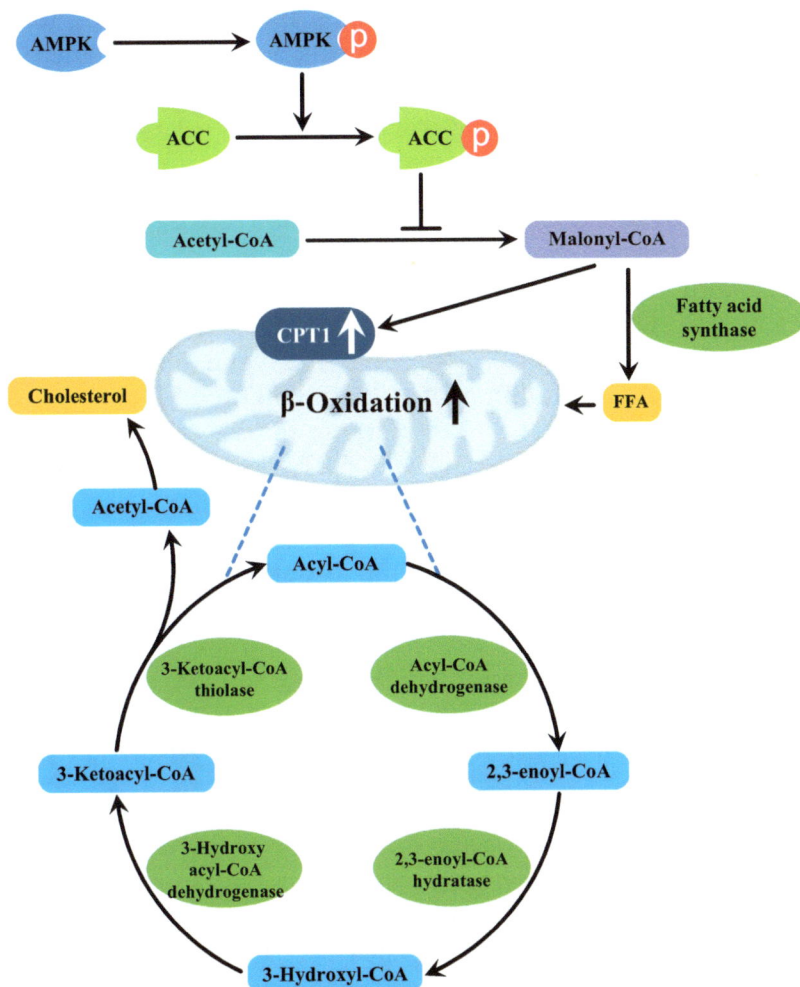

Fig. (7). Role of AMPK in the regulation of β-oxidation of fatty acids.

Adenosine Monophosphate (AMP) Kinase Activators

Adenosine monophosphate kinase (AMPK) is an enzyme ubiquitously expressed in several tissues throughout the human body. AMPK is described as a metabolic master switch that is involved in the regulation and activation of numerous target proteins in metabolism. The active role of AMPK has been well demonstrated in exercising skeletal myocytes. The activation of AMPK in muscle has been found to increase transportation of glucose [289] and also reported to upregulate muscle fatty acid oxidation [290]. Acyl-CoA carboxylase (ACC) is a well-studied downstream target of AMPK, wherein activated AMPK inactivates ACC *via* phosphorylation and inhibits active ACC [291]. ACC is a key enzyme in the biosynthesis of fatty acids, and catalyzes the biosynthesis of malonyl-CoA, an inhibitor of CPT1 (Fig. **7**). CPT1 regulates transportation of fatty acids into mitochondria, where it is oxidized to produce ketone bodies in the liver, and used as energy in other organs [292]. Therefore, the major outcome of AMPK activation in muscle is that it increases the level of CPT1 resulting in oxidation of fatty acid.

As summarized in Table **9**, *Adenophora triphylla* (root extract), and *Citrus sunki* (peel extract) have been reported to activate the level of AMPK and PPARα and inhibit the expression of FAS, ACC and HMG-CoA reductase in liver and adipocytes of HFD C57BL/6 mice [218, 293]. Further, *Vigna nakashimae* (Seeds extract) have been observed to decrease the gene expression of ACC2 by upregulating the phosphorylation of AMPK in HFD fed SD rats [294]. Extracts of *Allium nigrum* have been observed to increase fatty acid oxidation *via* increasing activation of AMPK, FOXO1, ACO and CPT1, resulting in downregulation of CD36 in adipose tissues and HFD mice [282]. Further, *Angelica keiskei*, also known as Ashitaba, has been shown to exhibit lipid accumulation inhibitory activity in 3T3L1 and HepG2 cells, and observed to reduce weight gain *via* increasing lipid oxidative proteins such as AMPK, CPT1 and PPARα in HFD mice [221]. The leaf extracts of *Corchorus olitorius* L. has been observed to activate β-oxidation of fatty acid in HFD fed obese mice *via* downregulating the gene expression of gp91phox (NOX2) in the regulation of oxidative stress, thereby upregulating genes of β-oxidation including PPARα and CPT1 in the liver tissue of HFD mice [295].

PPARα (peroxisome proliferator activated receptor α) has also been reported to mediate expression and activation of many genes that modulates lipid oxidation. *Salacia oblonga* (root extract) has been reported to activate PPARα, resulting in improved hyperlipidemia and hepatic steatosis in obese animal models [296]. Mangiferrin (root) from *Salacia oblonga* was found to upregulate hepatic PPARα activity and decrease weight gain in Zucker fatty rats [297]. Furthermore, administration of gemfibrozil (*Bombax ceiba* L.) and *Berberine cortidis* (rhizome extract) have been observed to inactivate the gene expression of ACC and FAS *via* AMPK activation, thereby triggering weight loss in male Wister albino rats [298]. Secoiridoids (*Fraxinus excelsior* L.) has been reported to ameliorate lipid metabolism through β-oxidation, decreasing fat storage and body weight gain in HFD mice [299]. Punicic acid from *Punica granatum* L. has been observed to enhance β-oxidation through upregulating PPARα, SCD1, CPT1, acyl-coenzyme A dehydrogenase, whereas it suppresses the expression of the inflammatory cytokines TNFα and NFκB activation in HFD obese mice [300].

Table 9. List of plant products involved in lipolysis and fatty acid oxidation.

Name of the Plant	Active Extracts and Compounds	Biological Role	References
Adenophora triphylla	Root extract	Increases adiponectin secretion through activation of AMPK, and PPARα and inhibits expression of HMG-CoA reductase in HFD C57BL/6 mice.	[218]
Allium nigrum	Crude extract	Upregulates lipolysis and fatty acid oxidation *via* activation of AMPK, FOXO1, Sirt1, ATGL, HSL, perilipin, ACO, CPT-1, and UCP1 in the adipose tissues, and downregulates CD36 in HFD mice.	[282]
Angelica keiskei	Ashitaba extract	Inhibits lipid accumulation in 3T3L1 and HepG2 cells, reduces weight gain *via* AMPK, increases lipid oxidation *via* increasing CPT1 and PPARα in in HFD mice.	[221]
Bombax ceiba L.	Gemfibrozil	Inactivates ACC *via* AMPK activation, stimulates thermogenesis and inhibits FAS in male Wister albino rats.	[298]
Brassica rapa L.	Root	Stimulates lipolysis associated genes including β3-adrenergic receptor, ATGL, HSL and UCP proteins in adipocytes of experimental animals and 3T3L1 cells.	[280]
Citrus sunki	Peel extract	Phosphorylation levels of AMPK and ACC are decreased in HFD mice.	[293]
Corchorus olitorius L.	Crude extract	Activates β-oxidation in HFD fed obese mice *via* down regulating gene expression of gp91phox (NOX2) involved in the regulation of oxidative stress and upregulates genes of β-oxidation including PPARα and CPT1 in liver tissue of HFD mice.	[295]
Cortidis rhizoma	Berberine	AMPK activation, decrease in body weight in *db/db* mice	[223]
Curcuma longa L.	Curcumin	Enhances expression of lipolysis genes such as ATGL and reduces gene of perilipin level *via* increased activation of AMPK in adipocytes, also curcumin suppresses the expression of inflammatory cytokines including MCP1 and NFκB in 3T3L1 adipocytes.	[283, 284]
Cyamopsis tetragonoloba L.	Beans extract	Decreases adipose TG level with enhancement of HSL activity in HFD fed Wister rats	[281]
Fraxinus excelsior L.	Secoiridoids	Ameliorates fatty acid metabolism through β-oxidation, decreases fat storage in HFD mice.	[299]
Nelumbo nucifera	Whole plant extract	Suppresses the expression of lipogenic proteins such as FAS, ACC and HMG-CoA reductase through upregulation of active AMPK in the hepatocytes of HFD fed C57BL/6 and SD mice.	[32, 33]

(Table 9) cont.....

Name of the Plant	Active Extracts and Compounds	Biological Role	References
Panax ginseng	Ginsam (root)	Secretes GLP1, decreases food intake, body weight and fat mass, enhances expression of PPARα and AMPK phosphorylation in hepatic and skeletal muscle tissues, extracts markedly stimulate lipolysis *via* upregulation of PKA dependent activation of HSL in HFD fed obese mice.	[24, 25]
Prunus mume	Fruit	Increases CPT1 expression through suppressing FAS, ACC and SREBP1c in the liver and muscle of mice, thereby reducing TG accumulation and protecting the animal from dysregulated metabolism of energy, lipid and glucose, potentiates hypothalamic leptin and insulin signaling in HFD fed ovariectomized rats.	[228]
Punica granatum L	Punicic acid	Enhances β-oxidation through upregulating PPARα and its responsive genes SCD1, CPT1, acyl-coenzyme A dehydrogenase and suppresses expression of the inflammatory cytokine TNFα and NFκB activation in HFD obese mice.	[300]
Salacia oblonga	Mangiferin (root)	As hepatic PPARα activator, it reduces body weight in Zucker obese Rats.	[297]
Vigna nakashimae	Seeds extract	Enhances phosphorylation of AMPK and ACC and induces fatty acid oxidation in HFD obese mice.	[294]

Sirtuin 1 as a Novel Target of Obesity

Sirtuin 1 (SIRT1), belongs to the sirtuins family of enzymes and the silent information regulator 2 (Sir2). Sirtuins have been envisaged as central players in the regulation of crucial mechanisms including lipid and insulin metabolism. SIRT1 have been reported to regulate their targets along with other proteins through reversible deacetylation [301, 302]. SIRT1 has also been reported to be associated with long expectancy of life and reduced intake of food along with augmentation of mobilization of lipids and induction of lipolysis. Binding of SIRT1 triggers suppression of PPARγ regulated genes including mediators of lipid storage proteins [303]. Additionally, interaction of SIRT1 with PPARγ coactivator 1α (PGC1α) triggers activation of mitochondrial genes involved in fatty acid oxidation [304]. Hence, Sirtuin 1 is becoming one of the target molecules for management of obesity.

Resveratrol, a natural stilbene type of phenolic compound, was observed to enhance the expression of SIRT1, while decreasing the gene expression of forkhead box O1 (FoxO1) and PPARγ2 levels. Further, resveratrol has been reported to inhibit differentiation of adipocytes through downregulation of early and late adipogenic markers such as C/EBPβ, C/EBPα and PPARγ mainly mediated by SIRT1. Cells treated with higher concentrations of resveratrol regulate the expression of SIRT1 and ATGL genes, and enhances the release of glycerol [305]. In addition to resveratrol, its glucouronide metabolites have also been reported to upregulate SIRT1 gene expression [306].

MULTIFUNCTIONAL ROLE OF NATURAL ANTIOBESITY COMPOUNDS

Plant based compounds retaining their synergistic multi targeted properties might be a useful therapeutic strategy for obesity. Many natural compounds exhibiting multiple activities have been identified based on the mechanism of adipocyte biology [304]. Some natural biomaterials possessing multi-functional antiobesity activities have been discovered. *Camellia sinensis* L. (Green tea) and *Garcina cambogia* (Malabar tamarind), *Curcuma longa* L. (Turmaric), *Panax ginseng* (Chinese ginseng), *Hibiscus sabdariffa* (Sorrel) and *Nelumbo nucifera* (Indian lotus) and *Hoodia gordonii* (Succulent plant) are among the best examples known for their multifunctional role in obesity management (illustrated in Table **10**).

Garcina cambogia has been well documented for its antiobesity potential and is widely cultivated in the South of India and other Asian countries [139]. The main bioactive principle of this plant is (-)-hydroxycitric acid (HCA) which has been reported to act by preventing the metabolism of carbohydrates and fat through suppressing the activity of lipogenesis, increased body fat expenditure and decreased appetite [307]. Moreover, extracts of *G. cambogia* have been reported to inhibit differentiation of adipocytes and synthesis of fatty acids by decreasing ATP dependent activation of citrate lyase activity, thereby increasing the cardio protective serum Apo A1 and HDL-cholesterol activity. For more than two decades, it is available commercially as an antiobesity drug exhibiting no side effects [308, 309].

Curcuma longa L. is a widely used medicinal and culinary plant. Curcumin isolated from this plant has been reported to enhance the expression of genes involved in lipolysis such as ATGL and a reduction in the expression of perilipin through activation of AMPK in adipocytes. Curcumin has also been observed to suppress the expression of inflammatory cytokines including MCP1 and NFκB in 3T3L1 adipocytes, resulting in a decrease in fat accumulation and weight gain [283, 284]. Different ginsenoids isolated from *P. ginseng*, also known as Chinese ginseng have been reported to increase the secretion of GLP1 levels in intestinal L cells using HFD fed obese mice, leading to decreased appetite [310]. Moreover, it has been observed to enhance activation of PPARγ and AMPK in hepatic and skeletal muscle tissues, displaying significant levels of lipolysis in HFD fed obese mice [24, 25].

The anthocyanin rich aqueous extract of *Hibiscus sabdariffa* has been observed to exhibit potential antiadipogenic effects including antihyperglycemic activity, inhibition of gastric and pancreatic lipase activity, reduction in plasma level, suppression of lipid accumulation in adipose tissue and energy expenditure through thermogenesis [227]. The *Nelumbo nucifera* (leaf extract) also exhibits multiple antiobesity effects such as inhibition of lipase activity, suppression of lipogenesis *via* inhibition of FAS, ACC and HMG-CoA activity, decreased lipid accumulation in cultured human adipocytes and increased energy expenditure, thereby aiding in body weight reduction [32, 33, 311].

Table 10. List of multi targeted natural products.

Name of the Plant	Active Extract and Compounds	Activity	References
Adenophora triphylla	Root extract	Increases adiponectin *via* activation of AMPK, and PPARα, and inhibits expression of HMG-CoA reductase in HFD C57Bl/6 mice.	[218]
Aegle marmelos L.	Halfordinol, Esculetin and Umbelliferone	Decreases adipocyte lipid accumulation. Ameliorates hyperlipidemia in HFD male SD rat.	[26]
Allium fistulosum L.	Root extract	Reduces body weight, adipose tissue and adipocyte size through down regulation of lipogenesis in HFD mice	[220]
Allium nigrum	Extract	Upregulates lipolysis and fatty acid oxidation *via* activation of AMPK, FOXO1, Sirt1, ATGL, HSL, perilipin, ACO, CPT1, and UCP1 in the adipose tissues, and downregulates CD36 in HFD mice.	[282]
Allium sativum	Crude extract	Inhibits fat storage *via* decreasing the activity of SREBP1c, ACC, FAS and HMG-CoA reductase HFD mice.	[312]
Alnus hirsute	Platyphyllonol-5-O-β- D-xylopyranoside	Attenuates adipocytes differentiation *via* modulation of lipogenic induction factors such as PPARγ and C/EBPα in differentiating 3T3L1 adipocytes.	[197]
Alpinia galanga	Galangin	Decreases lipid peroxidation, serum lipids, liver weight, and accumulation of hepatic TG in female obese rats.	[27]

(Table 10) cont.....

Name of the Plant	Active Extract and Compounds	Activity	References
Angelica gigas Nakai	Decursin	Improves glucose tolerance and significantly reduces secretion adipocytokines such as resistin, IL6 and MCP1 in HFD rats.	[313]
Angelica keiskei	Ashitaba extract (4-hydroxyderricin and xanthoangelol)	Inhibits lipid accumulation in 3T3L1 and HepG2 cells; reduces weight gain *via* AMPK and downregulating PPARγ, SREBP1c, CEBPα, and FAS; increases lipid oxidation *via* increasing CPT1 and PPARα in HFD mice.	[221]
Anredera cordifolia	Leaves extract	Suppresses lipid accumulation and downregulates PPARγ, CEBPα, SREBP. Also increases phosphorylation of AMPK in HFD mice.	[196]
Aster pseudoglehni L.	Leaves Extract	Suppresses expression of adipogenic related genes including PPARγ, C/EBPα, and SREBP1c in HFD mice.	[222]
Bombax ceiba L.	Gemfibrozil	Inactivates ACC *via* AMPK activation, stimulates thermogenesis and inhibits FAS in male Wister albino rats.	[298]
Brassica rapa L.	Root	Stimulates lipolysis associated genes including β3-adrenergic receptor, ATGL, HSL and UCP proteins in adipocytes of experimental animals and 3T3L1 cells.	[280]
Buddleja officinalis	Crude extract	Reduces body weight gain and inhibits adipocyte differentiation.	[314]
Camellia japonica L.	Leaves extract	Modulates synthesis of lipid *via* reduction in SREBP1c levels, regulates hepatic TG synthesis in HFD fed SD rats.	[194]
Camellia sinensis L.	Leaves extract and Chakasaponin II	Attenuates lipid accumulation through decreasing expression of SREBP1c, FAS and CEBPα. Chakasaponin II from flower bud, restricted mRNA levels of NPY. Decreases gene level expression of adipogenic factors such as PPARγ, C/EBPα, SREBP-1c, adipocyte FABP4, LPL and FAS in experimental animals.	[21 - 23, 119]
Cirsium brevicaule	Leaves extract	Inhibits activation of FAS and suppresses lipid accumulation by affecting adipogenic markers such as SREBP1c, C/EBPα and PPARγ in HFD fed mice.	[195]
Citrus reticulata	Peel extract	Reduces lipogenic components such as SREBP1c, FAS and ACC in the liver and decreases the size of adipocytes in HFD mice.	[315]

(Table 10) cont.....

Name of the Plant	Active Extract and Compounds	Activity	References
Citrus sunki	Peel extract	Phosphorylation levels of AMPK and ACC are decreased in HFD mice.	[316]
Coprinus comatus Cap	Ethanolic extract	Decrease in lipid accumulation *via* decreasing level of PPARγ and CEBPα, LPL and aP2, increases adiponectin and pAkt in in 3T3L1 adipocyte, reduces the body weight *via* downregulating PPARγ and Akt in HFD fed rats.	[216]
Corchorus olitorius L.	Leaves	Activates β-oxidation in HFD fed obese mice *via* down regulating gene expression of gp91phox (NOX2) involved in the regulation of oxidative stress and upregulates genes of β-oxidation including PPARα and CPT1 in liver tissue of HFD mice.	[295]
Curcuma longa L.	Curcumin	Enhances expression of lipolysis genes such as ATGL and reduces expression of perilipin and acts *via* increased activation of AMPK in adipocytes. Also, curcumin suppresses the expression of inflammatory cytokines including MCP1 and NFκB in 3T3L1 adipocytes.	[283, 284]
Cyamopsis tetragonoloba L.	Beans extract	Decreases adipose TG level with enhancement of HSL activity in HFD fed Wister rats	[281]
Cyclopia maculata	Mangifefrin and Hesperidin	Inhibits intracellular TG and fat accumulation *via* decreasing PPARγ2 expression in differentiating 3T3L1 adipocytes.	[203]
Dimocarpus longans	Crude extracts	Reduces dietary fat absorption, and normalizes hepatic mediated PPARγ gene regulation through suppression of pancreatic activity and SREBP1c and FAS gene expression in high caloric diet induced SD rats.	[198]
Dioscoreae tokoronis	Root	Decreases total TG, total plasma cholesterol and VLDL and inhibits expression of SREBP1 as well as FAS in adipocytes and hepatocytes of HFD fed mice.	[226]
Ecklonia cava	Dieckol	Inhibits lipid accumulation in 3T3L1 adipocytes, HFD fed zebrafish and mice *via* cell cycle arrest and AMPKα activation	[317]
Euonymus alatus	Quercetin	Attenuates lipid inflammation through decreasing PPARγ, (MAPKs) JNK and p38; increases adiponectin in 3T3L1 adipocyte and high fructose consumption in rats.	[201]

(Table 10) cont.....

Name of the Plant	Active Extract and Compounds	Activity	References
Fraxinus excelsior L.	Secoiridoids	Ameliorates fatty acid metabolism through β-oxidation, inhibits adipocyte differentiation during development of animal and restricts fat storage in HFD mice.	[299]
Garcina cambogia	Fruit extract	Suppresses lipogenesis and appetite, increases body fat expenditure, Inhibits the enzyme ATP-mediated activation citrate lyase and increases serum levels of apo A1 and HDL-cholesterol.	[307 - 309]
Hibiscus sabdariffa L.	Leaf extract	Secretes GLP1, decreases food intake, body weight and fat mass, attenuates progress of liver steatosis *via* downregulating expression of SREBP1c and PPARγ, reduces mRNA level inflammatory factors such as IL1β, TNFα mRNA and lipid peroxidation and increases catalase mRNA in HFD C57BL/6NH SD mice.	[227]
Humulus lupulus L.	Whole plant extract	Decreases fatty acid synthesis *via* reduction of liver specific SREBP1c expression in the HFD fed rats.	[318, 319]
Ipomoea batatas L.	Fruit	Reduces hepatic fat synthesis *via* limiting the expression of SREBP-lc, Acyl-CoA synthase, Glycerol-3-phosphate acyltransferase, HMG-CoA reductase and FAS in liver tissue of mice.	[320]
Lithocarpus polystachyus	Leaves	Reduces body fatness with reduction in circulatory level of leptin and insulin, ameliorates the state of oxidative stress, increases serum adiponectin, reduces circulating levels of CRP and resistin and blocks expression of PPARγ and C/EBPα in HFD rats.	[321]
Lithospermum erythrorhizon	Acetylshikonin	Suppresses adipocyte differentiation and adipogenic transcription factor in HFD mice.	[228]
Lonicera japoinica	Luteolin	Increases insulin action, decreases inflammatory cytokines (MCP1, TNFα and IL6) and induces expression of PPARγ2 and GLUT4, adiponectin and leptin in in 3T3L1 adipocytes.	[199]

(Table 10) cont.....

Name of the Plant	Active Extract and Compounds	Activity	References
Momordica charantia	Triterpenoid extract	Secretes GLP1, decrease food intake, body weight and fat mass, reduces preadipocyte differentiation through G2/M cell cycle arrest; inhibits lipid accumulation and increases adiponectin level in 3T3L1 adipocyte.	[206]
Morus alba L.	Mulberry leaves extract	Increases lipid accumulation *via* expression of CEBPα and PPARγ, increases adiponectin secretion in 3T3L1 adipocytes.	[215]
Nelumbo nucifera	Whole plant extract	Extracts enriched with flavonoids inhibit both adipocyte differentiation and pancreatic lipase activity, decreases lipid accumulation *via* attenuation of PPARγ, GLUT4, and leptin expression in cultured human adipocytes, inhibits lipase activity and suppresses the expression of lipogenic proteins such as FAS, ACC and HMG-CoA reductase through upregulation of active AMPK in the hepatocytes of HFD fed C57Bl/6 and SD mice.	[32, 33, 311]
Orthosiphon aristatus	Betulinic acid	Suppresses hypothalamic expression of PTP1B and improves the antiobesity effect of leptin in obese rats fed with HFD.	[163]
Panax ginseng	Ginsam (root)	Secretes GLP1, decrease food intake, body weight and fat mass, enhanced expression of PPARγ and AMPK phosphorylation in hepatic and skeletal muscle tissues, stimulates lipolysis *via* upregulation of PKA dependent activation of HSL in HFD fed obese mice.	[24, 25]
Petasites japonicus	Flower buds extract	Blocks lipid storage *via* attenuation of adipogenic transcription factors such as PPARγ2, CEBPα and SREBP1c in HFD mice.	[229]
Pinus koraiensis	Leaves extract	Suppresses fat accumulation and intracellular TG storage through downregulation of lipogenic factor including PPARγ and CEBPα in the differentiated 3T3L1 adipocytes, attenuates expression of FABP and GPDH during adipocyte differentiation in HFD male SD rats.	[204]
Polygonum aviculare L.	Crude extract	Reduces the elevated mRNA expression of SREBP1c, PPARγ, FAS and aP2 in the WAT of obese mice.	[230]

(Table 10) cont.....

Name of the Plant	Active Extract and Compounds	Activity	References
Prunus mume	Fruit	Increases CPT1 expression through suppressing FAS, ACC and SREBP1c in the liver and muscles of animal, thereby reducing TG accumulation and protect the animal from dysregulated metabolism of energy, lipid and glucose, potentiates hypothalamic leptin and insulin signaling in HFD fed rats.	[228]
Punica granatum L	Punicic acid	Enhances β-oxidation through upregulating PPARα and its responsive genes SCD1, CPT1, acyl-coenzyme A dehydrogenase, PPARγ dependent expression of CD36 and FABP4 in WAT and suppresses expression of the inflammatory cytokine TNFα and NFκB activation in HFD obese mice.	[300]
Radix astragali	Cycloastragenol	Suppresses accumulation of lipid droplet in 3T3L1 adipocytes and HepG2.	[231]
Rhizoma coptidis	Berberine	Reduced body weight causes significant improvement in glucose tolerance in *db/db* mice and reduced lipid accumulation in 3T3L1 adipocytes *via* AMPK dependent manner.	[223, 322]
Rosmarinus officinalis L.	Leaves	Decreases circulating level of TNFα, IL1β and leptin, upregulates levels of adiponectin, the extract stimulates gene expression PGC1α and diminishes serum TG, total cholesterol and insulin levels in lean (*Le, fa/+*) and obese (*Ob, fa/fa*) female Zucker rats.	[200]
Salicornia herbacea L.	Isorhamnetin 3-O---D-glucopyranoside	Suppresses adipogenesis and downregulates expression of PPARγ, C/EBP1α, SREBP1c and adipocyte related proteins through upregulation of phospho AMPK in differentiated 3T3L1 preadipocytes.	[205]
Sasa quelpaertensis	Leaves extract	Attenuates lipid synthesis and storage through downregulating the expression levels of C/EBPα, PPARγ, SREBP1c, FAS and aP2, increases mRNA expression of adiponectin in mature adipocytes, enhances activation of AMPK and ACC in HFD fed C57Bl/6 mice.	[293]
Schisandra chinensis	Peel extract	Suppresses transcriptional expression of genes such as C/EBPβ, C/EBPα, PPARγ and blocks late phase adipogenesis marker aP2 during differentiation of 3T3L1 and downregulates activity of Akt and GSK3β, reduces progression of adipogenesis in diet induced obese mice.	[232]

(Table 10) cont.....

Name of the Plant	Active Extract and Compounds	Activity	References
Syzygium aromaticum	Flower buds extract	Decreases lipogenesis and attenuates expression of lipid metabolism proteins such as SREBP1, FAS, CD36 and PPARγ in the liver and WAT in HFD C57Bl/6 mice.	[323]
Tecomella undulata	Bark extract	Regulates adipogenesis by reducing adipocytes markers such as PPARγ, C/EBP, E2F1, leptin and LPL levels, increases the activation of SIRT1 and adiponectin in differentiated adipocytes and exhibits betterment in lipid and glucose levels in diet induced obese mice.	[217]
Vaccinium corymbosum L.	Peel extract	Inhibits lipid accumulation *via* diminishing expression of PPARγ, C/EBPβ and C/EBPα genes during progression of adipocytes, also reduces expression of genes including aP2 and FAS in HFD induced obese mice.	[233]
Vigna nakashimae	Seeds extract	Suppresses mRNA level expression of PPARγ and its downstream genes such as C/EBP and SREBP1c through enhancing phosphorylation of AMPK and ACC and induces fatty acid oxidation in HFD obese mice.	[294]
Zanthoxylum bungeanum	Fruit	Modulates loss of WAT and decreases serum lipid profile such as TG and cholesterol levels, reduces accumulation fat *via* downregulation of lipogenic genes and proteins including PPARγ, C/EBPα, SREBP1c and FAS in the hepatic tissue of obese C57Bl/6 mice	[234]
Zingiber zerumbet L.	6-Gingerol	inhibits adipogenesis, decreases PPARγ, CEBPα, Akt, GSK3β, fatty acid synthase (FAS) and adipocyte-specific fatty acid binding protein (aP2) in 3T3L1 cells.	[235]

CLINICAL TRIALS STUDY

Human clinical studies performed with plant extracts are summarized in Table **11**. Significant antiobesity effects such as decreasing body mass index (BMI), body weight (BW) and waist circumference (WC) in obese and healthy subjects were observed in most of the randomized clinical trials (RCT). Black Chinese tea, *Camellia sinensis*, *Carum carvi* L., *Nigella sativa* and Oolong tea showed significant decrease in waist circumference and weight loss, along with reduction in fasting blood glucose (FBS), total triglycerides and low-density lipoprotein cholesterol (LDL-c) levels [324 - 328]. Moreover, the antihyperlipidemic effects of these herbal plants were found to be statistically significant in the management of obesity. Few active compounds such as Epigallocatechin-3-gallate (EGCG) from *Camellia sinensis* was found to modulate body weight *via* increasing body lipid metabolism, oxidation and metabolic rate in randomized double-blind clinical studies [324]. Treatment with *Lycium barbarum* was shown to significantly increase fatty acid oxidation and caloric expenditure, thereby decreasing waist circumference, in comparison to pretreatment and RCT-placebo group. These effects were mainly due to an increase in lipid metabolism and higher activation of β-oxidation while decreasing PPARγ agonistic effect and fatty acid synthesis [329].

In a randomized clinical trial (n = 19), ephedrine/*Ephedra spp.* was observed to decrease body weight significantly through increasing thermogenic factors [330]. In another RCT (double-blind), supplementation of *Citrus aurantium* (bitter orange) extract to healthy subjects (n = 23), a significant reduction in body weight was observed and the effect was hypothesized to be due to the presence of sympathomimetic compound synephrine, which is a phenylephrine analog [331]. *Hibiscus sabdariffa* was observed to exhibit a significant level of increase in the HDL-cholesterol with reduction in plasma glucose and total cholesterol levels [332]. Supplementation of *Crocus sativas* L. extract to healthy and overweight women was found to show significant reduction in body weight and snacking frequency than placebo group [333]. *Caralluma fimbriata* showed a marked decrease in waist circumference and appetite in the randomized placebo-controlled trial (n = 50 adults) supplemented for 60 days [132].

Cissus quadrangularis (CQ), a juicy vine plant has been widely used in traditional Ayurvedic and African medicine for over a century. Supplementation with CQ in overweight and obese subjects showed a significant reduction in serum lipids and fasting blood glucose levels, with marked increase in HDL-cholesterol and plasma 5-HT (serotonin) levels, thereby reducing body fatness, weight gain and food consumption [132]. A combination of *Cissus quadrangularis* (CQ) with *Irvingia gabonensis* (IG) (CQ-IG 250 mg) in both overweight and obese subjects was observed to significantly decrease levels of body weight, body fat, waist size, serum profile of TC, LDL-cholesterol and fasting blood glucose. All these noticeable changes were observed in both subjects compared to placebo group from 4th week to 10th week of treatment [334]. In another RCT (double-blind), treatment with a combination of compounds such as *Camellia sinensis* and *Semen cassiae* (RCM-104) as a capsule to obese patients, a significant reduction in BMI and body weight was observed. These studies highlight the combinatorial therapy of multi plant extracts that have multifunctional effects in the control of obesity [335].

Table 11. List of natural products utilized for clinical trials.

Plant's Name	Study Details	Major Outcomes	References
Black Chinese Tea	RCT (double-blind) placebo-controlled study with 36 overweight Japanese adults for 12 weeks	Significantly reduced body mass index (BMI), body weight (BW), waist circumference (WC) and visceral fat area compared to baseline.	[328]
Camellia sinensis	RCT, obese subjects (n = 35), 4 cups/d green tea or 2cap and 4 cups water/day for 8 weeks	Significantly decreases BW and BMI and decreases LDL-c and LDL/HDL ratio.	[324]
Caralluma fimbriata	Randomized, placebo-controlled trial with 50 adults, supplemented with 1 g/day for 60 days	Markedly reduces WC, hunger levels in the treated group compared to placebo group.	[132]
Carum carvi (water extract)	RCT (triple-blind) placebo-controlled study with 70 obese women and overweight subjects for 3 months	Significantly reduced BMI, body fat (BF), waist to hip ratio (WHR), WC and enhanced body-muscle percentage, compared to before treatment and placebo group.	[327]
Cissus quadrangularis	RCT (double-blind) in overweight and obese patients, 300, 1028 mg/day	Marked decrease in body weight body fat, serum lipids and glucose and accompanied by a significant increase in HDL-c, plasma 5-HT and creatinine.	[336]
Citrus aurantium	RCT, healthy subjects (n = 23), 975 mg/day for 6 weeks	Reduces body weight *via* sympathomimetic effect of synephrine.	[331]
Combination of *Cissus quadrangularis/ Irvingia gabonensis* (CQ-IG 250 mg)	RCT (double-blind), placebo-controlled study with 72 obese and overweight subjects (33 male and 39 female) for 10 weeks	BW, BF, waist size, TC, LDL-c, and fasting blood glucose levels were significantly reduced in both treated groups.	[334]
Compound of *Camellia sinensis, Semen cassiae* (RCM-104)	RCT (double-blind), obese (n = 117), 4 capsule (500 mg) per time, 3 times/day for 12 week	Reduced weight, BMI and body fat with non-significant changes in food intake.	[335]
Crocus sativas L.	RCT (double-blind), placebo-controlled study of 60 healthy and overweight women for 8 weeks	Causes significant reduction of BW than placebo, snacking frequency was significantly reduced in treated groups compared to placebo.	[333]
Ephedra spp./ ephedrine	RCT (n=19) with unspecified subjects (n = 1,451), 60 – 150 mg/day for 8-27 weeks	Markedly reduces body weight through activation of thermogenic factors.	[330]

(Table 11) cont.....

Plant's Name	Study Details	Major Outcomes	References
Epigallocatechin-3-gallate (EGCG) of green tea	RCT (double-blind), obese male (n = 10), low EGCG (300 mg) and high EGCG (600 mg) for 3 days	Increase in fat oxidation.	[337]
Hibiscus sabdariffa	RCT, human, 100 mg/day for 1 month	Markedly reduced glucose and total cholesterol levels, with significant increase in HDL-cholesterol level.	[332]
Lycium barbarum L.	RCT (double-blind) placebo-controlled study with 15 human for 14 days	Significantly increased caloric expenditure and decreased waist circumference compared with pretreatment and placebo group.	[329]
Nigella sativa	Randomized Clinical Trial – (RCT) (double-blind) in obese male subjects (n = 50), two capsule of 750 mg twice daily for 3 month	Significant reduction of BW, waist circumference, insignificant reduction in blood pressure, TG and HDL-cholesterol.	[325]
Oolong tea	RCT, diet-induced obese or overweight (n = 102), 8 g for 6 week	Significant decrease in BW, decrease in subcutaneous fat content, decrease plasma levels of total cholesterol and glucose.	[326]
Trigonella foenum-graecum L.	RCT (double-blind), with healthy overweight male (n = 39), 1176 mg/day for 6 week	Decreased fat consumption, non-significant modulation in weight, appetite or oxidative parameters, decrease in plasma insulin and glucose ratio.	[338]

CONCLUSION

Obesity is predominantly a multifactorial disorder. Many proteins and enzymes that are actively involved in adipogenesis, appetite suppression, energy expenditure and lipid metabolism have been recognized as new targets, leading to investigations on their therapeutic potential for multi targeted drug development. Among the newer targets, GLP1 analogues, DPP4 inhibitors, leptin and adiponectin secretogogues, allosteric PTP1B inhibitors, partial PPARγ agonists, lipase inhibitors, AMPK activators and sirtuins modulators have been acknowledged as promising targets for obesity. Several strategies have been implemented to prevent body weight gain and its related complications. Many drugs that were approved for management of obesity have later been withdrawn owing to their serious adverse effects. Recently, considerable attention is being focused towards development of multi targeted drugs or network therapeutics, since single target drugs fail to exhibit satisfactory biological effects due to drug resistance problems.

Herbal medicines and their products are gaining attention in the present scenario towards identification of compounds for the control of obesity, since most of the plant products are multi-functional. Several bioactive agents represented in this chapter have potential advantages in the management of obesity, and its related metabolic complications such as hyperglycemia, insulin resistance, hyperlipidemia, liver steatosis and cardio vascular diseases. Moreover, these phytochemicals have an intricate mechanism of action in the regulation of multiple targets on adipocyte biology such as the inhibition of adipocyte differentiation, reduction of lipid formation and stimulation of lipolysis. Clinical studies have proven that *Garcinia cambogia* (inhibitor of citrate lyase), *Camellia sinensis* (stimulator of sympathetic tone) and *Hoodia gordonii* (modulator of neuropeptides) are found to be more effective in stimulating satiety, energy expenditure and lipid oxidation. Interestingly, isolated single molecules such as EGCG and EGC from black and green tea have been reported to suppress adipocyte differentiation, decrease cellular lipids, increase fatty acid oxidation and improve thermogenesis signifying its antiobesity activity. Functional and clinical characterization of these medicinal plants could provide a possible therapeutic application in the management of obesity.

CONSENT FOR PUBLICATION

Not applicable.

CONFLICT OF INTEREST

The author (editor) declares no conflict of interest, financial or otherwise.

ACKNOWLEDGEMENTS

None declared.

REFERENCES

[1]   Qatanani M, Lazar MA. Mechanisms of obesity-associated insulin resistance: many choices on the menu. Genes Dev 2007; 21(12): 1443-55.
[http://dx.doi.org/10.1101/gad.1550907] [PMID: 17575046]

[2]   Harley IT, Karp CL. Obesity and the gut microbiome: Striving for causality. Mol Metab 2012; 1(1-2): 21-31.
[http://dx.doi.org/10.1016/j.molmet.2012.07.002] [PMID: 24024115]

[3]   Schwartz S, Fabricatore AN, Diamond A. Weight reduction in diabetes. Adv Exp Med Biol 2012; 771: 438-58.
[PMID: 23393695]

[4]   O'Neill S, O'Driscoll L. Metabolic syndrome: a closer look at the growing epidemic and its associated pathologies. Obes Rev 2015; 16(1): 1-12.
[http://dx.doi.org/10.1111/obr.12229] [PMID: 25407540]

[5]   Terada T, Johnson JA, Norris C, *et al.* Severe Obesity Is Associated With Increased Risk of Early Complications and Extended Length of Stay Following Coronary Artery Bypass Grafting Surgery. J Am Heart Assoc 2016; 5(6): e003282.
[http://dx.doi.org/10.1161/JAHA.116.003282] [PMID: 27250114]

[6]   Konige M, Wang H, Sztalryd C. Role of adipose specific lipid droplet proteins in maintaining whole body energy homeostasis. Biochim Biophys Acta 2014; 1842(3): 393-401.
[http://dx.doi.org/10.1016/j.bbadis.2013.05.007] [PMID: 23688782]

[7]   LeBlanc E, O'Connor E, Whitlock EP, Patnode C, Kapka TU. Preventive Services Task Force Evidence Syntheses, formerly Systematic Evidence Reviews Screening for and Management of Obesity and Overweight in Adults Rockville (MD). US: Agency for Healthcare Research and Quality 2011.

[8]   Sjöström L, Narbro K, Sjöström CD, *et al.* Effects of bariatric surgery on mortality in Swedish obese subjects. N Engl J Med 2007; 357(8): 741-52.
[http://dx.doi.org/10.1056/NEJMoa066254] [PMID: 17715408]

[9]   Field BC, Chaudhri OB, Bloom SR. Obesity treatment: novel peripheral targets. Br J Clin Pharmacol 2009; 68(6): 830-43.
[http://dx.doi.org/10.1111/j.1365-2125.2009.03522.x] [PMID: 20002077]

[10]   Sargent BJ, Moore NA. New central targets for the treatment of obesity. Br J Clin Pharmacol 2009; 68(6): 852-60.
[http://dx.doi.org/10.1111/j.1365-2125.2009.03550.x] [PMID: 20002079]

[11]   Kang KT, Lee PL, Weng WC, Hsu WC. Body weight status and obstructive sleep apnea in children. Int J Obes 2012; 36(7): 920-4.
[http://dx.doi.org/10.1038/ijo.2012.5] [PMID: 22270381]

[12]   Rodgers RJ, Tschöp MH, Wilding JP. Anti-obesity drugs: past, present and future. Dis Model Mech 2012; 5(5): 621-6.
[http://dx.doi.org/10.1242/dmm.009621] [PMID: 22915024]

[13]   Kang JG, Park CY. Anti-Obesity Drugs: A Review about Their Effects and Safety. Diabetes Metab J 2012; 36(1): 13-25.
[http://dx.doi.org/10.4093/dmj.2012.36.1.13] [PMID: 22363917]

[14]   Hasani-Ranjbar S, Jouyandeh Z, Abdollahi M. A systematic review of anti-obesity medicinal plants - an update. J Diabetes Metab Disord 2013; 12(1): 28.
[http://dx.doi.org/10.1186/2251-6581-12-28] [PMID: 23777875]

[15]   Cragg GM, Newman DJ. Natural products: a continuing source of novel drug leads. Biochim Biophys Acta 2013; 1830(6): 3670-95.
[http://dx.doi.org/10.1016/j.bbagen.2013.02.008] [PMID: 23428572]

[16]   Han JC, Li F, Li CC. Collective synthesis of humulanolides using a metathesis cascade reaction. J Am Chem Soc 2014; 136(39): 13610-3.
[http://dx.doi.org/10.1021/ja5084927] [PMID: 25228021]

[17]   Elfawal MA, Towler MJ, Reich NG, Golenbock D, Weathers PJ, Rich SM. Dried whole plant Artemisia annua as an antimalarial therapy. PLoS One 2012; 7(12): e52746.
[http://dx.doi.org/10.1371/journal.pone.0052746] [PMID: 23289055]

[18]   Wani MC, Taylor HL, Wall ME, Coggon P, McPhail AT. Plant antitumor agents. VI. The isolation and structure of taxol, a novel antileukemic and antitumor agent from Taxus brevifolia. J Am Chem Soc 1971; 93(9): 2325-7.
[http://dx.doi.org/10.1021/ja00738a045] [PMID: 5553076]

[19]   Hamid K, Alqahtani A, Kim MS, *et al.* Tetracyclic triterpenoids in herbal medicines and their activities in diabetes and its complications. Curr Top Med Chem 2015; 15(23): 2406-30.
[http://dx.doi.org/10.2174/1568026615666150619141940] [PMID: 26088353]

[20]   Zhang S, Zhang ZY. PTP1B as a drug target: recent developments in PTP1B inhibitor discovery. Drug Discov Today 2007; 12(9-10): 373-81.
[http://dx.doi.org/10.1016/j.drudis.2007.03.011] [PMID: 17467573]

[21]   Kim HJ, Jeon SM, Lee MK, Jung UJ, Shin SK, Choi MS. Antilipogenic effect of green tea extract in C57BL/6J-Lep ob/ob mice. Phytother Res 2009; 23(4): 467-71.
[http://dx.doi.org/10.1002/ptr.2647] [PMID: 19051209]

[22]   Lee MS, Kim CT, Kim Y. Green tea (-)-epigallocatechin-3-gallate reduces body weight with regulation of multiple genes expression in adipose tissue of diet-induced obese mice. Ann Nutr Metab 2009; 54(2): 151-7.
[http://dx.doi.org/10.1159/000214834] [PMID: 19390166]

[23]   Wein S, Schrader E, Rimbach G, Wolffram S. Oral green tea catechins transiently lower plasma glucose concentrations in female db/db mice. J Med Food 2013; 16(4): 312-7.
[http://dx.doi.org/10.1089/jmf.2012.0205] [PMID: 23514230]

[24]   Lim S, Yoon JW, Choi SH, *et al.* Effect of ginsam, a vinegar extract from Panax ginseng, on body weight and glucose homeostasis in an obese insulin-resistant rat model. Metabolism 2009; 58(1): 8-15.
[http://dx.doi.org/10.1016/j.metabol.2008.07.027] [PMID: 19059525]

[25]   Park J, Jeon YD, Kim HL, Lim H, Jung Y, Youn DH, *et al.* Interaction of Veratrum nigrum with Panax ginseng against Obesity: A Sang-ban Relationship. Evid Based Complement Alternat Med 2013; 2013: 732126.

[26]   Karmase A, Birari R, Bhutani KK. Evaluation of anti-obesity effect of Aegle marmelos leaves. Phytomedicine 2013; 20(10): 805-12.
[http://dx.doi.org/10.1016/j.phymed.2013.03.014] [PMID: 23632084]

[27]   Kumar S, Alagawadi KR. Anti-obesity effects of galangin, a pancreatic lipase inhibitor in cafeteria diet fed female rats. Pharm Biol 2013; 51(5): 607-13.
[http://dx.doi.org/10.3109/13880209.2012.757327] [PMID: 23363068]

[28]   Rabbani GH, Butler T, Knight J, Sanyal SC, Alam K. Randomized controlled trial of berberine sulfate therapy for diarrhea due to enterotoxigenic Escherichia coli and Vibrio cholerae. J Infect Dis 1987; 155(5): 979-84.
[http://dx.doi.org/10.1093/infdis/155.5.979] [PMID: 3549923]

[29]   Turner N, Li JY, Gosby A, *et al.* Berberine and its more biologically available derivative, dihydroberberine, inhibit mitochondrial respiratory complex I: a mechanism for the action of berberine to activate AMP-activated protein kinase and improve insulin action. Diabetes 2008; 57(5): 1414-8.
[http://dx.doi.org/10.2337/db07-1552] [PMID: 18285556]

[30]   Xia X, Yan J, Shen Y, *et al.* Berberine improves glucose metabolism in diabetic rats by inhibition of hepatic gluconeogenesis. PLoS One 2011; 6(2): e16556.
[http://dx.doi.org/10.1371/journal.pone.0016556] [PMID: 21304897]

[31]   Tan MJ, Ye JM, Turner N, *et al.* Antidiabetic activities of triterpenoids isolated from bitter melon associated with activation of the AMPK pathway. Chem Biol 2008; 15(3): 263-73.
[http://dx.doi.org/10.1016/j.chembiol.2008.01.013] [PMID: 18355726]

[32]   Velusami CC, Agarwal A, Mookambeswaran V. Effect of Nelumbo nucifera Petal Extracts on Lipase, Adipogenesis, Adipolysis, and Central Receptors of Obesity. Evid Based Complement Alternat Med 2013; 2013: 145925.

[33]   You JS, Lee YJ, Kim KS, Kim SH, Chang KJ. Anti-obesity and hypolipidaemic effects of Nelumbo nucifera seed ethanol extract in human pre-adipocytes and rats fed a high-fat diet. J Sci Food Agric 2014; 94(3): 568-75.
[http://dx.doi.org/10.1002/jsfa.6297] [PMID: 23824592]

[34]   Thounaojam MC, Jadeja RN, Ramani UV, Devkar RV, Ramachandran AV. Sida rhomboidea. Roxb leaf extract down-regulates expression of PPARγ2 and leptin genes in high fat diet fed C57BL/6J Mice

and retards *in vitro* 3T3L1 pre-adipocyte differentiation. Int J Mol Sci 2011; 12(7): 4661-77.
[http://dx.doi.org/10.3390/ijms12074661] [PMID: 21845103]

[35]   Cherniack EP. Polyphenols: planting the seeds of treatment for the metabolic syndrome. Nutrition 2011; 27(6): 617-23.
[http://dx.doi.org/10.1016/j.nut.2010.10.013] [PMID: 21367579]

[36]   Murase T, Yokoi Y, Misawa K, *et al.* Coffee polyphenols modulate whole-body substrate oxidation and suppress postprandial hyperglycaemia, hyperinsulinaemia and hyperlipidaemia. Br J Nutr 2012; 107(12): 1757-65.
[http://dx.doi.org/10.1017/S0007114511005083] [PMID: 22017960]

[37]   Galgani J, Ravussin E. Energy metabolism, fuel selection and body weight regulation. Int J Obes 2008; 32 (Suppl. 7): S109-19.
[http://dx.doi.org/10.1038/ijo.2008.246] [PMID: 19136979]

[38]   Ducharme NA, Bickel PE. Lipid droplets in lipogenesis and lipolysis. Endocrinology 2008; 149(3): 942-9.
[http://dx.doi.org/10.1210/en.2007-1713] [PMID: 18202123]

[39]   Mandrup S, Lane MD. Regulating adipogenesis. J Biol Chem 1997; 272(9): 5367-70.
[http://dx.doi.org/10.1074/jbc.272.9.5367] [PMID: 9102400]

[40]   Guilherme A, Virbasius JV, Puri V, Czech MP. Adipocyte dysfunctions linking obesity to insulin resistance and type 2 diabetes. Nat Rev Mol Cell Biol 2008; 9(5): 367-77.
[http://dx.doi.org/10.1038/nrm2391] [PMID: 18401346]

[41]   Hotamisligil GS, Shargill NS, Spiegelman BM. Adipose expression of tumor necrosis factor-alpha: direct role in obesity-linked insulin resistance. Science 1993; 259(5091): 87-91.
[http://dx.doi.org/10.1126/science.7678183] [PMID: 7678183]

[42]   Han L, Li W, Narimatsu S, Liu L, Fu H, Okuda H, *et al.* Inhibitory effects of compounds isolated from fruit of Juglans mandshurica on pancreatic lipase. J Nat Med 2007; 61(2): 184-6.
[http://dx.doi.org/10.1007/s11418-006-0109-4]

[43]   Sharma N, Sharma VK, Seo SY. Screening of some medicinal plants for anti-lipase activity. J Ethnopharmacol 2005; 97(3): 453-6.
[http://dx.doi.org/10.1016/j.jep.2004.11.009] [PMID: 15740880]

[44]   Ballinger A, Peikin SR. Orlistat: its current status as an anti-obesity drug. Eur J Pharmacol 2002; 440(2-3): 109-17.
[http://dx.doi.org/10.1016/S0014-2999(02)01422-X] [PMID: 12007529]

[45]   Hadváry P, Lengsfeld H, Wolfer H. Inhibition of pancreatic lipase *in vitro* by the covalent inhibitor tetrahydrolipstatin. Biochem J 1988; 256(2): 357-61.
[http://dx.doi.org/10.1042/bj2560357] [PMID: 3223916]

[46]   Birari RB, Bhutani KK. Pancreatic lipase inhibitors from natural sources: unexplored potential. Drug Discov Today 2007; 12(19-20): 879-89.
[http://dx.doi.org/10.1016/j.drudis.2007.07.024] [PMID: 17933690]

[47]   Han LK, Zheng YN, Xu BJ, Okuda H, Kimura Y. Saponins from platycodi radix ameliorate high fat diet-induced obesity in mice. J Nutr 2002; 132(8): 2241-5.
[PMID: 12163669]

[48]   Han LK, Zheng YN, Yoshikawa M, Okuda H, Kimura Y. Anti-obesity effects of chikusetsusaponins isolated from Panax japonicus rhizomes. BMC Complement Altern Med 2005; 5: 9.
[http://dx.doi.org/10.1186/1472-6882-5-9] [PMID: 15811191]

[49]   Ono Y, Hattori E, Fukaya Y, Imai S, Ohizumi Y. Anti-obesity effect of Nelumbo nucifera leaves extract in mice and rats. J Ethnopharmacol 2006; 106(2): 238-44.
[http://dx.doi.org/10.1016/j.jep.2005.12.036] [PMID: 16495025]

[50]   Kishino E, Ito T, Fujita K, Kiuchi Y. A mixture of the Salacia reticulata (Kotala himbutu) aqueous extract and cyclodextrin reduces the accumulation of visceral fat mass in mice and rats with high-fat diet-induced obesity. J Nutr 2006; 136(2): 433-9.
[PMID: 16424124]

[51]   Seyedan A, Alshawsh MA, Alshagga MA, Koosha S, Mohamed Z. Medicinal Plants and Their Inhibitory Activities against Pancreatic Lipase: A Review. Evid Based Complement Alternat Med 2015; 2015: 13.
[http://dx.doi.org/10.1155/2015/973143]

[52]   Ekanem AP, Wang M, Simon JE, Moreno DA. Antiobesity properties of two African plants (Afromomum meleguetta and Spilanthes acmella) by pancreatic lipase inhibition. Phytother Res 2007; 21(12): 1253-5.
[http://dx.doi.org/10.1002/ptr.2239] [PMID: 17705140]

[53]   Chompoo J, Upadhyay A, Gima S, Fukuta M, Tawata S. Antiatherogenic properties of acetone extract of Alpinia zerumbet seeds. Molecules 2012; 17(6): 6237-48.
[http://dx.doi.org/10.3390/molecules17066237] [PMID: 22634836]

[54]   Raghavendra H, Mallikarjun N, Venugopal T. HS AK. Elemental composition, anticariogenic, pancreatic lipase inhibitory and cytotoxic activity of Artocarpus lakoocha Roxb pericarp. International Journal of Drug Development and Research 2012; 4(1): 330-6.

[55]   Souza SPd. Pereira LLS, Souza AA, Santos CDd. Inhibition of pancreatic lipase by extracts of Baccharis trimera (Less.) DC., Asteraceae: evaluation of antinutrients and effect on glycosidases. Rev Bras Farmacogn 2011; 21: 450-5.
[http://dx.doi.org/10.1590/S0102-695X2011005000049]

[56]   Ivanov SA, Nomura K, Malfanov IL, Sklyar IV, Ptitsyn LR. Isolation of a novel catechin from Bergenia rhizomes that has pronounced lipase-inhibiting and antioxidative properties. Fitoterapia 2011; 82(2): 212-8.
[http://dx.doi.org/10.1016/j.fitote.2010.09.013] [PMID: 20923698]

[57]   Adisakwattana S, Intrawangso J, Hemrid A, Chanathong B, Mäkynen K. Extracts of edible plants inhibit pancreatic lipase, cholesterol esterase and cholesterol micellization, and bind bile acids. Food Technol Biotechnol 2012; 50(1): 11.

[58]   Habtemariam S. Antihyperlipidemic components of Cassia auriculata aerial parts: identification through *in vitro* studies. Phytother Res 2013; 27(1): 152-5.
[http://dx.doi.org/10.1002/ptr.4711] [PMID: 22511465]

[59]   Kumar D, Karmase A, Jagtap S, Shekhar R, Bhutani KK. Pancreatic lipase inhibitory activity of cassiamin A, a bianthraquinone from Cassia siamea. Nat Prod Commun 2013; 8(2): 195-8.
[PMID: 23513727]

[60]   Sahib NG, Hamid AA, Kitts D, Purnama M, Saari N, Abas F. The effects of Morinda citrifolia, Momordica charantia and Centella asiatica extracts on lipoprotein lipase abd 3T3☐L1 preadipocytes. J Food Biochem 2011; 35(4): 1186-205.
[http://dx.doi.org/10.1111/j.1745-4514.2010.00444.x]

[61]   Kaewpiboon C, Lirdprapamongkol K, Srisomsap C, *et al.* Studies of the *in vitro* cytotoxic, antioxidant, lipase inhibitory and antimicrobial activities of selected Thai medicinal plants. BMC Complement Altern Med 2012; 12: 217.
[http://dx.doi.org/10.1186/1472-6882-12-217] [PMID: 23145786]

[62]   Kim YS, Lee Y, Kim J, Sohn E, Kim CS, Lee YM, *et al.* Inhibitory Activities of Cudrania tricuspidata Leaves on Pancreatic Lipase *in vitro* and Lipolysis *in vivo*. Evid Based Complement Alternat Med 2012; 2012: 878365.

[63]   Kwon CS, Sohn HY, Kim SH, *et al.* Anti-obesity effect of Dioscorea nipponica Makino with lipase-inhibitory activity in rodents. Biosci Biotechnol Biochem 2003; 67(7): 1451-6.

[http://dx.doi.org/10.1271/bbb.67.1451] [PMID: 12913286]

[64]   Lai HY, Ong SL, Rao NK. *In vitro* lipase inhibitory effect of thirty two selected plants in Malaysia. Asian Journal of Pharmaceutical and Clinical Research 2014; 7(3): 19-24.

[65]   Marrelli M, Loizzo MR, Nicoletti M, Menichini F, Conforti F. Inhibition of key enzymes linked to obesity by preparations from Mediterranean dietary plants: effects on α-amylase and pancreatic lipase activities. Plant Foods Hum Nutr 2013; 68(4): 340-6.
[http://dx.doi.org/10.1007/s11130-013-0390-9] [PMID: 24122547]

[66]   Moreno S, Scheyer T, Romano CS, Vojnov AA. Antioxidant and antimicrobial activities of rosemary extracts linked to their polyphenol composition. Free Radic Res 2006; 40(2): 223-31.
[http://dx.doi.org/10.1080/10715760500473834] [PMID: 16390832]

[67]   Conforti F, Perri V, Menichini F, *et al.* Wild Mediterranean dietary plants as inhibitors of pancreatic lipase. Phytother Res 2012; 26(4): 600-4.
[http://dx.doi.org/10.1002/ptr.3603] [PMID: 21972081]

[68]   Teixeira LS, Lima AS, Boleti AP, *et al.* Effects of Passiflora nitida Kunth leaf extract on digestive enzymes and high caloric diet in rats. J Nat Med 2014; 68(2): 316-25.
[http://dx.doi.org/10.1007/s11418-013-0800-1] [PMID: 24078292]

[69]   Zheng CD, Duan YQ, Gao JM, Ruan ZG. Screening for anti-lipase properties of 37 traditional Chinese medicinal herbs. J Chin Med Assoc 2010; 73(6): 319-24.
[http://dx.doi.org/10.1016/S1726-4901(10)70068-X] [PMID: 20603090]

[70]   Morikawa T, Chaipech S, Matsuda H, *et al.* Anti-hyperlipidemic constituents from the bark of Shorea roxburghii. J Nat Med 2012; 66(3): 516-24.
[http://dx.doi.org/10.1007/s11418-011-0619-6] [PMID: 22261856]

[71]   Lee YM, Kim YS, Lee Y, *et al.* Inhibitory activities of pancreatic lipase and phosphodiesterase from Korean medicinal plant extracts. Phytother Res 2012; 26(5): 778-82.
[http://dx.doi.org/10.1002/ptr.3644] [PMID: 22069182]

[72]   Moreno DA, Ilic N, Poulev A, Brasaemle DL, Fried SK, Raskin I. Inhibitory effects of grape seed extract on lipases. Nutrition 2003; 19(10): 876-9.
[http://dx.doi.org/10.1016/S0899-9007(03)00167-9] [PMID: 14559324]

[73]   Han LK, Nose R, Li W, *et al.* Reduction of fat storage in mice fed a high-fat diet long term by treatment with saponins prepared from Kochia scoparia fruit. Phytother Res 2006; 20(10): 877-82.
[http://dx.doi.org/10.1002/ptr.1981] [PMID: 16892459]

[74]   Kim HY, Kang MH. Screening of Korean medicinal plants for lipase inhibitory activity. Phytother Res 2005; 19(4): 359-61.
[http://dx.doi.org/10.1002/ptr.1592] [PMID: 16041737]

[75]   Shimoda H, Seki E, Aitani M. Inhibitory effect of green coffee bean extract on fat accumulation and body weight gain in mice. BMC Complement Altern Med 2006; 6: 9.
[http://dx.doi.org/10.1186/1472-6882-6-9] [PMID: 16545124]

[76]   Lin JK, Lin-Shiau SY. Mechanisms of hypolipidemic and anti-obesity effects of tea and tea polyphenols. Mol Nutr Food Res 2006; 50(2): 211-7.
[http://dx.doi.org/10.1002/mnfr.200500138] [PMID: 16404708]

[77]   Thielecke F, Boschmann M. The potential role of green tea catechins in the prevention of the metabolic syndrome - a review. Phytochemistry 2009; 70(1): 11-24.
[http://dx.doi.org/10.1016/j.phytochem.2008.11.011] [PMID: 19147161]

[78]   Nakai M, Fukui Y, Asami S, *et al.* Inhibitory effects of oolong tea polyphenols on pancreatic lipase *in vitro.* J Agric Food Chem 2005; 53(11): 4593-8.
[http://dx.doi.org/10.1021/jf047814+] [PMID: 15913331]

[79]   Sergent T, Vanderstraeten J, Winand J, Beguin P, Schneider Y-J. Phenolic compounds and plant

extracts as potential natural anti-obesity substances. Food Chem 2012; 135(1): 68-73.
[http://dx.doi.org/10.1016/j.foodchem.2012.04.074]

[80]   Dalar A, Konczak I. Phenolic contents, antioxidant capacities and inhibitory activities against key metabolic syndrome relevant enzymes of herbal teas from Eastern Anatolia. Ind Crops Prod 2013; 44: 383-90.
[http://dx.doi.org/10.1016/j.indcrop.2012.11.037]

[81]   Slanc P, Doljak B, Kreft S, Lunder M, Janes D, Strukelj B. Screening of selected food and medicinal plant extracts for pancreatic lipase inhibition. Phytother Res 2009; 23(6): 874-7.
[http://dx.doi.org/10.1002/ptr.2718] [PMID: 19107742]

[82]   Yoshizumi K, Hirano K, Ando H, *et al.* Lupane-type saponins from leaves of Acanthopanax sessiliflorus and their inhibitory activity on pancreatic lipase. J Agric Food Chem 2006; 54(2): 335-41.
[http://dx.doi.org/10.1021/jf052047f] [PMID: 16417288]

[83]   Yuda N, Tanaka M, Suzuki M, Asano Y, Ochi H, Iwatsuki K. Polyphenols extracted from black tea (Camellia sinensis) residue by hot-compressed water and their inhibitory effect on pancreatic lipase *in vitro*. J Food Sci 2012; 77(12): H254-61.
[http://dx.doi.org/10.1111/j.1750-3841.2012.02967.x] [PMID: 23106349]

[84]   Ado MA, Abas F, Mohammed AS, Ghazali HM. Anti- and pro-lipase activity of selected medicinal, herbal and aquatic plants, and structure elucidation of an anti-lipase compound. Molecules 2013; 18(12): 14651-69.
[http://dx.doi.org/10.3390/molecules181214651] [PMID: 24287996]

[85]   Ninomiya K, Matsuda H, Shimoda H, *et al.* Carnosic acid, a new class of lipid absorption inhibitor from sage. Bioorg Med Chem Lett 2004; 14(8): 1943-6.
[http://dx.doi.org/10.1016/j.bmcl.2004.01.091] [PMID: 15050633]

[86]   Neary NM, Goldstone AP, Bloom SR. Appetite regulation: from the gut to the hypothalamus. Clin Endocrinol (Oxf) 2004; 60(2): 153-60.
[http://dx.doi.org/10.1046/j.1365-2265.2003.01839.x] [PMID: 14725674]

[87]   Atkinson TJ. Central and peripheral neuroendocrine peptides and signalling in appetite regulation: considerations for obesity pharmacotherapy. Obes Rev 2008; 9(2): 108-20.
[http://dx.doi.org/10.1111/j.1467-789X.2007.00412.x] [PMID: 18257752]

[88]   Chantre P, Lairon D. Recent findings of green tea extract AR25 (Exolise) and its activity for the treatment of obesity. Phytomedicine 2002; 9(1): 3-8.
[http://dx.doi.org/10.1078/0944-7113-00078] [PMID: 11924761]

[89]   Neary MT, Batterham RL. Gut hormones: implications for the treatment of obesity. Pharmacol Ther 2009; 124(1): 44-56.
[http://dx.doi.org/10.1016/j.pharmthera.2009.06.005] [PMID: 19560488]

[90]   Moran TH, Dailey MJ. Minireview: Gut peptides: targets for antiobesity drug development? Endocrinology 2009; 150(6): 2526-30.
[http://dx.doi.org/10.1210/en.2009-0003] [PMID: 19372201]

[91]   Moran TH, Smedh U, Kinzig KP, Scott KA, Knipp S, Ladenheim EE. Peptide YY(3-36) inhibits gastric emptying and produces acute reductions in food intake in rhesus monkeys. Am J Physiol Regul Integr Comp Physiol 2005; 288(2): R384-8.
[http://dx.doi.org/10.1152/ajpregu.00535.2004] [PMID: 15388494]

[92]   Atkinson RL. Current status of the field of obesity. Trends Endocrinol Metab 2014; 25(6): 283-4.
[http://dx.doi.org/10.1016/j.tem.2014.03.003] [PMID: 24735507]

[93]   Astrup A, Carraro R, Finer N, *et al.* NN8022-1807 Investigators. Safety, tolerability and sustained weight loss over 2 years with the once-daily human GLP-1 analog, liraglutide. Int J Obes 2012; 36(6): 843-54.
[http://dx.doi.org/10.1038/ijo.2011.158] [PMID: 21844879]

[94]   Flint A, Kapitza C, Zdravkovic M. The once-daily human GLP-1 analogue liraglutide impacts appetite and energy intake in patients with type 2 diabetes after short-term treatment. Diabetes Obes Metab 2013; 15(10): 958-62.
[http://dx.doi.org/10.1111/dom.12108] [PMID: 23551925]

[95]   Wilding JP, Hardy K. Glucagon-like peptide-1 analogues for type 2 diabetes. BMJ 2011; 342: d410.
[http://dx.doi.org/10.1136/bmj.d410] [PMID: 21325387]

[96]   Witkamp RF. Current and future drug targets in weight management. Pharm Res 2011; 28(8): 1792-818.
[http://dx.doi.org/10.1007/s11095-010-0341-1] [PMID: 21181547]

[97]   Liu C, Zhang M, Hu MY, *et al.* Increased glucagon-like peptide-1 secretion may be involved in antidiabetic effects of ginsenosides. J Endocrinol 2013; 217(2): 185-96.
[http://dx.doi.org/10.1530/JOE-12-0502] [PMID: 23444389]

[98]   Liu C, Hu MY, Zhang M, *et al.* Association of GLP-1 secretion with anti-hyperlipidemic effect of ginsenosides in high-fat diet fed rats. Metabolism 2014; 63(10): 1342-51.
[http://dx.doi.org/10.1016/j.metabol.2014.06.015] [PMID: 25060691]

[99]   Xie JT, Mehendale SR, Li X, *et al.* Anti-diabetic effect of ginsenoside Re in ob/ob mice. Biochim Biophys Acta 2005; 1740(3): 319-25.
[http://dx.doi.org/10.1016/j.bbadis.2004.10.010] [PMID: 15949698]

[100] Park S, Ahn IS, Kwon DY, Ko BS, Jun WK. Ginsenosides Rb1 and Rg1 suppress triglyceride accumulation in 3T3-L1 adipocytes and enhance beta-cell insulin secretion and viability in Min6 cells *via* PKA-dependent pathways. Biosci Biotechnol Biochem 2008; 72(11): 2815-23.
[http://dx.doi.org/10.1271/bbb.80205] [PMID: 18997435]

[101] González-Abuín N, Martínez-Micaelo N, Margalef M, *et al.* A grape seed extract increases active glucagon-like peptide-1 levels after an oral glucose load in rats. Food Funct 2014; 5(9): 2357-64.
[http://dx.doi.org/10.1039/C4FO00447G] [PMID: 25088664]

[102] Suh HW, Lee KB, Kim KS, *et al.* A bitter herbal medicine Gentiana scabra root extract stimulates glucagon-like peptide-1 secretion and regulates blood glucose in db/db mouse. J Ethnopharmacol 2015; 172: 219-26.
[http://dx.doi.org/10.1016/j.jep.2015.06.042] [PMID: 26129938]

[103] Zhang S, Ma Y, Li J, Ma J, Yu B, Xie X. Molecular matchmaking between the popular weight-loss herb Hoodia gordonii and GPR119, a potential drug target for metabolic disorder. Proc Natl Acad Sci USA 2014; 111(40): 14571-6.
[http://dx.doi.org/10.1073/pnas.1324130111] [PMID: 25246581]

[104] Choi E-K, Kim K-S, Yang HJ, Shin M-H, Suh H-W, Lee K-B, *et al.* Hexane fraction of Citrus aurantium L. stimulates glucagon-like peptide-1 (GLP-1) secretion *via* membrane depolarization in NCI-H716 cells. Biochip J 2012; 6(1): 41-7.
[http://dx.doi.org/10.1007/s13206-012-6106-7]

[105] Kim K-H, Kim K-S, Shin MH, Jang EG, Kim EY, Lee J-H, *et al.* Aqueous extracts of Anemarrhena asphodeloides stimulate glucagon-like peptide-1 secretion in enteroendocrine NCI-H716 cells. Biochip J 2013; 7(2): 188-93.
[http://dx.doi.org/10.1007/s13206-013-7213-9]

[106] Shin MH, Choi EK, Kim KS, Kim KH, Jang YP, Ahn KS, *et al.* Hexane Fractions of Bupleurum falcatum L. Stimulates Glucagon-Like Peptide-1 Secretion through G beta gamma -Mediated Pathway. Evid Based Complement Alternat Med 2014; 2014: 982165.

[107] Chakrabarti R, Bhavtaran S, Narendra P, Varghese N, Vanchhawng L, Mohamed Sham Shihabudeen H, *et al.* Dipeptidyl peptidase-IV inhibitory activity of Berberis aristata. J Nat Prod 2011; 4: 158-63.

[108] Singh AK, Jatwa R, Joshi J. Cytoprotective and dipeptidyl peptidase IV (Dpp-Iv/Cd26) inhibitory roles of ocimum sanctum and momordica charantia extract. Asian J Pharm Clin Res 2014; 7(1): 115-

20.

[109] Yogisha S, Raveesha K IV. Dipeptidyl Peptidase IV inhibitory activity of Mangifera indica. J Nat Prod 2010; 3: 76-9.

[110] Reeve JR Jr, Eysselein VE, Rosenquist G, *et al.* Evidence that CCK-58 has structure that influences its biological activity. Am J Physiol 1996; 270(5 Pt 1): G860-8.
       [PMID: 8967499]

[111] Kobelt P, Tebbe JJ, Tjandra I, *et al.* CCK inhibits the orexigenic effect of peripheral ghrelin. Am J Physiol Regul Integr Comp Physiol 2005; 288(3): R751-8.
       [http://dx.doi.org/10.1152/ajpregu.00094.2004] [PMID: 15550621]

[112] Fink DJ, Datta S, Mata M. Isoform specific reductions in Na+,K(+)-ATPase catalytic (alpha) subunits in the nerve of rats with streptozotocin-induced diabetes. J Neurochem 1994; 63(5): 1782-6.
       [http://dx.doi.org/10.1046/j.1471-4159.1994.63051782.x] [PMID: 7931333]

[113] Pasman WJ, Heimerikx J, Rubingh CM, *et al.* The effect of Korean pine nut oil on *in vitro* CCK release, on appetite sensations and on gut hormones in post-menopausal overweight women. Lipids Health Dis 2008; 7: 10.
       [http://dx.doi.org/10.1186/1476-511X-7-10] [PMID: 18355411]

[114] Hughes GM, Boyland EJ, Williams NJ, *et al.* The effect of Korean pine nut oil (PinnoThin) on food intake, feeding behaviour and appetite: a double-blind placebo-controlled trial. Lipids Health Dis 2008; 7: 6.
       [http://dx.doi.org/10.1186/1476-511X-7-6] [PMID: 18307772]

[115] Adan RA, Vanderschuren LJ, la Fleur SE. Anti-obesity drugs and neural circuits of feeding. Trends Pharmacol Sci 2008; 29(4): 208-17.
       [http://dx.doi.org/10.1016/j.tips.2008.01.008] [PMID: 18353447]

[116] Obici S. Minireview: Molecular targets for obesity therapy in the brain. Endocrinology 2009; 150(6): 2512-7.
       [http://dx.doi.org/10.1210/en.2009-0409] [PMID: 19372196]

[117] Weigle DS. Pharmacological therapy of obesity: past, present, and future. J Clin Endocrinol Metab 2003; 88(6): 2462-9.
       [http://dx.doi.org/10.1210/jc.2003-030151] [PMID: 12788841]

[118] Kim JH, Hahm DH, Yang DC, Kim JH, Lee HJ, Shim I. Effect of crude saponin of Korean red ginseng on high-fat diet-induced obesity in the rat. J Pharmacol Sci 2005; 97(1): 124-31.
       [http://dx.doi.org/10.1254/jphs.FP0040184] [PMID: 15655288]

[119] Hamao M, Matsuda H, Nakamura S, *et al.* Anti-obesity effects of the methanolic extract and chakasaponins from the flower buds of Camellia sinensis in mice. Bioorg Med Chem 2011; 19(20): 6033-41.
       [http://dx.doi.org/10.1016/j.bmc.2011.08.042] [PMID: 21925888]

[120] Ingalls AM, Dickie MM, Snell GD. Obese, a new mutation in the house mouse. Obes Res 1996; 4(1): 101.
       [http://dx.doi.org/10.1002/j.1550-8528.1996.tb00519.x] [PMID: 8787944]

[121] Pelleymounter MA, Cullen MJ, Baker MB, *et al.* Effects of the obese gene product on body weight regulation in ob/ob mice. Science 1995; 269(5223): 540-3.
       [http://dx.doi.org/10.1126/science.7624776] [PMID: 7624776]

[122] Farooqi IS, O'Rahilly S. New advances in the genetics of early onset obesity. Int J Obes 2005; 29(10): 1149-52.
       [http://dx.doi.org/10.1038/sj.ijo.0803056] [PMID: 16155585]

[123] Considine RV, Sinha MK, Heiman ML, *et al.* Serum immunoreactive-leptin concentrations in normal-weight and obese humans. N Engl J Med 1996; 334(5): 292-5.
       [http://dx.doi.org/10.1056/NEJM199602013340503] [PMID: 8532024]

[124] Tartaglia LA, Dembski M, Weng X, *et al.* Identification and expression cloning of a leptin receptor, OB-R. Cell 1995; 83(7): 1263-71.
[http://dx.doi.org/10.1016/0092-8674(95)90151-5] [PMID: 8548812]

[125] Münzberg H, Myers MG Jr. Molecular and anatomical determinants of central leptin resistance. Nat Neurosci 2005; 8(5): 566-70.
[http://dx.doi.org/10.1038/nn1454] [PMID: 15856064]

[126] Myers MG Jr. Leptin receptor signaling and the regulation of mammalian physiology. Recent Prog Horm Res 2004; 59: 287-304.
[http://dx.doi.org/10.1210/rp.59.1.287] [PMID: 14749507]

[127] Morris DL, Rui L. Recent advances in understanding leptin signaling and leptin resistance. Am J Physiol Endocrinol Metab 2009; 297(6): E1247-59.
[http://dx.doi.org/10.1152/ajpendo.00274.2009] [PMID: 19724019]

[128] Ozcan L, Ergin AS, Lu A, *et al.* Endoplasmic reticulum stress plays a central role in development of leptin resistance. Cell Metab 2009; 9(1): 35-51.
[http://dx.doi.org/10.1016/j.cmet.2008.12.004] [PMID: 19117545]

[129] van Heerden FR. Hoodia gordonii: a natural appetite suppressant. J Ethnopharmacol 2008; 119(3): 434-7.
[http://dx.doi.org/10.1016/j.jep.2008.08.023] [PMID: 18804523]

[130] MacLean DB, Luo LG. Increased ATP content/production in the hypothalamus may be a signal for energy-sensing of satiety: studies of the anorectic mechanism of a plant steroidal glycoside. Brain Res 2004; 1020(1-2): 1-11.
[http://dx.doi.org/10.1016/j.brainres.2004.04.041] [PMID: 15312781]

[131] Loftus TM, Jaworsky DE, Frehywot GL, *et al.* Reduced food intake and body weight in mice treated with fatty acid synthase inhibitors. Science 2000; 288(5475): 2379-81.
[http://dx.doi.org/10.1126/science.288.5475.2379] [PMID: 10875926]

[132] Kuriyan R, Raj T, Srinivas SK, Vaz M, Rajendran R, Kurpad AV. Effect of Caralluma fimbriata extract on appetite, food intake and anthropometry in adult Indian men and women. Appetite 2007; 48(3): 338-44.
[http://dx.doi.org/10.1016/j.appet.2006.09.013] [PMID: 17097761]

[133] Kao YH, Hiipakka RA, Liao S. Modulation of endocrine systems and food intake by green tea epigallocatechin gallate. Endocrinology 2000; 141(3): 980-7.
[http://dx.doi.org/10.1210/endo.141.3.7368] [PMID: 10698173]

[134] Moon HS, Chung CS, Lee HG, Kim TG, Choi YJ, Cho CS. Inhibitory effect of (-)-epigallocatechi--3-gallate on lipid accumulation of 3T3-L1 cells. Obesity (Silver Spring) 2007; 15(11): 2571-82.
[http://dx.doi.org/10.1038/oby.2007.309] [PMID: 18070748]

[135] Naka T, Nagao T, Sakamoto J, Maruyama S, Sakagami H, Ohkawa S. Modulation of branching morphogenesis of fetal mouse submandibular gland by sodium ascorbate and epigallocatechin gallate. In Vivo 2005; 19(5): 883-8.
[PMID: 16097443]

[136] Wolfram S, Raederstorff D, Preller M, *et al.* Epigallocatechin gallate supplementation alleviates diabetes in rodents. J Nutr 2006; 136(10): 2512-8.
[PMID: 16988119]

[137] Kim SO, Yun SJ, Jung B, *et al.* Hypolipidemic effects of crude extract of adlay seed (Coix lachrymajobi var. mayuen) in obesity rat fed high fat diet: relations of TNF-alpha and leptin mRNA expressions and serum lipid levels. Life Sci 2004; 75(11): 1391-404.
[http://dx.doi.org/10.1016/j.lfs.2004.03.006] [PMID: 15234196]

[138] Saito M, Ueno M, Ogino S, Kubo K, Nagata J, Takeuchi M. High dose of Garcinia cambogia is effective in suppressing fat accumulation in developing male Zucker obese rats, but highly toxic to the

testis. Food Chem Toxicol 2005; 43(3): 411-9.
[http://dx.doi.org/10.1016/j.fct.2004.11.008] [PMID: 15680676]

[139] Heymsfield SB, Allison DB, Vasselli JR, Pietrobelli A, Greenfield D, Nunez C. Garcinia cambogia (hydroxycitric acid) as a potential antiobesity agent: a randomized controlled trial. JAMA 1998; 280(18): 1596-600.
[http://dx.doi.org/10.1001/jama.280.18.1596] [PMID: 9820262]

[140] van Heerden FR, Marthinus Horak R, Maharaj VJ, Vleggaar R, Senabe JV, Gunning PJ. An appetite suppressant from Hoodia species. Phytochemistry 2007; 68(20): 2545-53.
[http://dx.doi.org/10.1016/j.phytochem.2007.05.022] [PMID: 17603088]

[141] Lee RA, Balick MJ. Indigenous use of Hoodia gordonii and appetite suppression. Explore (NY) 2007; 3(4): 404-6.
[http://dx.doi.org/10.1016/j.explore.2007.05.005] [PMID: 17681262]

[142] Baintner K, Kiss P, Pfüller U, Bardocz S, Pusztai A. Effect of orally and intraperitoneally administered plant lectins on food consumption of rats. Acta Physiol Hung 2003; 90(2): 97-107.
[http://dx.doi.org/10.1556/APhysiol.90.2003.2.2] [PMID: 12903908]

[143] Tonks NK, Diltz CD, Fischer EH. Purification of the major protein-tyrosine-phosphatases of human placenta. J Biol Chem 1988; 263(14): 6722-30.
[PMID: 2834386]

[144] Frangioni JV, Beahm PH, Shifrin V, Jost CA, Neel BG. The nontransmembrane tyrosine phosphatase PTP-1B localizes to the endoplasmic reticulum *via* its 35 amino acid C-terminal sequence. Cell 1992; 68(3): 545-60.
[http://dx.doi.org/10.1016/0092-8674(92)90190-N] [PMID: 1739967]

[145] Tonks NK, Neel BG. Combinatorial control of the specificity of protein tyrosine phosphatases. Curr Opin Cell Biol 2001; 13(2): 182-95.
[http://dx.doi.org/10.1016/S0955-0674(00)00196-4] [PMID: 11248552]

[146] Vaisse C, Halaas JL, Horvath CM, Darnell JE Jr, Stoffel M, Friedman JM. Leptin activation of Stat3 in the hypothalamus of wild-type and ob/ob mice but not db/db mice. Nat Genet 1996; 14(1): 95-7.
[http://dx.doi.org/10.1038/ng0996-95] [PMID: 8782827]

[147] Zabolotny JM, Bence-Hanulec KK, Stricker-Krongrad A, *et al.* PTP1B regulates leptin signal transduction *in vivo.* Dev Cell 2002; 2(4): 489-95.
[http://dx.doi.org/10.1016/S1534-5807(02)00148-X] [PMID: 11970898]

[148] Klaman LD, Boss O, Peroni OD, *et al.* Increased energy expenditure, decreased adiposity, and tissue-specific insulin sensitivity in protein-tyrosine phosphatase 1B-deficient mice. Mol Cell Biol 2000; 20(15): 5479-89.
[http://dx.doi.org/10.1128/MCB.20.15.5479-5489.2000] [PMID: 10891488]

[149] Jiang CS, Liang LF, Guo YW. Natural products possessing protein tyrosine phosphatase 1B (PTP1B) inhibitory activity found in the last decades. Acta Pharmacol Sin 2012; 33(10): 1217-45.
[http://dx.doi.org/10.1038/aps.2012.90] [PMID: 22941286]

[150] He ZZ, Yan JF, Song ZJ, *et al.* Chemical constituents from the aerial parts of Artemisia minor. J Nat Prod 2009; 72(6): 1198-201.
[http://dx.doi.org/10.1021/np800643n] [PMID: 19476336]

[151] Na M, Cui L, Min BS, *et al.* Protein tyrosine phosphatase 1B inhibitory activity of triterpenes isolated from Astilbe koreana. Bioorg Med Chem Lett 2006; 16(12): 3273-6.
[http://dx.doi.org/10.1016/j.bmcl.2006.03.036] [PMID: 16580200]

[152] Chen C, Zhang Y, Huang C. Berberine inhibits PTP1B activity and mimics insulin action. Biochem Biophys Res Commun 2010; 397(3): 543-7.
[http://dx.doi.org/10.1016/j.bbrc.2010.05.153] [PMID: 20515652]

[153] Chen RM, Hu LH, An TY, Li J, Shen Q. Natural PTP1B inhibitors from Broussonetia papyrifera.

Bioorg Med Chem Lett 2002; 12(23): 3387-90.
[http://dx.doi.org/10.1016/S0960-894X(02)00757-6] [PMID: 12419367]

[154] Muthusamy VS, Saravanababu C, Ramanathan M, *et al.* Inhibition of protein tyrosine phosphatase 1B and regulation of insulin signalling markers by caffeoyl derivatives of chicory (Cichorium intybus) salad leaves. Br J Nutr 2010; 104(6): 813-23.
[http://dx.doi.org/10.1017/S0007114510001480] [PMID: 20444318]

[155] Muthusamy VS, Anand S, Sangeetha KN, Sujatha S, Arun B, Lakshmi BS. Tannins present in Cichorium intybus enhance glucose uptake and inhibit adipogenesis in 3T3-L1 adipocytes through PTP1B inhibition. Chem Biol Interact 2008; 174(1): 69-78.
[http://dx.doi.org/10.1016/j.cbi.2008.04.016] [PMID: 18534569]

[156] Zhang W, Hong D, Zhou Y, *et al.* Ursolic acid and its derivative inhibit protein tyrosine phosphatase 1B, enhancing insulin receptor phosphorylation and stimulating glucose uptake. Biochim Biophys Acta 2006; 1760(10): 1505-12.
[http://dx.doi.org/10.1016/j.bbagen.2006.05.009] [PMID: 16828971]

[157] Shilpa K, Sangeetha KN, Muthusamy VS, Sujatha S, Lakshmi BS. Probing key targets in insulin signaling and adipogenesis using a methanolic extract of Costus pictus and its bioactive molecule, methyl tetracosanoate. Biotechnol Lett 2009; 31(12): 1837-41.
[http://dx.doi.org/10.1007/s10529-009-0105-3] [PMID: 19693444]

[158] Maeda A, Kai K, Ishii M, Ishii T, Akagawa M. Safranal, a novel protein tyrosine phosphatase 1B inhibitor, activates insulin signaling in C2C12 myotubes and improves glucose tolerance in diabetic KK-Ay mice. Mol Nutr Food Res 2014; 58(6): 1177-89.
[http://dx.doi.org/10.1002/mnfr.201300675] [PMID: 24668740]

[159] Quang TH, Ngan NT, Yoon CS, *et al.* Protein Tyrosine Phosphatase 1B Inhibitors from the Roots of Cudrania tricuspidata. Molecules 2015; 20(6): 11173-83.
[http://dx.doi.org/10.3390/molecules200611173] [PMID: 26091075]

[160] Li JM, Li YC, Kong LD, Hu QH. Curcumin inhibits hepatic protein-tyrosine phosphatase 1B and prevents hypertriglyceridemia and hepatic steatosis in fructose-fed rats. Hepatology 2010; 51(5): 1555-66.
[http://dx.doi.org/10.1002/hep.23524] [PMID: 20222050]

[161] Zhang J, Shen Q, Lu J-C, Li J-Y, Liu W-Y, Yang J-J, *et al.* Phenolic compounds from the leaves of Cyclocarya paliurus (Batal.) Ijinskaja and their inhibitory activity against PTP1B. Food Chem 2010; 119(4): 1491-6.
[http://dx.doi.org/10.1016/j.foodchem.2009.09.031]

[162] Na M, Jang J, Njamen D, *et al.* Protein tyrosine phosphatase-1B inhibitory activity of isoprenylated flavonoids isolated from Erythrina mildbraedii. J Nat Prod 2006; 69(11): 1572-6.
[http://dx.doi.org/10.1021/np0601861] [PMID: 17125223]

[163] Choi YJ, Park SY, Kim JY, *et al.* Combined treatment of betulinic acid, a PTP1B inhibitor, with Orthosiphon stamineus extract decreases body weight in high-fat-fed mice. J Med Food 2013; 16(1): 2-8.
[http://dx.doi.org/10.1089/jmf.2012.2384] [PMID: 23256448]

[164] Baumgartner RR, Steinmann D, Heiss EH, *et al.* Bioactivity-guided isolation of 1,2,3,4,6-Penta-O-galloyl-D-glucopyranose from Paeonia lactiflora roots as a PTP1B inhibitor. J Nat Prod 2010; 73(9): 1578-81.
[http://dx.doi.org/10.1021/np100258e] [PMID: 20806783]

[165] Bustanji Y, Taha MO, Al-Masri IM, Mohammad MK. Docking simulations and *in vitro* assay unveil potent inhibitory action of papaverine against protein tyrosine phosphatase 1B. Biol Pharm Bull 2009; 32(4): 640-5.
[http://dx.doi.org/10.1248/bpb.32.640] [PMID: 19336898]

[166] Ramírez-Espinosa JJ, Rios MY, López-Martínez S, *et al.* Antidiabetic activity of some pentacyclic

acid triterpenoids, role of PTP-1B: *in vitro*, in silico, and *in vivo* approaches. Eur J Med Chem 2011; 46(6): 2243-51.
[http://dx.doi.org/10.1016/j.ejmech.2011.03.005] [PMID: 21453996]

[167] Nazaruk J, Borzym-Kluczyk M. The role of triterpenes in the management of diabetes mellitus and its complications. Phytochem Rev 2015; 14(4): 675-90.
[http://dx.doi.org/10.1007/s11101-014-9369-x] [PMID: 26213526]

[168] Tamrakar AK, Yadav PP, Tiwari P, Maurya R, Srivastava AK. Identification of pongamol and karanjin as lead compounds with antihyperglycemic activity from Pongamia pinnata fruits. J Ethnopharmacol 2008; 118(3): 435-9.
[http://dx.doi.org/10.1016/j.jep.2008.05.008] [PMID: 18572336]

[169] Yadav PP, Ahmad G, Maurya R. An efficient route for commercially viable syntheses of furan- and thiophene-anellated β-hydroxychalcones. Tetrahedron Lett 2005; 46(34): 5621-4.
[http://dx.doi.org/10.1016/j.tetlet.2005.06.111]

[170] Kim YC, Oh H, Kim BS, *et al. In vitro* protein tyrosine phosphatase 1B inhibitory phenols from the seeds of Psoralea corylifolia. Planta Med 2005; 71(1): 87-9.
[http://dx.doi.org/10.1055/s-2005-837759] [PMID: 15678382]

[171] Choi YH, Zhou W, Oh J, *et al.* Rhododendric acid A, a new ursane-type PTP1B inhibitor from the endangered plant Rhododendron brachycarpum G. Don. Bioorg Med Chem Lett 2012; 22(19): 6116-9.
[http://dx.doi.org/10.1016/j.bmcl.2012.08.029] [PMID: 22940448]

[172] Sasaki T, Li W, Morimura H, *et al.* Chemical constituents from Sambucus adnata and their protein-tyrosine phosphatase 1B inhibitory activities. Chem Pharm Bull (Tokyo) 2011; 59(11): 1396-9.
[http://dx.doi.org/10.1248/cpb.59.1396] [PMID: 22041077]

[173] Na M, Kim BY, Osada H, Ahn JS. Inhibition of protein tyrosine phosphatase 1B by lupeol and lupenone isolated from Sorbus commixta. J Enzyme Inhib Med Chem 2009; 24(4): 1056-9.
[http://dx.doi.org/10.1080/14756360802693312] [PMID: 19548777]

[174] Thiyagarajan G, Muthukumaran P, Sarath Kumar B, Muthusamy VS, Lakshmi BS. Selective Inhibition of PTP1B by Vitalboside A from Syzygium cumini Enhances Insulin Sensitivity and Attenuates Lipid Accumulation Via Partial Agonism to PPARγ: In Vitro and In Silico Investigation. Chem Biol Drug Des 2016; 88(2): 302-12.
[http://dx.doi.org/10.1111/cbdd.12757] [PMID: 26989847]

[175] Na M, Thuong PT, Hwang IH, *et al.* Protein tyrosine phosphatase 1B inhibitory activity of 24-norursane triterpenes isolated from Weigela subsessilis. Phytother Res 2010; 24(11): 1716-9.
[http://dx.doi.org/10.1002/ptr.3203] [PMID: 20564495]

[176] Vintonyak VV, Antonchick AP, Rauh D, Waldmann H. The therapeutic potential of phosphatase inhibitors. Curr Opin Chem Biol 2009; 13(3): 272-83.
[http://dx.doi.org/10.1016/j.cbpa.2009.03.021] [PMID: 19410499]

[177] Krishnan N, Koveal D, Miller DH, *et al.* Targeting the disordered C terminus of PTP1B with an allosteric inhibitor. Nat Chem Biol 2014; 10(7): 558-66.
[http://dx.doi.org/10.1038/nchembio.1528] [PMID: 24845231]

[178] Wiesmann C, Barr KJ, Kung J, *et al.* Allosteric inhibition of protein tyrosine phosphatase 1B. Nat Struct Mol Biol 2004; 11(8): 730-7.
[http://dx.doi.org/10.1038/nsmb803] [PMID: 15258570]

[179] Johnson TO, Ermolieff J, Jirousek MR. Protein tyrosine phosphatase 1B inhibitors for diabetes. Nat Rev Drug Discov 2002; 1(9): 696-709.
[http://dx.doi.org/10.1038/nrd895] [PMID: 12209150]

[180] Baskaran SK, Goswami N, Selvaraj S, Muthusamy VS, Lakshmi BS. Molecular dynamics approach to probe the allosteric inhibition of PTP1B by chlorogenic and cichoric acid. J Chem Inf Model 2012; 52(8): 2004-12.

[http://dx.doi.org/10.1021/ci200581g] [PMID: 22747429]

[181] Kwon JH, Chang MJ, Seo HW, *et al.* Triterpenoids and a sterol from the stem-bark of Styrax japonica and their protein tyrosine phosphatase 1B inhibitory activities. Phytother Res 2008; 22(10): 1303-6.
[http://dx.doi.org/10.1002/ptr.2484] [PMID: 18693295]

[182] Jin T, Yu H, Huang XF. Selective binding modes and allosteric inhibitory effects of lupane triterpenes on protein tyrosine phosphatase 1B. Sci Rep 2016; 6: 20766.
[http://dx.doi.org/10.1038/srep20766] [PMID: 26865097]

[183] Brey CW, Nelder MP, Hailemariam T, Gaugler R, Hashmi S. Krüppel-like family of transcription factors: an emerging new frontier in fat biology. Int J Biol Sci 2009; 5(6): 622-36.
[http://dx.doi.org/10.7150/ijbs.5.622] [PMID: 19841733]

[184] Zuo Y, Qiang L, Farmer SR. Activation of CCAAT/enhancer-binding protein (C/EBP) alpha expression by C/EBP beta during adipogenesis requires a peroxisome proliferator-activated receptor-gamma-associated repression of HDAC1 at the C/ebp alpha gene promoter. J Biol Chem 2006; 281(12): 7960-7.
[http://dx.doi.org/10.1074/jbc.M510682200] [PMID: 16431920]

[185] Wang YX. PPARs: diverse regulators in energy metabolism and metabolic diseases. Cell Res 2010; 20(2): 124-37.
[http://dx.doi.org/10.1038/cr.2010.13] [PMID: 20101262]

[186] Tontonoz P, Hu E, Graves RA, Budavari AI, Spiegelman BM. mPPAR gamma 2: tissue-specific regulator of an adipocyte enhancer. Genes Dev 1994; 8(10): 1224-34.
[http://dx.doi.org/10.1101/gad.8.10.1224] [PMID: 7926726]

[187] Savage DB. PPAR gamma as a metabolic regulator: insights from genomics and pharmacology. Expert Rev Mol Med 2005; 7(1): 1-16.
[http://dx.doi.org/10.1017/S1462399405008793] [PMID: 15673477]

[188] Mouchiroud L, Eichner LJ, Shaw RJ, Auwerx J. Transcriptional coregulators: fine-tuning metabolism. Cell Metab 2014; 20(1): 26-40.
[http://dx.doi.org/10.1016/j.cmet.2014.03.027] [PMID: 24794975]

[189] Ji C, Chan C, Kaplowitz N. Predominant role of sterol response element binding proteins (SREBP) lipogenic pathways in hepatic steatosis in the murine intragastric ethanol feeding model. J Hepatol 2006; 45(5): 717-24.
[http://dx.doi.org/10.1016/j.jhep.2006.05.009] [PMID: 16879892]

[190] Leavens KF, Easton RM, Shulman GI, Previs SF, Birnbaum MJ. Akt2 is required for hepatic lipid accumulation in models of insulin resistance. Cell Metab 2009; 10(5): 405-18.
[http://dx.doi.org/10.1016/j.cmet.2009.10.004] [PMID: 19883618]

[191] Ono H, Shimano H, Katagiri H, *et al.* Hepatic Akt activation induces marked hypoglycemia, hepatomegaly, and hypertriglyceridemia with sterol regulatory element binding protein involvement. Diabetes 2003; 52(12): 2905-13.
[http://dx.doi.org/10.2337/diabetes.52.12.2905] [PMID: 14633850]

[192] Zeng T, Zhang CL, Song FY, *et al.* PI3K/Akt pathway activation was involved in acute ethanol-induced fatty liver in mice. Toxicology 2012; 296(1-3): 56-66.
[http://dx.doi.org/10.1016/j.tox.2012.03.005] [PMID: 22459179]

[193] Kim HJ, Bae IY, Ahn CW, Lee S, Lee HG. Purification and identification of adipogenesis inhibitory peptide from black soybean protein hydrolysate. Peptides 2007; 28(11): 2098-103.
[http://dx.doi.org/10.1016/j.peptides.2007.08.030] [PMID: 17935831]

[194] Chen Q, Wu X, Liu L, Shen J. Polyphenol-rich extracts from Oiltea camellia prevent weight gain in obese mice fed a high-fat diet and slowed the accumulation of triacylglycerols in 3T3-L1 adipocytes. J Funct Foods 2014; 9: 148-55.
[http://dx.doi.org/10.1016/j.jff.2014.03.034]

[195] Inafuku M, Nugara RN, Kamiyama Y, Futenma I, Inafuku A, Oku H. Cirsium brevicaule A. GRAY leaf inhibits adipogenesis in 3T3-L1 cells and C57BL/6 mice. Lipids Health Dis 2013; 12: 124.
[http://dx.doi.org/10.1186/1476-511X-12-124] [PMID: 23945333]

[196] Kim H, Choung SY. Anti-obesity effects of Boussingaulti gracilis Miers var. pseudobaselloides Bailey *via* activation of AMP-activated protein kinase in 3T3-L1 cells. J Med Food 2012; 15(9): 811-7.
[http://dx.doi.org/10.1089/jmf.2011.2126] [PMID: 22871035]

[197] Lee M, Song JY, Chin YW, Sung SH. Anti-adipogenic diarylheptanoids from Alnus hirsuta f. sibirica on 3T3-L1 cells. Bioorg Med Chem Lett 2013; 23(7): 2069-73.
[http://dx.doi.org/10.1016/j.bmcl.2013.01.127] [PMID: 23465614]

[198] Yang DJ, Chang YY, Hsu CL, *et al.* Antiobesity and hypolipidemic effects of polyphenol-rich longan (Dimocarpus longans Lour.) flower water extract in hypercaloric-dietary rats. J Agric Food Chem 2010; 58(3): 2020-7.
[http://dx.doi.org/10.1021/jf903355q] [PMID: 20088600]

[199] Ding L, Jin D, Chen X. Luteolin enhances insulin sensitivity via activation of PPARγ transcriptional activity in adipocytes. J Nutr Biochem 2010; 21(10): 941-7.
[http://dx.doi.org/10.1016/j.jnutbio.2009.07.009] [PMID: 19954946]

[200] Romo Vaquero M, Yáñez-Gascón MJ, García Villalba R, *et al.* Inhibition of gastric lipase as a mechanism for body weight and plasma lipids reduction in Zucker rats fed a rosemary extract rich in carnosic acid. PLoS One 2012; 7(6): e39773.
[http://dx.doi.org/10.1371/journal.pone.0039773] [PMID: 22745826]

[201] Vazquez Prieto MA, Bettaieb A, Rodriguez Lanzi C, *et al.* Catechin and quercetin attenuate adipose inflammation in fructose-fed rats and 3T3-L1 adipocytes. Mol Nutr Food Res 2015; 59(4): 622-33.
[http://dx.doi.org/10.1002/mnfr.201400631] [PMID: 25620282]

[202] Murase T, Nagasawa A, Suzuki J, Hase T, Tokimitsu I. Beneficial effects of tea catechins on diet-induced obesity: stimulation of lipid catabolism in the liver. Int J Obes relat Metab Disor 2002; 26(11): 1459-64.
[http://dx.doi.org/10.1038/sj.ijo.0802141]

[203] Dudhia Z, Louw J, Muller C, *et al.* Cyclopia maculata and Cyclopia subternata (honeybush tea) inhibits adipogenesis in 3T3-L1 pre-adipocytes. Phytomedicine 2013; 20(5): 401-8.
[http://dx.doi.org/10.1016/j.phymed.2012.12.002] [PMID: 23428403]

[204] Ko HS, Lee HJ, Lee HJ, Sohn EJ, Yun M, Lee MH, *et al.* Essential Oil of Pinus koraiensis Exerts Antiobesic and Hypolipidemic Activity via Inhibition of Peroxisome Proliferator-Activated Receptors Gamma Signaling. Evid Based Complement Alternat Med 2013; 2013: 947037.

[205] Kong CS, Seo Y. Antiadipogenic activity of isohamnetin 3-O-β-D-glucopyranoside from Salicornia herbacea. Immunopharmacol Immunotoxicol 2012; 34(6): 907-11.
[http://dx.doi.org/10.3109/08923973.2012.670643] [PMID: 22978277]

[206] Popovich DG, Lee Y, Li L, Zhang W. Momordica charantia seed extract reduces pre-adipocyte viability, affects lactate dehydrogenase release, and lipid accumulation in 3T3-L1 cells. J Med Food 2011; 14(3): 201-8.
[http://dx.doi.org/10.1089/jmf.2010.1150] [PMID: 21332398]

[207] Andrade-Oliveira V, Camara NO, Moraes-Vieira PM. Adipokines as drug targets in diabetes and underlying disturbances. J Diabetes Res 2015; 2015: 681612.

[208] Bik W, Baranowska B. Adiponectin - a predictor of higher mortality in cardiovascular disease or a factor contributing to longer life? Neuroendocrinol Lett 2009; 30(2): 180-4.
[PMID: 19675525]

[209] Duntas LH, Popovic V, Panotopoulos G. Adiponectin: novelties in metabolism and hormonal regulation. Nutr Neurosci 2004; 7(4): 195-200.
[http://dx.doi.org/10.1080/10284150400009998] [PMID: 15682645]

[210]   Kadowaki T, Yamauchi T. Adiponectin and adiponectin receptors. Endocr Rev 2005; 26(3): 439-51.
        [http://dx.doi.org/10.1210/er.2005-0005] [PMID: 15897298]

[211]   Scherer PE, Williams S, Fogliano M, Baldini G, Lodish HF. A novel serum protein similar to C1q,
        produced exclusively in adipocytes. J Biol Chem 1995; 270(45): 26746-9.
        [http://dx.doi.org/10.1074/jbc.270.45.26746] [PMID: 7592907]

[212]   Kadowaki T, Yamauchi T, Kubota N. The physiological and pathophysiological role of adiponectin
        and adiponectin receptors in the peripheral tissues and CNS. FEBS Lett 2008; 582(1): 74-80.
        [http://dx.doi.org/10.1016/j.febslet.2007.11.070] [PMID: 18054335]

[213]   Bauche IB, El Mkadem SA, Pottier AM, *et al.* Overexpression of adiponectin targeted to adipose
        tissue in transgenic mice: impaired adipocyte differentiation. Endocrinology 2007; 148(4): 1539-49.
        [http://dx.doi.org/10.1210/en.2006-0838] [PMID: 17204560]

[214]   Okada-Iwabu M, Yamauchi T, Iwabu M, *et al.* A small-molecule AdipoR agonist for type 2 diabetes
        and short life in obesity. Nature 2013; 503(7477): 493-9.
        [http://dx.doi.org/10.1038/nature12656] [PMID: 24172895]

[215]   Naowaboot J, Chung CH, Pannangpetch P, *et al.* Mulberry leaf extract increases adiponectin in murine
        3T3-L1 adipocytes. Nutr Res 2012; 32(1): 39-44.
        [http://dx.doi.org/10.1016/j.nutres.2011.12.003] [PMID: 22260862]

[216]   Park HJ, Yun J, Jang S-H, *et al. Coprinus comatus* cap inhibits adipocyte differentiation *via* regulation
        of PPARγ and Akt signaling pathway. PLoS One 2014; 9(9): e105809.
        [http://dx.doi.org/10.1371/journal.pone.0105809] [PMID: 25181477]

[217]   Alvala R, Alvala M, Sama V, Dharmarajan S, Ullas JV, B MR. Scientific evidence for traditional
        claim of anti-obesity activity of Tecomella undulata bark. J Ethnopharmacol 2013; 148(2): 441-8.
        [http://dx.doi.org/10.1016/j.jep.2013.04.033] [PMID: 23628454]

[218]   Choi H-J, Chung MJ, Ham S-S. Antiobese and hypocholesterolaemic effects of an Adenophora
        triphylla extract in HepG2 cells and high fat diet-induced obese mice. Food Chem 2010; 119(2): 437-
        44.
        [http://dx.doi.org/10.1016/j.foodchem.2009.06.039]

[219]   Choi KM, Lee YS, Kim W, *et al.* Sulforaphane attenuates obesity by inhibiting adipogenesis and
        activating the AMPK pathway in obese mice. J Nutr Biochem 2014; 25(2): 201-7.
        [http://dx.doi.org/10.1016/j.jnutbio.2013.10.007] [PMID: 24445045]

[220]   Sung YY, Yoon T, Kim SJ, Yang WK, Kim HK. Anti-obesity activity of Allium fistulosum L. extract
        by down-regulation of the expression of lipogenic genes in high-fat diet-induced obese mice. Mol Med
        Rep 2011; 4(3): 431-5.
        [PMID: 21468588]

[221]   Zhang T, Yamashita Y, Yasuda M, Yamamoto N, Ashida H. Ashitaba (Angelica keiskei) extract
        prevents adiposity in high-fat diet-fed C57BL/6 mice. Food Funct 2015; 6(1): 135-45.
        [http://dx.doi.org/10.1039/C4FO00525B] [PMID: 25406632]

[222]   Lee HM, Yang G, Ahn TG, Kim MD, Nugroho A, Park HJ, *et al.* Antiadipogenic Effects of Aster
        glehni Extract: In Vivo and In Vitro Effects. Evid Based Complement Alternat Med 2013; p. 859624.

[223]   Lee YS, Kim WS, Kim KH, *et al.* Berberine, a natural plant product, activates AMP-activated protein
        kinase with beneficial metabolic effects in diabetic and insulin-resistant states. Diabetes 2006; 55(8):
        2256-64.
        [http://dx.doi.org/10.2337/db06-0006] [PMID: 16873688]

[224]   Fang XK, Gao J, Zhu DN. Kaempferol and quercetin isolated from Euonymus alatus improve glucose
        uptake of 3T3-L1 cells without adipogenesis activity. Life Sci 2008; 82(11-12): 615-22.
        [http://dx.doi.org/10.1016/j.lfs.2007.12.021] [PMID: 18262572]

[225]   Shin DW, Kim SN, Lee SM, *et al.* (-)-Catechin promotes adipocyte differentiation in human bone

marrow mesenchymal stem cells through PPAR gamma transactivation. Biochem Pharmacol 2009; 77(1): 125-33.
[http://dx.doi.org/10.1016/j.bcp.2008.09.033] [PMID: 18951882]

[226]   Song MY, Lv N, Kim EK, *et al*. Antiobesity activity of aqueous extracts of Rhizoma Dioscoreae Tokoronis on high-fat diet-induced obesity in mice. J Med Food 2009; 12(2): 304-9.
[http://dx.doi.org/10.1089/jmf.2008.1010] [PMID: 19459730]

[227]   Villalpando-Arteaga EV, Mendieta-Condado E, Esquivel-Solís H, *et al*. Hibiscus sabdariffa L. aqueous extract attenuates hepatic steatosis through down-regulation of PPAR-γ and SREBP-1c in diet-induced obese mice. Food Funct 2013; 4(4): 618-26.
[http://dx.doi.org/10.1039/c3fo30270a] [PMID: 23389749]

[228]   Ko BS. Prunus mume and Lithospermum erythrorhizon Extracts Synergistically Prevent Visceral Adiposity by Improving Energy Metabolism through Potentiating Hypothalamic Leptin and Insulin Signalling in Ovariectomized Rats. Evid Based Complement Alternat Med 2013; 2013: 750986.

[229]   Watanabe T, Hata K, Hiwatashi K, Hori K, Suzuki N, Itoh H. Suppression of murine preadipocyte differentiation and reduction of visceral fat accumulation by a Petasites japonicus ethanol extract in mice fed a high-fat diet. Biosci Biotechnol Biochem 2010; 74(3): 499-503.
[http://dx.doi.org/10.1271/bbb.90684] [PMID: 20208359]

[230]   Sung YY, Yoon T, Yang WK, Kim SJ, Kim DS, Kim HK. The Antiobesity Effect of Polygonum aviculare L. Ethanol Extract in High-Fat Diet-Induced Obese Mice. Evid Based Complement Alternat Med 2013; 2013: 626397.

[231]   Wang S, Zhai C, Liu Q, *et al*. Cycloastragenol, a triterpene aglycone derived from Radix astragali, suppresses the accumulation of cytoplasmic lipid droplet in 3T3-L1 adipocytes. Biochem Biophys Res Commun 2014; 450(1): 306-11.
[http://dx.doi.org/10.1016/j.bbrc.2014.05.117] [PMID: 24942874]

[232]   Park HJ, Cho J-Y, Kim MK, Koh P-O, Cho K-W, Kim CH, *et al*. Anti-obesity effect of Schisandra chinensis in 3T3-L1 cells and high fat diet-induced obese rats. Food Chem 2012; 134(1): 227-34.
[http://dx.doi.org/10.1016/j.foodchem.2012.02.101] [PMID: 23265481]

[233]   Song Y, Park HJ, Kang SN, *et al*. Blueberry peel extracts inhibit adipogenesis in 3T3-L1 cells and reduce high-fat diet-induced obesity. PLoS One 2013; 8(7): e69925.
[http://dx.doi.org/10.1371/journal.pone.0069925] [PMID: 23936120]

[234]   Gwon SY, Ahn JY, Kim TW, Ha TY. Zanthoxylum piperitum DC ethanol extract suppresses fat accumulation in adipocytes and high fat diet-induced obese mice by regulating adipogenesis. J Nutr Sci Vitaminol (Tokyo) 2012; 58(6): 393-401.
[http://dx.doi.org/10.3177/jnsv.58.393] [PMID: 23419397]

[235]   Tzeng TF, Liu IM. 6-gingerol prevents adipogenesis and the accumulation of cytoplasmic lipid droplets in 3T3-L1 cells. Phytomedicine 2013; 20(6): 481-7.
[http://dx.doi.org/10.1016/j.phymed.2012.12.006] [PMID: 23369342]

[236]   Ahmadian M, Suh JM, Hah N, *et al*. PPARγ signaling and metabolism: the good, the bad and the future. Nat Med 2013; 19(5): 557-66.
[http://dx.doi.org/10.1038/nm.3159] [PMID: 23652116]

[237]   Cariou B, Charbonnel B, Staels B. Thiazolidinediones and PPARγ agonists: time for a reassessment. Trends Endocrinol Metab 2012; 23(5): 205-15.
[http://dx.doi.org/10.1016/j.tem.2012.03.001] [PMID: 22513163]

[238]   Higgins LS, Depaoli AM. Selective peroxisome proliferator-activated receptor gamma (PPARgamma) modulation as a strategy for safer therapeutic PPARgamma activation. Am J Clin Nutr 2010; 91(1): 267S-72S.
[http://dx.doi.org/10.3945/ajcn.2009.28449E] [PMID: 19906796]

[239]   Guasch L, Sala E, Valls C, *et al*. Structural insights for the design of new PPARgamma partial

agonists with high binding affinity and low transactivation activity. J Comput Aided Mol Des 2011; 25(8): 717-28.
[http://dx.doi.org/10.1007/s10822-011-9446-9] [PMID: 21691811]

[240] Zoete V, Grosdidier A, Michielin O. Peroxisome proliferator-activated receptor structures: ligand specificity, molecular switch and interactions with regulators. Biochim Biophys Acta 2007; 1771(8): 915-25.
[http://dx.doi.org/10.1016/j.bbalip.2007.01.007] [PMID: 17317294]

[241] Farce A, Renault N, Chavatte P. Structural insight into PPARgamma ligands binding. Curr Med Chem 2009; 16(14): 1768-89.
[http://dx.doi.org/10.2174/092986709788186165] [PMID: 19442144]

[242] Bruning JB, Chalmers MJ, Prasad S, *et al.* Partial agonists activate PPARgamma using a helix 12 independent mechanism. Structure 2007; 15(10): 1258-71.
[http://dx.doi.org/10.1016/j.str.2007.07.014] [PMID: 17937915]

[243] Lu B, Moser AH, Shigenaga JK, Feingold KR, Grunfeld C. Type II nuclear hormone receptors, coactivator, and target gene repression in adipose tissue in the acute-phase response. J Lipid Res 2006; 47(10): 2179-90.
[http://dx.doi.org/10.1194/jlr.M500540-JLR200] [PMID: 16847310]

[244] Lee W, Ham J, Kwon HC, Kim YK, Kim SN. Anti-diabetic effect of amorphastilbol through PPARα/γ dual activation in db/db mice. Biochem Biophys Res Commun 2013; 432(1): 73-9.
[http://dx.doi.org/10.1016/j.bbrc.2013.01.083] [PMID: 23376064]

[245] Kim T, Lee W, Jeong KH, *et al.* Total synthesis and dual PPARα/γ agonist effects of amorphastilbol and its synthetic derivatives. Bioorg Med Chem Lett 2012; 22(12): 4122-6.
[http://dx.doi.org/10.1016/j.bmcl.2012.04.062] [PMID: 22579420]

[246] Weidner C, Wowro SJ, Freiwald A, *et al.* Amorfrutin B is an efficient natural peroxisome proliferator-activated receptor gamma (PPARγ) agonist with potent glucose-lowering properties. Diabetologia 2013; 56(8): 1802-12.
[http://dx.doi.org/10.1007/s00125-013-2920-2] [PMID: 23680913]

[247] Weidner C, de Groot JC, Prasad A, *et al.* Amorfrutins are potent antidiabetic dietary natural products. Proc Natl Acad Sci USA 2012; 109(19): 7257-62.
[http://dx.doi.org/10.1073/pnas.1116971109] [PMID: 22509006]

[248] Chacko BK, Chandler RT, D'Alessandro TL, *et al.* Anti-inflammatory effects of isoflavones are dependent on flow and human endothelial cell PPARgamma. J Nutr 2007; 137(2): 351-6.
[PMID: 17237310]

[249] Zou G, Gao Z, Wang J, *et al.* Deoxyelephantopin inhibits cancer cell proliferation and functions as a selective partial agonist against PPARgamma. Biochem Pharmacol 2008; 75(6): 1381-92.
[http://dx.doi.org/10.1016/j.bcp.2007.11.021] [PMID: 18164690]

[250] Atanasov AG, Blunder M, Fakhrudin N, *et al.* Polyacetylenes from Notopterygium incisum--new selective partial agonists of peroxisome proliferator-activated receptor-gamma. PLoS One 2013; 8(4): e61755.
[http://dx.doi.org/10.1371/journal.pone.0061755] [PMID: 23630612]

[251] Shen P, Liu MH, Ng TY, Chan YH, Yong EL. Differential effects of isoflavones, from Astragalus membranaceus and Pueraria thomsonii, on the activation of PPARalpha, PPARgamma, and adipocyte differentiation *in vitro.* J Nutr 2006; 136(4): 899-905.
[PMID: 16549448]

[252] Mueller M, Jungbauer A. Culinary plants, herbs and spices-A rich source of PPARγ ligands. Food Chem 2009; 117: 660-7.
[http://dx.doi.org/10.1016/j.foodchem.2009.04.063]

[253] Atanasov AG, Wang JN, Gu SP, *et al.* Honokiol: a non-adipogenic PPARγ agonist from nature.

Biochim Biophys Acta 2013; 1830(10): 4813-9.
[http://dx.doi.org/10.1016/j.bbagen.2013.06.021] [PMID: 23811337]

[254] Jungbauer A, Medjakovic S. Anti-inflammatory properties of culinary herbs and spices that ameliorate the effects of metabolic syndrome. Maturitas 2012; 71(3): 227-39.
[http://dx.doi.org/10.1016/j.maturitas.2011.12.009] [PMID: 22226987]

[255] Ouarghidi A, Martin GJ, Powell B, Esser G, Abbad A. Botanical identification of medicinal roots collected and traded in Morocco and comparison to the existing literature. J Ethnobiol Ethnomed 2013; 9(1): 59.
[http://dx.doi.org/10.1186/1746-4269-9-59] [PMID: 23945196]

[256] Puhl AC, Bernardes A, Silveira RL, *et al.* Mode of peroxisome proliferator-activated receptor γ activation by luteolin. Mol Pharmacol 2012; 81(6): 788-99.
[http://dx.doi.org/10.1124/mol.111.076216] [PMID: 22391103]

[257] Choi SS, Cha BY, Lee YS, *et al.* Magnolol enhances adipocyte differentiation and glucose uptake in 3T3-L1 cells. Life Sci 2009; 84(25-26): 908-14.
[http://dx.doi.org/10.1016/j.lfs.2009.04.001] [PMID: 19376135]

[258] Fakhrudin N, Ladurner A, Atanasov AG, *et al.* Computer-aided discovery, validation, and mechanistic characterization of novel neolignan activators of peroxisome proliferator-activated receptor gamma. Mol Pharmacol 2010; 77(4): 559-66.
[http://dx.doi.org/10.1124/mol.109.062141] [PMID: 20064974]

[259] Sohn EJ, Kim CS, Kim YS, *et al.* Effects of magnolol (5,5'-diallyl-2,2'-dihydroxybiphenyl) on diabetic nephropathy in type 2 diabetic Goto-Kakizaki rats. Life Sci 2007; 80(5): 468-75.
[http://dx.doi.org/10.1016/j.lfs.2006.09.037] [PMID: 17070554]

[260] Alberdi G, Rodríguez VM, Miranda J, *et al.* Changes in white adipose tissue metabolism induced by resveratrol in rats. Nutr Metab (Lond) 2011; 8(1): 29.
[http://dx.doi.org/10.1186/1743-7075-8-29] [PMID: 21569266]

[261] Beaudoin MS, Snook LA, Arkell AM, Simpson JA, Holloway GP, Wright DC. Resveratrol supplementation improves white adipose tissue function in a depot-specific manner in Zucker diabetic fatty rats. Am J Physiol Regul Integr Comp Physiol 2013; 305(5): R542-51.
[http://dx.doi.org/10.1152/ajpregu.00200.2013] [PMID: 23824959]

[262] Ge H, Zhang JF, Guo BS, *et al.* Resveratrol inhibits macrophage expression of EMMPRIN by activating PPARgamma. Vascul Pharmacol 2007; 46(2): 114-21.
[http://dx.doi.org/10.1016/j.vph.2006.08.412] [PMID: 17055343]

[263] Kim SN, Choi HY, Lee W, Park GM, Shin WS, Kim YK. Sargaquinoic acid and sargahydroquinoic acid from Sargassum yezoense stimulate adipocyte differentiation through PPARalpha/gamma activation in 3T3-L1 cells. FEBS Lett 2008; 582(23-24): 3465-72.
[http://dx.doi.org/10.1016/j.febslet.2008.09.011] [PMID: 18804110]

[264] Saito M, Yoneshiro T, Matsushita M. Food Ingredients as Anti-Obesity Agents. Trends Endocrinol Metab 2015; 26(11): 585-7.
[http://dx.doi.org/10.1016/j.tem.2015.08.009] [PMID: 26421678]

[265] Cannon B, Nedergaard J. Brown adipose tissue: function and physiological significance. Physiol Rev 2004; 84(1): 277-359.
[http://dx.doi.org/10.1152/physrev.00015.2003] [PMID: 14715917]

[266] Saito M. Brown adipose tissue as a regulator of energy expenditure and body fat in humans. Diabetes Metab J 2013; 37(1): 22-9.
[http://dx.doi.org/10.4093/dmj.2013.37.1.22] [PMID: 23441053]

[267] Whiting S, Derbyshire E, Tiwari BK. Capsaicinoids and capsinoids. A potential role for weight management? A systematic review of the evidence. Appetite 2012; 59(2): 341-8.
[http://dx.doi.org/10.1016/j.appet.2012.05.015] [PMID: 22634197]

[268] Yoneshiro T, Aita S, Kawai Y, Iwanaga T, Saito M. Nonpungent capsaicin analogs (capsinoids) increase energy expenditure through the activation of brown adipose tissue in humans. Am J Clin Nutr 2012; 95(4): 845-50.
[http://dx.doi.org/10.3945/ajcn.111.018606] [PMID: 22378725]

[269] Ma S, Yu H, Zhao Z, *et al.* Activation of the cold-sensing TRPM8 channel triggers UCP1-dependent thermogenesis and prevents obesity. J Mol Cell Biol 2012; 4(2): 88-96.
[http://dx.doi.org/10.1093/jmcb/mjs001] [PMID: 22241835]

[270] Kurogi M, Kawai Y, Nagatomo K, Tateyama M, Kubo Y, Saitoh O. Auto-oxidation products of epigallocatechin gallate activate TRPA1 and TRPV1 in sensory neurons. Chem Senses 2015; 40(1): 27-46.
[http://dx.doi.org/10.1093/chemse/bju057] [PMID: 25422365]

[271] Thavanesan N. The putative effects of green tea on body fat: an evaluation of the evidence and a review of the potential mechanisms. Br J Nutr 2011; 106(9): 1297-309.
[http://dx.doi.org/10.1017/S0007114511003849] [PMID: 21810286]

[272] Yoneshiro T, Aita S, Matsushita M, *et al.* Recruited brown adipose tissue as an antiobesity agent in humans. J Clin Invest 2013; 123(8): 3404-8.
[http://dx.doi.org/10.1172/JCI67803] [PMID: 23867622]

[273] Langin D. Adipose tissue lipolysis as a metabolic pathway to define pharmacological strategies against obesity and the metabolic syndrome. Pharmacol Res 2006; 53(6): 482-91.
[http://dx.doi.org/10.1016/j.phrs.2006.03.009] [PMID: 16644234]

[274] Auwerx J, Schoonjans K, Fruchart JC, Staels B. Transcriptional control of triglyceride metabolism: fibrates and fatty acids change the expression of the LPL and apo C-III genes by activating the nuclear receptor PPAR. Atherosclerosis 1996; 124 (Suppl.): S29-37.
[http://dx.doi.org/10.1016/0021-9150(96)05854-6] [PMID: 8831913]

[275] Brasaemle DL, Dolios G, Shapiro L, Wang R. Proteomic analysis of proteins associated with lipid droplets of basal and lipolytically stimulated 3T3-L1 adipocytes. J Biol Chem 2004; 279(45): 46835-42.
[http://dx.doi.org/10.1074/jbc.M409340200] [PMID: 15337753]

[276] Lafontan M, Langin D. Lipolysis and lipid mobilization in human adipose tissue. Prog Lipid Res 2009; 48(5): 275-97.
[http://dx.doi.org/10.1016/j.plipres.2009.05.001] [PMID: 19464318]

[277] Arner P, Langin D. Lipolysis in lipid turnover, cancer cachexia, and obesity-induced insulin resistance. Trends Endocrinol Metab 2014; 25(5): 255-62.
[http://dx.doi.org/10.1016/j.tem.2014.03.002] [PMID: 24731595]

[278] Bartness TJ, Shrestha YB, Vaughan CH, Schwartz GJ, Song CK. Sensory and sympathetic nervous system control of white adipose tissue lipolysis. Mol Cell Endocrinol 2010; 318(1-2): 34-43.
[http://dx.doi.org/10.1016/j.mce.2009.08.031] [PMID: 19747957]

[279] Ohkoshi E, Miyazaki H, Shindo K, Watanabe H, Yoshida A, Yajima H. Constituents from the leaves of Nelumbo nucifera stimulate lipolysis in the white adipose tissue of mice. Planta Med 2007; 73(12): 1255-9.
[http://dx.doi.org/10.1055/s-2007-990223] [PMID: 17893829]

[280] An S, Han JI, Kim MJ, *et al.* Ethanolic extracts of Brassica campestris spp. rapa roots prevent high-fat diet-induced obesity *via* beta(3)-adrenergic regulation of white adipocyte lipolytic activity. J Med Food 2010; 13(2): 406-14.
[http://dx.doi.org/10.1089/jmf.2009.1295] [PMID: 20132043]

[281] Pande S, Srinivasan K. Potentiation of hypolipidemic and weight-reducing influence of dietary tender cluster bean (Cyamopsis tetragonoloba) when combined with capsaicin in high-fat-fed rats. J Agric Food Chem 2012; 60(33): 8155-62.

[http://dx.doi.org/10.1021/jf301211c] [PMID: 22835261]

[282]   Chen Y-C, Kao T-H, Tseng C-Y, Chang W-T, Hsu C-L. Methanolic extract of black garlic ameliorates diet-induced obesity *via* regulating adipogenesis, adipokine biosynthesis, and lipolysis. J Funct Foods 2014; 9: 98-108.
[http://dx.doi.org/10.1016/j.jff.2014.02.019]

[283]   Bradford PG. Curcumin and obesity. Biofactors 2013; 39(1): 78-87.
[http://dx.doi.org/10.1002/biof.1074] [PMID: 23339049]

[284]   Ho JN, Park SJ, Choue R, Lee J. Standardized Ethanol Extract of Curcuma longa L. Fermented by Aspergillus oryzae Promotes Lipolysis *via* Activation of cAMP□Dependent PKA in 3T3□L1 Adipocytes. J Food Biochem 2013; 37(5): 595-603.

[285]   Isken F, Klaus S, Petzke KJ, Loddenkemper C, Pfeiffer AF, Weickert MO. Impairment of fat oxidation under high- *vs.* low-glycemic index diet occurs before the development of an obese phenotype. Am J Physiol Endocrinol Metab 2010; 298(2): E287-95.
[http://dx.doi.org/10.1152/ajpendo.00515.2009] [PMID: 19934403]

[286]   Kerner J, Hoppel C. Fatty acid import into mitochondria. Biochim Biophys Acta 2000; 1486(1): 1-17.
[http://dx.doi.org/10.1016/S1388-1981(00)00044-5] [PMID: 10856709]

[287]   Duplus E, Forest C. Is there a single mechanism for fatty acid regulation of gene transcription? Biochem Pharmacol 2002; 64(5-6): 893-901.
[http://dx.doi.org/10.1016/S0006-2952(02)01157-7] [PMID: 12213584]

[288]   Eaton S, Bartlett K, Pourfarzam M. Mammalian mitochondrial beta-oxidation. Biochem J 1996; 320(Pt 2): 345-57.
[http://dx.doi.org/10.1042/bj3200345] [PMID: 8973539]

[289]   Hayashi T, Hirshman MF, Fujii N, Habinowski SA, Witters LA, Goodyear LJ. Metabolic stress and altered glucose transport: activation of AMP-activated protein kinase as a unifying coupling mechanism. Diabetes 2000; 49(4): 527-31.
[http://dx.doi.org/10.2337/diabetes.49.4.527] [PMID: 10871188]

[290]   Ruderman NB, Saha AK, Vavvas D, Witters LA. Malonyl-CoA, fuel sensing, and insulin resistance. Am J Physiol 1999; 276(1 Pt 1): E1-E18.
[PMID: 9886945]

[291]   Saha AK, Ruderman NB. Malonyl-CoA and AMP-activated protein kinase: an expanding partnership. Mol Cell Biochem 2003; 253(1-2): 65-70.
[http://dx.doi.org/10.1023/A:1026053302036] [PMID: 14619957]

[292]   Flier JS. Obesity wars: molecular progress confronts an expanding epidemic. Cell 2004; 116(2): 337-50.
[http://dx.doi.org/10.1016/S0092-8674(03)01081-X] [PMID: 14744442]

[293]   Kang SW, Kang SI, Shin HS, *et al.* Sasa quelpaertensis Nakai extract and its constituent p-coumaric acid inhibit adipogenesis in 3T3-L1 cells through activation of the AMPK pathway. Food Chem Toxicol 2013; 59: 380-5.
[http://dx.doi.org/10.1016/j.fct.2013.06.033] [PMID: 23810795]

[294]   Son Y, Nam J-S, Jang M-K, Jung I-A, Cho S-I, Jung M-H. Antiobesity activity of Vigna nakashimae extract in high-fat diet-induced obesity. Biosci Biotechnol Biochem 2013; 77(2): 332-8.
[http://dx.doi.org/10.1271/bbb.120755] [PMID: 23391927]

[295]   Wang L, Yamasaki M, Katsube T, Sun X, Yamasaki Y, Shiwaku K. Antiobesity effect of polyphenolic compounds from molokheiya (Corchorus olitorius L.) leaves in LDL receptor-deficient mice. Eur J Nutr 2011; 50(2): 127-33.
[http://dx.doi.org/10.1007/s00394-010-0122-y] [PMID: 20617439]

[296]   Huang TH, Peng G, Li GQ, Yamahara J, Roufogalis BD, Li Y. Salacia oblonga root improves postprandial hyperlipidemia and hepatic steatosis in Zucker diabetic fatty rats: activation of PPAR-α.

Toxicol Appl Pharmacol 2006; 210(3): 225-35.
[http://dx.doi.org/10.1016/j.taap.2005.05.003] [PMID: 15975614]

[297] Rong X, Kim MS, Su N, *et al.* An aqueous extract of Salacia oblonga root, a herb-derived peroxisome proliferator-activated receptor-alpha activator, by oral gavage over 28 days induces gender-dependent hepatic hypertrophy in rats. Food Chem Toxicol 2008; 46(6): 2165-72.
[http://dx.doi.org/10.1016/j.fct.2008.02.022] [PMID: 18397819]

[298] Gupta P, Goyal R, Chauhan Y, Sharma PL. Possible modulation of FAS and PTP-1B signaling in ameliorative potential of Bombax ceiba against high fat diet induced obesity. BMC Complement Altern Med 2013; 13: 281.
[http://dx.doi.org/10.1186/1472-6882-13-281] [PMID: 24160453]

[299] Ibarra A, Bai N, He K, *et al.* Fraxinus excelsior seed extract FraxiPure™ limits weight gains and hyperglycemia in high-fat diet-induced obese mice. Phytomedicine 2011; 18(6): 479-85.
[http://dx.doi.org/10.1016/j.phymed.2010.09.010] [PMID: 21036576]

[300] Vroegrijk IO, van Diepen JA, van den Berg S, *et al.* Pomegranate seed oil, a rich source of punicic acid, prevents diet-induced obesity and insulin resistance in mice. Food Chem Toxicol 2011; 49(6): 1426-30.
[http://dx.doi.org/10.1016/j.fct.2011.03.037] [PMID: 21440024]

[301] Baur JA. Resveratrol, sirtuins, and the promise of a DR mimetic. Mech Ageing Dev 2010; 131(4): 261-9.
[http://dx.doi.org/10.1016/j.mad.2010.02.007] [PMID: 20219519]

[302] Jiang WJ. Sirtuins: novel targets for metabolic disease in drug development. Biochem Biophys Res Commun 2008; 373(3): 341-4.
[http://dx.doi.org/10.1016/j.bbrc.2008.06.048] [PMID: 18577374]

[303] Picard F, Kurtev M, Chung N, *et al.* Sirt1 promotes fat mobilization in white adipocytes by repressing PPAR-gamma. Nature 2004; 429(6993): 771-6. [gamma].
[http://dx.doi.org/10.1038/nature02583] [PMID: 15175761]

[304] Rayalam S, Yang J-Y, Ambati S, Della-Fera MA, Baile CA. Resveratrol induces apoptosis and inhibits adipogenesis in 3T3-L1 adipocytes. Phytother Res 2008; 22(10): 1367-71.
[http://dx.doi.org/10.1002/ptr.2503] [PMID: 18688788]

[305] Shan T, Ren Y, Wang Y. Sirtuin 1 affects the transcriptional expression of adipose triglyceride lipase in porcine adipocytes. J Anim Sci 2013; 91(3): 1247-54.
[http://dx.doi.org/10.2527/jas.2011-5030] [PMID: 23296834]

[306] Carpéné C, Gomez-Zorita S, Gupta R, *et al.* Combination of low dose of the anti-adipogenic agents resveratrol and phenelzine in drinking water is not sufficient to prevent obesity in very-high-fat diet-fed mice. Eur J Nutr 2014; 53(8): 1625-35.
[http://dx.doi.org/10.1007/s00394-014-0668-1] [PMID: 24531732]

[307] Kim K-Y, Lee HN, Kim YJ, Park T. Garcinia cambogia extract ameliorates visceral adiposity in C57BL/6J mice fed on a high-fat diet. Biosci Biotechnol Biochem 2008; 72(7): 1772-80.
[http://dx.doi.org/10.1271/bbb.80072] [PMID: 18603810]

[308] Altiner A, Ates A, Gursel E, Bilal T. Effect of the antiobesity agent Garcinia cambogia extract on serum lipoprotein (a), Apolipoproteins A1 and B, and total Cholesterol levels in female rats fed atherogenic diet. J Anim Plant Sci 2012; 22(4): 872-7.

[309] Márquez F, Babio N, Bulló M, Salas-Salvadó J. Evaluation of the safety and efficacy of hydroxycitric acid or Garcinia cambogia extracts in humans. Crit Rev Food Sci Nutr 2012; 52(7): 585-94.
[http://dx.doi.org/10.1080/10408398.2010.500551] [PMID: 22530711]

[310] Kim K, Park M, Lee YM, Rhyu MR, Kim HY. Ginsenoside metabolite compound K stimulates glucagon-like peptide-1 secretion in NCI-H716 cells *via* bile acid receptor activation. Arch Pharm Res 2014; 37(9): 1193-200.

[http://dx.doi.org/10.1007/s12272-014-0362-0] [PMID: 24590628]

[311] Ahn JH, Kim ES, Lee C, *et al.* Chemical constituents from Nelumbo nucifera leaves and their anti-obesity effects. Bioorg Med Chem Lett 2013; 23(12): 3604-8.
[http://dx.doi.org/10.1016/j.bmcl.2013.04.013] [PMID: 23642481]

[312] Lai YS, Chen WC, Ho CT, *et al.* Garlic essential oil protects against obesity-triggered nonalcoholic fatty liver disease through modulation of lipid metabolism and oxidative stress. J Agric Food Chem 2014; 62(25): 5897-906.
[http://dx.doi.org/10.1021/jf500803c] [PMID: 24857364]

[313] Hwang JT, Kim SH, Hur HJ, *et al.* Decursin, an active compound isolated from Angelica gigas, inhibits fat accumulation, reduces adipocytokine secretion and improves glucose tolerance in mice fed a high-fat diet. Phytother Res 2012; 26(5): 633-8.
[http://dx.doi.org/10.1002/ptr.3612] [PMID: 21972114]

[314] Roh C, Park MK, Shin HJ, Jung U, Kim JK. Buddleja officinalis Maximowicz extract inhibits lipid accumulation on adipocyte differentiation in 3T3-L1 cells and high-fat mice. Molecules 2012; 17(7): 8687-95.
[http://dx.doi.org/10.3390/molecules17078687] [PMID: 22825621]

[315] Lee YS, Cha BY, Saito K, *et al.* Effects of a Citrus depressa Hayata (shiikuwasa) extract on obesity in high-fat diet-induced obese mice. Phytomedicine 2011; 18(8-9): 648-54.
[http://dx.doi.org/10.1016/j.phymed.2010.11.005] [PMID: 21216135]

[316] Kang S-I, Shin H-S, Kim H-M, *et al.* Immature *Citrus sunki* peel extract exhibits antiobesity effects by β-oxidation and lipolysis in high-fat diet-induced obese mice. Biol Pharm Bull 2012; 35(2): 223-30.
[http://dx.doi.org/10.1248/bpb.35.223] [PMID: 22293353]

[317] Choi HS, Jeon HJ, Lee OH, Lee BY. Dieckol, a major phlorotannin in Ecklonia cava, suppresses lipid accumulation in the adipocytes of high-fat diet-fed zebrafish and mice: Inhibition of early adipogenesis via cell-cycle arrest and AMPKα activation. Mol Nutr Food Res 2015; 59(8): 1458-71.
[http://dx.doi.org/10.1002/mnfr.201500021] [PMID: 25944759]

[318] Sumiyoshi M, Kimura Y. Hop (Humulus lupulus L.) extract inhibits obesity in mice fed a high-fat diet over the long term. Br J Nutr 2013; 109(1): 162-72.
[http://dx.doi.org/10.1017/S000711451200061X] [PMID: 22715886]

[319] Yui K, Kiyofuji A, Osada K. Effects of xanthohumol-rich extract from the hop on fatty acid metabolism in rats fed a high-fat diet. J Oleo Sci 2014; 63(2): 159-68.
[http://dx.doi.org/10.5650/jos.ess13136] [PMID: 24420065]

[320] Ju JH, Yoon HS, Park HJ, *et al.* Anti-obesity and antioxidative effects of purple sweet potato extract in 3T3-L1 adipocytes *in vitro*. J Med Food 2011; 14(10): 1097-106.
[http://dx.doi.org/10.1089/jmf.2010.1450] [PMID: 21861722]

[321] Zhou CJ, Huang S, Liu JQ, *et al.* Sweet tea leaves extract improves leptin resistance in diet-induced obese rats. J Ethnopharmacol 2013; 145(1): 386-92.
[http://dx.doi.org/10.1016/j.jep.2012.09.057] [PMID: 23147498]

[322] Cao S, Zhou Y, Xu P, *et al.* Berberine metabolites exhibit triglyceride-lowering effects *via* activation of AMP-activated protein kinase in Hep G2 cells. J Ethnopharmacol 2013; 149(2): 576-82.
[http://dx.doi.org/10.1016/j.jep.2013.07.025] [PMID: 23899453]

[323] Jung CH, Ahn J, Jeon TI, Kim TW, Ha TY. Syzygium aromaticum ethanol extract reduces high-fat diet-induced obesity in mice through downregulation of adipogenic and lipogenic gene expression. Exp Ther Med 2012; 4(3): 409-14.
[http://dx.doi.org/10.3892/etm.2012.609] [PMID: 23181109]

[324] Basu A, Du M, Sanchez K, *et al.* Green tea minimally affects biomarkers of inflammation in obese subjects with metabolic syndrome. Nutrition 2011; 27(2): 206-13.
[http://dx.doi.org/10.1016/j.nut.2010.01.015] [PMID: 20605696]

[325] Datau EA, Wardhana , Surachmanto EE, Pandelaki K, Langi JA, Fias . Efficacy of Nigella sativa on serum free testosterone and metabolic disturbances in central obese male. Acta Med Indones 2010; 42(3): 130-4.
[PMID: 20724766]

[326] He RR, Chen L, Lin BH, Matsui Y, Yao XS, Kurihara H. Beneficial effects of oolong tea consumption on diet-induced overweight and obese subjects. Chin J Integr Med 2009; 15(1): 34-41.
[http://dx.doi.org/10.1007/s11655-009-0034-8] [PMID: 19271168]

[327] Kazemipoor M, Radzi CW, Hajifaraji M, Haerian BS, Mosaddegh MH, Cordell GA. Antiobesity effect of caraway extract on overweight and obese women: a randomized, triple-blind, placebo-controlled clinical trial. Evid Based Complement Alternat Med 2013; 2013: 928582.
[http://dx.doi.org/10.1155/2013/928582]

[328] Kubota K, Sumi S, Tojo H, Sumi-Inoue Y. Improvements of mean body mass index and body weight in preobese and overweight Japanese adults with black Chinese tea (Pu-Erh) water extract. Nutr Res (NY) 2011; 31(6): 421-8.

[329] Amagase H, Nance DM. Lycium barbarum increases caloric expenditure and decreases waist circumference in healthy overweight men and women: pilot study. J Am Coll Nutr 2011; 30(5): 304-9.
[http://dx.doi.org/10.1080/07315724.2011.10719973] [PMID: 22081616]

[330] Shekelle PG, Hardy ML, Morton SC, *et al.* Efficacy and safety of ephedra and ephedrine for weight loss and athletic performance: a meta-analysis. JAMA 2003; 289(12): 1537-45.
[PMID: 12672771]

[331] Bent S, Padula A, Neuhaus J. Safety and efficacy of citrus aurantium for weight loss. Am J Cardiol 2004; 94(10): 1359-61.
[http://dx.doi.org/10.1016/j.amjcard.2004.07.137] [PMID: 15541270]

[332] Gurrola-Díaz CM, García-López PM, Sánchez-Enríquez S, Troyo-Sanromán R, Andrade-González I, Gómez-Leyva JF. Effects of Hibiscus sabdariffa extract powder and preventive treatment (diet) on the lipid profiles of patients with metabolic syndrome (MeSy). Phytomedicine 2010; 17(7): 500-5.
[http://dx.doi.org/10.1016/j.phymed.2009.10.014] [PMID: 19962289]

[333] Gout B, Bourges C, Paineau-Dubreuil S. Satiereal, a Crocus sativus L extract, reduces snacking and increases satiety in a randomized placebo-controlled study of mildly overweight, healthy women. Nutr Res 2010; 30(5): 305-13.
[http://dx.doi.org/10.1016/j.nutres.2010.04.008] [PMID: 20579522]

[334] Oben JE, Ngondi JL, Momo CN, Agbor GA, Sobgui CS. The use of a Cissus quadrangularis/Irvingia gabonensis combination in the management of weight loss: a double-blind placebo-controlled study. Lipids Health Dis 2008; 7: 12.
[http://dx.doi.org/10.1186/1476-511X-7-12] [PMID: 18377661]

[335] Lenon GB, Li KX, Chang YH, Yang AW, Da Costa C, Li CG, *et al.* Efficacy and Safety of a Chinese Herbal Medicine Formula (RCM-104) in the Management of Simple Obesity: A Randomized, Placebo-Controlled Clinical Trial. Evid Based Complement Alternat Med 2012; 2012: 435702.

[336] Oben JE, Enyegue DM, Fomekong GI, Soukontoua YB, Agbor GA. The effect of Cissus quadrangularis (CQR-300) and a Cissus formulation (CORE) on obesity and obesity-induced oxidative stress. Lipids Health Dis 2007; 6: 4.
[http://dx.doi.org/10.1186/1476-511X-6-4] [PMID: 17274828]

[337] Thielecke F, Rahn G, Böhnke J, *et al.* Epigallocatechin-3-gallate and postprandial fat oxidation in overweight/obese male volunteers: a pilot study. Eur J Clin Nutr 2010; 64(7): 704-13.
[http://dx.doi.org/10.1038/ejcn.2010.47] [PMID: 20372175]

[338] Chevassus H, Gaillard JB, Farret A, *et al.* A fenugreek seed extract selectively reduces spontaneous fat intake in overweight subjects. Eur J Clin Pharmacol 2010; 66(5): 449-55.
[http://dx.doi.org/10.1007/s00228-009-0770-0] [PMID: 20020282]

CHAPTER 6

Anti-Obesity Molecules from Plants and their Mode of Action

Megha Valsaraj, Navaneetha Saseendran, Arun Subash Koorapally and **Anu Augustine**[*]

Department of Biotechnology and Microbiology, Kannur University, Thalassery Campus, India

Abstract: Obesity is a chronic condition that is causally related to serious medical illnesses. Plants, especially those used in Ayurveda, can provide biologically active molecules and lead structures for the development of drugs with enhanced activity and reduced toxicity. Natural products, particularly medicinal plants, are believed to harbor potential anti-obesity agents that can act through various mechanisms, either by preventing weight gain, or by promoting weight loss. Their mechanisms of action include inhibition of key lipid and carbohydrate hydrolyzing and metabolizing enzymes, modification of serum lipoprotein and apolipoproteins, blockage of intestinal absorption, disruption of adipogenesis and adipogenic factors, suppression of appetite *etc*. The chapter gives an account of medicinal plants used in antiobesity drug formulations in Ayurveda and their mechanisms of action, like *Holoptelea integrifolia, Averrhoa bilimbi, Terminalia chebula, Picrorhiza kurroa, Acorus calamus etc*. The knowledge and detailed study about these plants will help to control obesity and to increase awareness on the importance of medicinal plants in addressing the issue.

Keywords: Acorus calamus, Apolipoprotein, Averrhoea bilimbi and Terminalia chebula, Cholesterol, Chylomicrons, HDL, HMGR, Holoptelea integrifolia, LCAT, LDL, LPL, Lekhaneyagana, Obesity, Picrorhiza kurroa, VLDL.

GENERAL INTRODUCTION

"Obesity is a multifactorial, chronic disorder that has reached epidemic proportions in most industrialized countries and is threatening to become a global epidemic" [1]. It also makes people prone to coronary artery disease, hypertension, hyperlipidemia, diabetes mellitus, cancers, cerebrovascular accidents, osteoarthritis and restrictive pulmonary disease [2]. In fact, obesity and related cardiovascular diseases claim more lives than the other four leading causes, like cancer, respiratory diseases, accidents, and diabetes [3, 4]. Obesity is a challenging clinical condition to treat, because of the complex environmental

---

[*] **Corresponding author Anu Augustine:** Department of Biotechnology and Microbiology, Kannur University, Thalassery Campus, India; Fax: 91-490 2345317; E-mail: anuaugus@rediffmail.com

Atta-ur-Rahman & M. Iqbal Choudhary (Eds.)

component involved in its pathogenesis. Efforts to develop innovative antiobesity drugs have been recently intensified [5]. "Moreover, due to absolute etiology of obesity, non-availability of drugs for its treatment, short-term efficacy and limiting contraindication and side effects of available drugs, the treatment is not satisfactory and thus there is demand for new safer ones" [6, 7].

Ayurveda, means "the science of life" (or living), which represents a way of life that merges the art of healing through peace with nature and the environment. The approach of Ayurveda to life and living is universal and its range is infinite, while its application is universal and far reaching [8]. '*Charakasamhitha*', an authentic book of Ayurveda mentions a pharmacological classification of plants, "*lekhaneyagana*", which helps to remove excess fat from body [9]. The active compounds and the exact mechanism of weight reduction have not been revealed [10].

35-50% of Indian population suffers from major obesity disorders. A study about such phytochemicals with antiobesity action and scientific validation of the findings in such studies is of utmost importance in the diagnosis and treatment of obesity disorders [10 - 12]. Most of the medicinal plants that have anticholesterol property, albeit being used as ethanomedicine, are yet to be properly validated. Detailed investigations and characterization of such plants will eventually help develop better and safer drugs for obesity and atherosclerosis [13].

The World Health Organization (2008) has recommended evaluation of the effectiveness of plants for conditions where we lack safe modern drugs [14]. The chapter deals with the definition of obesity and its causes, lipoproteins, enzymes involved, role of medicinal plants in controlling obesity and experimental studies in animal models.

Obesity

When abnormal fat accumulation interferes with normal activities and impairs the health of an individual, it may be termed obesity. Obesity is a chronic disease that is usually related to serious medical illnesses. In the United States alone, the consequences of obesity account for an estimated 300,000 deaths per year [15]. The medical expenses and cost of lost productivity due to obesity are greater than $100 billion per year and are increasing alarmingly. Over weight and obesity are linked to more deaths worldwide than underweight [16].

Definition and Assessment of Obesity

The most widely used and accepted method to gauge obesity is the body mass index (BMI), which is equal to weight/height^2 (in kg/m^2) (Fig. **1**). Other approaches to quantifying obesity include densitometry (under-water weighing), anthropometry (skin-fold thickness), computed tomography (CT), magnetic resonance imaging (MRI) and electrical impedance. There is a strong curvilinear relation between BMI and relative body fat mass [17]. However, the current practical definition of obesity is based on the relationship between BMI and health outcome.

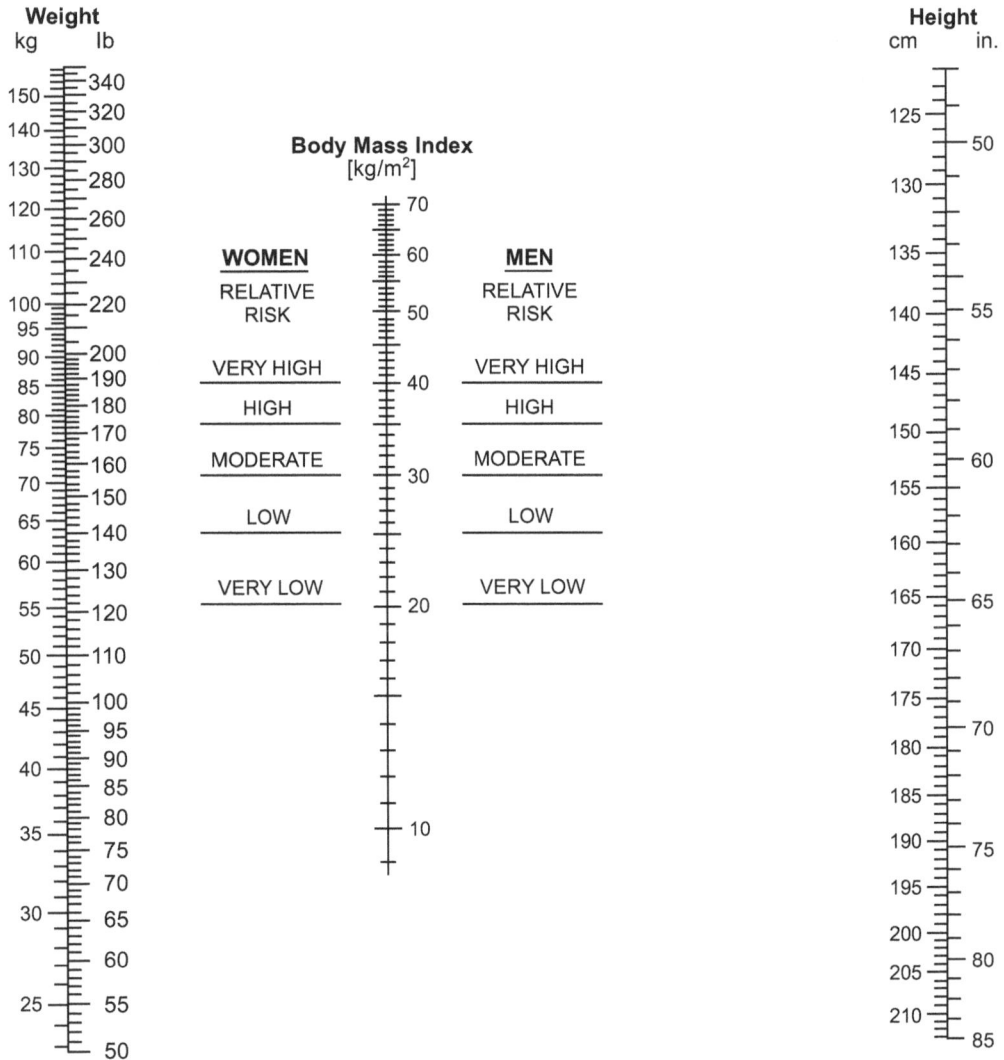

Fig. (1). Nomogram for determining BMI. To use this nomogram, place a ruler or other straight edge between the body weight (without clothes) in kilograms or pounds located on the left-hand line and the height in cm or inches located on the right-hand line. The body mass index is read from the middle of the scale and is in metric units. (Copyright 1979, George A. Bray, M.D).

Genetic and Environmental Factors Causing Obesity

About 40-80% of the variance in BMI can be attributed to genetic factors. There is considerable evidence that genes have significant role in obesity related diseases. Some of the genes that are associated with obesity phenotypes include *ACDC* (Adipocyte, C1Q and collagen domain containing, adiponectin), *LEP* (Leptin), *NR3C1* (Nuclear receptor subfamily 3), *etc* [18]. Obesity is a heritable trait and risk factor for many common diseases such as heart diseases, type 2 diabetes, and hyper tension. The heritability is estimated to be as high as 30-40% for factors relevant to energy balance such as resting metabolic rate, fat distribution, energy expenditure after overeating, basal rates of lipolysis and lipoprotein lipase activity. More than 200 genetic markers have been traced in connection with obesity-related variables in humans *e.g.*, BMI, waist-to-hip ratio, fat mass, skin-fold thickness *etc* [15].

Rapid increase in the prevalence of obesity can be attributed to more environmental factors, broadly conceptualized to include physical and social factors, than to biological change. One of the environmental changes that have been identified to be a potential environmental contributor is the habit of eating away from home, particularly at "junk food" outlets. Also, nutritional analysis of food products sold indicated that they are typically high in energy density [19].

Endocrine and Metabolic Factors

Our understanding of the relation between obesity and metabolic risk factors is growing rapidly. Any impairment of the metabolic and endocrine system causes obesity and the complex interactions between the metabolic and endocrine systems are found to be contributing factors to obesity [15]. It is based on the discovery of multiple products released in abnormal amounts from adipocytes in the presence of obesity. Each of these products adds to one or another of the metabolic risk factors [20]. Some of the factors most implicated in the development of metabolic syndrome are Nonesterified Fatty Acids (NEFAs), Inflammatory cytokines, PAI-1, Adiponectin, and Leptin Resistin [21].

Hypothyroidism, Cushing syndrome and Polycystic ovarian syndrome in women, Hypogonadism in men and hypothalamic lesions like infections or severe trauma and tumors are some of the obesity-causing disease conditions [22].

Psychological Factors

Externality (obesity being socially contagious) and depression are mostly observed to be causative personality characteristics related to obesity and research evidence strongly suggests that obesity is not a unitary syndrome [15].

Psychological factors include the interconnection of mind to brain, especially as they relate to food choice and eating habits, cognitive factors involved in motivation, self-regulation, and self-efficacy, discrimination and perceptions of prejudice as well as increased prevalence of psychiatric symptoms, such as depression and anxiety, among the obese [23].

The interrelation between obesity and one's emotional fluctuations is now extensively recognized. Several patients take off their depressive symptoms by eating and putting on weight. As time passes, this becomes a continuous process and ultimately leads to obesity [22].

Control of Appetite and Energy Expenditure

Appetite is the desire to eat and this usually initiates food intake. During heavy exercise or during pregnancy, some patients eat more and are not able to get back to their former eating habits. The type of food consumed is one of the major factors contributing to obesity.

Gut hormones, local paracrine behavior and peripheral endocrine effects mediated through the bloodstream play a central role in transferring information on nutritional status to important appetite supervising centres within the central nervous system (CNS), such as the brainstem and the hypothalamus [24]. Following a meal, cholecystokinin, bombesin, somatostatin and enterostatin are released from the small intestine.

Obesity Management

In order to prevent obesity, several pharmacological and surgical interventions are available, but in many cases it may not be desirable [25]. Drug treatment for obesity has only short-term benefits. It is often associated with rebound weight gain after the termination of drug use, the potential for drug abuse and side effects from the medication [26]. Pharmacologic choices include Sibutramine, Orlistat, Phentermine, Diethylpropion, and Fluoxetine or Bupropion. Diethylpropion and Phentermine have potential for abuse and are only permitted for short-term use. Sibutramine and Orlistat are approved medications for long-term use in the treatment of obesity. However, proper care should be taken while applying these agents in patients with a history of cardiovascular disorders [27].

Role of Medicinal Plants in Obesity Treatment

Diet-based therapies and herbal supplements to reduce weight are among the most common, complementary and alternative medicine [CAM] modalities. Some of the targeted approaches to probe the antiobesity potential of medicinal plants are the inhibition of key lipid and carbohydrate hydrolyzing and metabolizing enzymes, disruption of adipogenesis and modulation of its factors and appetite suppression. The potential antiobesity effects of natural herbs have been studied both *in vitro* and *in vivo*. Studies show that plant products which exhibit antiobesity properties can act through different mechanisms such as anti-adipogenesis or by suppressing appetite.

Ayurveda is a medical system of India, handed down to the modern world as the most ancient of all systems of medicine. *Charakasamhita* is an early ayurvedic text on internal medicine. Charaka (700 BC) states that medicine is of two types; one is promotive of vigour in the healthy and the other destructive to diseases [28].

Charaka made the first attempt to classify drugs into 50 groups (based on their action and uses). The "*lekhaneyagana*" means 'to lessen excess of fat from our body'. It helps to eliminate or scrape the waste material adhering to or blocking different body channels. The *lekhaneyagana* includes 10 medicinal plants, *Cyperus rotundus, Saussurea lappa, Curcuma longa, Coccinium fenestratum, Holoptelea integrifolia, Acorus calamus, Aconitum heterophyllum, Plumbago rosea, Picrorrhiza kurroa* and *Terminalia chebula*.

Garcinia gummigutta, Hordeum vulgare, Coccinia indica, Embelia ribes, Boerhaavia diffusa, Commiphora mukul, Punica granatum and *Averrhoa bilimbi* have been already reported to have anti-cholesterol property and routinely used in slimming pills which are comparatively safer than commonly prescribed antiobesity drugs like Statins, Fibrates, Bile acid sequesters, Cholesterol ester transfer proteins (CETP) inhibitors, etc [29].

Mechanism of Action of Anti obesity Agents from Plants

Some medicinal plants prevent the intestinal lipid absorption and non-absorbed fat will be excreted through oily faeces. Certain bioactive components can increase the metabolic rate which enhances thermogenesis and helps burn calories and excess body fat. Another mechanism of hypolipidemic effect is the prevention of adipocyte differentiation which in turn inhibits adipogenesis and fat cell formation. Yet another mechanism is based on enhanced lipolysis brought about through β-oxidation or Nor-adrenaline secretion in fat cells. Other antiobesity ingredients may suppress appetite and induce satiety, allowing appetite control [30, 31].

Modifying Serum Lipoprotein

Clinical studies have recognized that elevated cholesterol and TG (Triglyceride) levels and low levels of HDL-c are associated with increased cardiovascular disease (CVD) risk [32]. Various medicinal plants and herbal supplements have proved to be effective against obesity and related disorders. Garlic reduces atherosclerosis by virtue of *Allicin* [33]. Steroids like Z-Guggulusterone and E-Guggulusterone found in *Commiphora mukul* possess lipid lowering activity and modify serum lipoproteins [34]. "Fibre extracts of *Cissus quadrangularis* have been shown to possess anti-lipase property that reduces absorption of dietary fats, reduces serum lipids and enhances satiation" [35].

Modifying Serum Apolipoproteins

A high level of total blood cholesterol, particularly in the form of LDL cholesterol (Low density lipoprotein-c), is a major risk factor for developing coronary heart disease [36]. Measurement of apolipoprotein levels (apo B& apo A) has methodological advantages over measurement of LDL-c [37]. Apo B and apo A-I can be measured directly, accurately and precisely. Moreover, measurement of apo B and apo A-I does not require fasting blood samples and is internationally standardized [38].

Consumption of Chinese tea-flavor liquor (TFL) has defensive effects on cardiovascular disease. TFL can be used to significantly reduce apolipoprotein A1 in healthy human subjects [39]. In humans, plant sterol esters lower plasma lipids and most carotenoids positively modify apolipoproteins [40].

Enzyme Inhibition

HMG-CoA Reductase

Studies show that Monascus-fermented soybean extracts used to treat hyperlipidemic rats show a significant reduction in HMGR (major enzyme involved in cholesterol biosynthesis) activity compared to control counterparts. Similar results were observed with Korean soybean paste (Doenjang), which is fermented by diverse microorganisms including fungi and baccilli [41]. Sung *et al* also identified the active components responsible for HMG-CoA reductase inhibition to be Genistein, Glycitein, Daidzein, and Aglycone forms of Isoflavones [41, 42].

Lecithin: Cholesterol Acyltransferase (LCAT)

The enzyme LCAT (involved in reverse cholesterol transport) is synthesized in the liver and circulates in plasma in its active form. The lipid lowering activity of *Phyllanthus niruri* has been studied in hyper lipidemic rats. The activity of this plant is mediated through inhibition of hepatic cholesterol biosynthesis; increased faecal bile acid excretion and enhanced plasma LCAT activity [43]. "The oral administration of extract of *Gymnema sylvestre* leaves significantly increases the blood LCAT activity" [44]. Previous studies have shown that treatment with *Anthocephalus indicus* extract for 30 days significantly increased the level of LCAT in plasma of Alloxan induced diabetic rats [45].

Lipoprotein Lipase

Inhibition of digestion and absorption of dietary fat has been used as target in obesity treatment [46]. LPL has also been targeted in obesity as it has been found that these obese subjects possess an increased LPL level. Release of free fatty acids (FFA) happens due to the hydrolysis of blood triglycerides, catalyzed by LPL. This increases the storage of triglycerides in adipose tissue. So it is expected that the assimilation of FFA can be reduced by inhibition of LPL and thus help in controlling obesity [47, 48]

A very low concentration of the *Nomame herba* extract resulted in 50% inhibition of lipase activity. The feeding of *N. herba* extract inhibited weight gain and plasma triglyceride levels in lean rats fed with a high fat diet, without affecting food intake. "Hence, it was concluded from this study that the extract might be a powerful lipase inhibitor and could be used as a weight control agent in obese subjects" [49]. *Exolise* (A standardized *Camellia sinensis* based drug), with active component Catechin, can be a natural antiobesity agent, through its antilipase activity and increase in thermogenesis [50].

Inhibitors of Adipogenesis and Adipogenic Factors

In humans and animals white adipose tissue (WAT) serves as the major energy reserve. Excess amount of energy is stored as triglycerides in this white adipose tissue. An excess of WAT has been thought to be one of the major causes of obesity [51]. It is known that the growth of the adipose tissue involves the development of new adipocytes from precursor cells leading to an increase in the size of the adipocyte. Treatments that can regulate the size and the number of adipocytes promote the expression of signals involved in energy balance and inhibit or enhance specific adipokines that are proved to express antiobesity-related bioactivities [52]. The proliferation and differentiation of primary human visceral preadipocyte is inhibited by a compound present in green tea, epigallocatechin gallate (EGCG) [53].

Extracts of *Centella asiatica, Morinda citrifolia,* and *Momordica charantia* inhibited the proliferation of 3T3-L1 adipose cell line in a dose-dependent method with *Momordica charantia* having the most toxic effect [31]. Perilla oil, which is abundant in (*n*-3) polyunsaturated fatty acids, in rats, was found to hinder the excessive growth of visceral adipose tissue by a down regulation of adipocyte differentiation [54].

Blocking Intestinal Absorption

Obesity can result from an imbalance between energy intake and energy expenditure. Since dietary fat constitutes 35-45% of energy intake, a further therapeutic approach, that is, the inhibition of absorption of fat from the gut, is used for the treatment of obesity.

Wang *et al* (2006) in their study provides direct evidence that Epigallocatechin gallate (EGCG) and Caffeine, when intraluminally administered, inhibit the intestinal absorption of lipids. EGCG interferes with luminal lipid hydrolysis and micellar solubilization; critical steps involved in the intestinal absorption of dietary fat;whereas Caffeine adversely affected the intracellular processing and secretion of lipids from the enterocyte *via* chylomicrons [55]. Studies in New Zealand White rabbits showed that increasing dietary stanols (campestanol and sitostanol) results in reduced intestinal cholesterol absorption [56].

Appetite Suppressants

The reductive synthesis of long chain fatty acids is catalyzed by Fatty Acid Synthase (FAS) from Acetyl Co-enzyme A and Malonyl-CoA. It is proven that the mice treated with FAS inhibitors showed a reduction in food intake and body weight due to inhibition of FAS. This makes the inhibition of FAS a potential therapeutic target of appetite suppression and weight loss induction [57].

Details of Plants Selected for Study

Holoptelea Integrifolia

Holoptelea integrifolia (Family: Ulmaceae) commonly known as 'Indian elm' (Fig. **2A**) is a large deciduous tree, growing up to 18 m tall. Its bark and leaves are also known for medicinal importance [58]. Globally the species are distributed in Sri Lanka, India, Myanmar, China and Malaysia. *H. integrifolia* contains several classes of secondary metabolites like alkaloids, terpeniods, glycosides, steroids, sterols, saponins, tannins and flavonoids. The leaves and stem bark of this plant were used traditionally in antiviral, antioxidant, antimicrobial, antiobesity preparations and in the management of cancer [59, 60].

Averrhoa bilimbi Linn.

A. bilimbi (Family: Oxalidaceae) commonly known as '*Bilimbi*' (Fig. **2B**)., is a small sized tree. The species are distributed in Sri Lanka, India and China. *A.*

bilimbi fruit is widely used in traditional medicine as a cure for diabetes, obesity, cough, cold, itches, boils, fever, mumps, pimples, inflammation, rheumatism, syphilis, diabetes, whooping cough and hypertension [61, 62]. *A. bilimbi* has been widely reported to have multiple ethnopharmacological properties such as anti-inflammatory, anti-scorbutic, astringent, anti-bacterial, and postpartum protective properties [63].

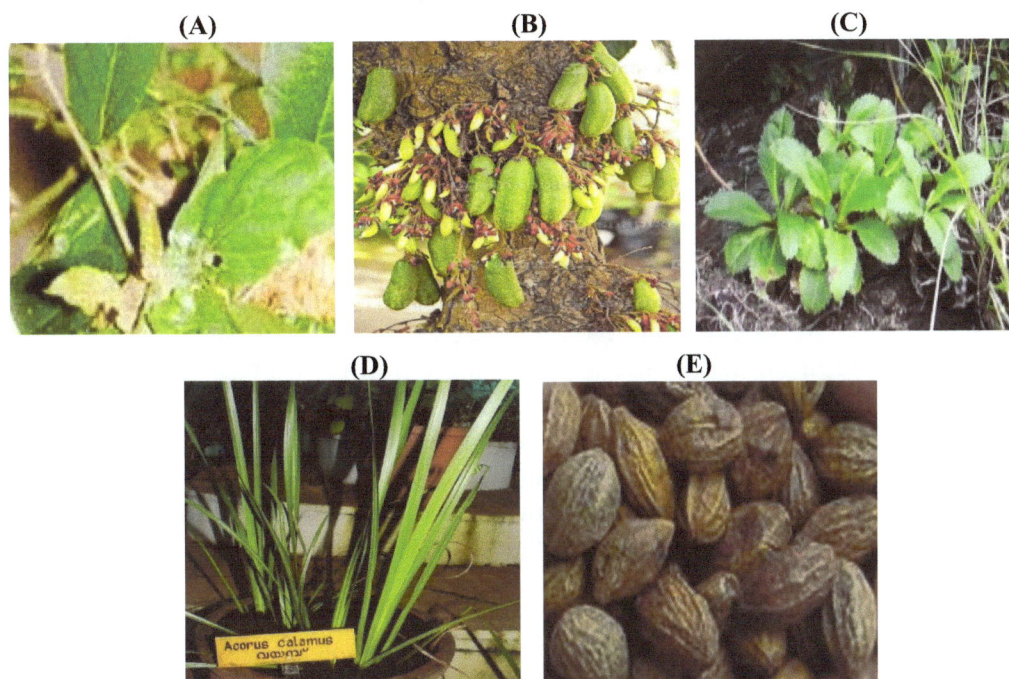

Fig. (2). Image showing plants selected for the study (A) *H. integrifolia* (B) *A. bilimbi* fruit (C) *P. kurroa* (D) *A. calamus* (E) *T. chebula* fruit.

Terminalia chebula Retz.

T. chebula (Family: Combretaceae) is a native plant of India and South East Asia, commonly known as "Black myrobalans" (Fig. **2E**) Fruits of *T. chebula* were used traditionally for their purgative activity and to cure bleeding. These fruits are also used for the treatment of burns, digestive disorders, diabetes, eye diseases, weak eye sight, fever, skin diseases and kidney dysfunction along with other herbs [64].

Acorus calamus Linn.

A. calamus (Family: Araceae) also known as sweet flag (Fig. **2D**), is a semi aquatic perennial herb with creeping and branched aromatic rhizome. This species is widely distributed in the North temperate hemisphere and tropical Asia. The ethyl acetate and methanol extracts of *A. calamus* show protective effects against oxidative damage induced by noise stress in rat brains. The essential oils isolated from *A. calamus* showed anti-hypercholesterolemia, anti-inflammatory and antioxidative activity [65, 66].

Picrorhiza kurroa Royle ex Benth

P. kurroa (Family: Scrophulariaceae), popularly known as 'kutki' (Fig. **2C**), is a mild hairy perennial herb distributed in the Himalayan range across Pakistan, India and Nepal. The subterranean part of the plants is used as bitter tonic, stomachic, laxative and is useful in gastrointestinal and urinary disorders, obesity and inflammatory affections.

Experimental Model and Findings

The consumption of high-fat diet leads to obesity, especially abdominal obesity, as it facilitates the development of a positive energy balance, leading to an increase in visceral fat deposition. Obesity induction *via* dietary means in animal models has been considered the most authentic reference available among researchers due to its high similarity in mimicking the usual route of obesity occurrence in humans. It is generally known that high-fat diet is one of the major factors causing obesity, and that the long-term intake of high-fat diet evokes a significant increase in abdominal fat weight in mammals.

The use of obese experimental model developed by a high fat diet for 4 weeks produces a dyslipidemic profile, elevates serum lipids, apolipoproteins and results in significant body weight gain.

Methodology

The plants/parts were collected, identified, authenticated and deposited in herbarium of Centre for Medicinal Plants Research (CMPR), Kottakkal, India. The finely powdered sample was used for soxhlet extraction using methanol. The homogenate was then filtered using Millipore filtration system 2 (Millipore, USA) and solvent was removed using a rotary evaporator at 40 °C. The methanol fraction was loaded on to a silica gel column (18 x 500 mm) and then eluted with methanol: water solvent, to get different fractions (100, 70, 50 and 30% methanol [67].

Animals

Sprague Dawley (SD) strain rats (4-6 weeks old), both sexes, body weight 160 ± 10 gm were used for experiments. The animals were selected such that the weight difference within and between groups does not exceed ± 20% of the average body weight of the sample population. They were housed in polypropylene cages (48 X 35 X 22 cm) at controlled temperature (22 ± 3 °C) and humidity (50 ±10%) and were kept in 12 hour light cycle. Rats were fed with standard diet and the water *adlibitum* and acclimated 7 days before they were used.

Acute Oral Toxicity

Acute oral toxicity tests of plant extracts were performed as per OECD-425 guidelines (acute class method). Toxicity test (Limit 5000 mg/kg) was performed as per AOT425 statpgm software. The animals were fasted overnight (10 hour), provided only water after which extract was administered to the groups orally at the dose level, single dose, 5000 mg/kg body weight by gastric intubation and were observed for 14 days. The animals were observed for toxic symptoms such as behavioral changes, locomotion, convulsions and mortality for 72 hours (OECD, USEPA, Washington, DC).

Establishment of Experimental Model

All rats were provided with normal diet for two weeks after the initiation of this preliminary rearing, and thereafter they were divided into two groups of normal fed (NF) and high fat (HF)-fed. NF-fed and HF-fed groups were provided with normal diet and high fat diet respectively until the end of the experiment (Table 1). Obesity in rats was induced by high fat diet for 4 weeks [68, 69]. After 4 weeks, blood samples were drawn from the tail vein and used for the measurement of serum lipid levels. The rats were considered to be obese only if their T-c and TG doubled, HDL-c value reduced to about half and LDL-c value increased about 6 times [70]. Control rats were fed freely with the standard diet. Diet induced obese rat models received high fat diet for 4 weeks.

Table 1. High fat diet Ingredients.

S/N	Ingredients	HF Diet%-gm/100 gm diet
1	Basic diet	82.8
2	Lard	10
3	Cholesterol	2
4	Bile salt	0.5
5	Propylthiouracil.	0.2
6	AIN-76[a] Vitamin mix	3.5
7	AIN-76[a] Mineral mix	1

[a] AIN-76-American Institute of Nutrition formulation 76.

Drug Treatment

Rats were randomly divided into 2 groups: normal control (NC) group (n = 10), and high-fat (HF) group including high fat diet (HFD) group (n=50), five plant extracts treated group (n=10/group) and mevinolin treated positive control (MEVN) group (n = 10). The rats in the NC group were fed with basic diet and 0.2 ml saline. The rats in extract treated groups were fed with a high-fat diet and orally given extract once a day (between 10.00 am -12. 00 pm) using feeding needles (Instech Solomon Laboratories, Inc. USA), dissolved in 0.2 ml saline) for 4 weeks, at a dosage of 200 and 400 mg/kg bodyweight. Mevinolin (statin-known HMG-CoA reductase) (3.0 mg/kg BW) was used as positive control (Xu *et al.*, 2009).The doses were chosen according to the acute toxicological study results [71].

From the start of rearing to the beginning of extract administration, the body weight and the feed intake of all rats were measured twice a week. After the beginning of extract administration, these were measured every day. Rats were allowed *ad libitum* to access the feed stuff and water during the experimental period. Faeces were collected from each group for the last 2 weeks of the experimental period, weighed, freeze-dried, and subjected to fat analysis.

Effect of Plant Extracts on Serum Lipids

A principal contributor to morbidity due to obesity is the alteration in serum lipid and lipoprotein levels. Elevated plasma cholesterol concentrations as well as triglyceride levels are associated with an increased risk of cardiovascular diseases. The total serum cholesterol of normal, high-fat diet extract and Mevinolin treated group are shown in Fig. (**3**). It is found that all treatments are able to positively modify (reduce) the total cholesterol. Analyzing the trend among plants, it was found that *P. kurroa* shows maximum reduction in serum lipid levels and is comparable to the positive control Mevinolin.

Effect of Plant Extracts on HDL Cholesterol Levels

Increased concentrations of HDL-cholesterol is closely associated with decreased risk of cardiovascular disease.

The HDL-cholesterol of normal, HFD, extracts and mevinolin treated group are shown in Fig. (**4**). The extracts from *T. chebula* and *H. integrifolia* cause a marked increase in cardioprotective lipid, HDL-c. On the other hand low doses of *P. kurroa* and *A. bilimbi* extract were not able to significantly improve serum HDL concentration.

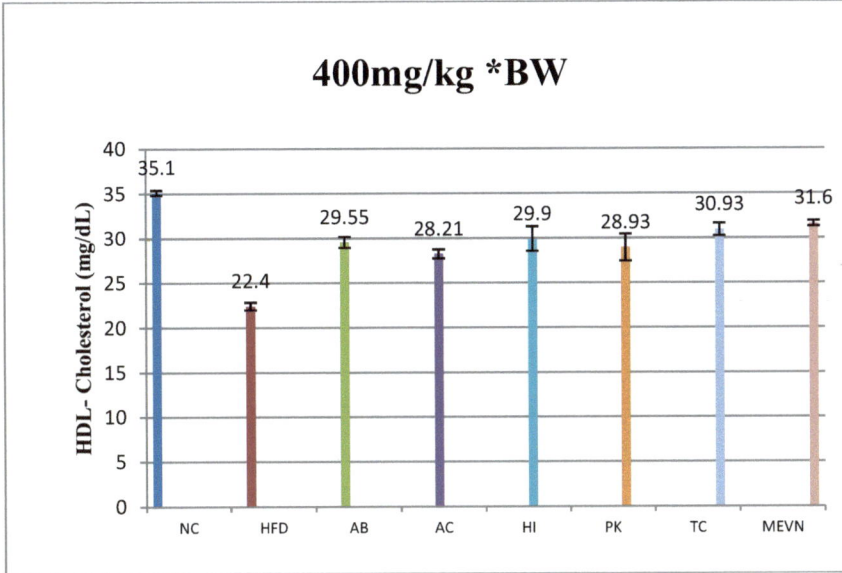

Fig. (3). Figure showing the effect of extract treatments on total serum cholesterol in diet induced obese rats. NC, Normal control group; HFD, High fat diet group, AB, *A. bilimbi* extract treated group; AC, *A. calamus* extract treated group; HI, *H. integrifolia* extract treated group; PK, *P kurroa* extract treated group; TC, *T.chebula* extract treated group and MEVN,mevinolin treated positive control group.*BW: Body Weight. The values are mean ± s.d for ten rats.

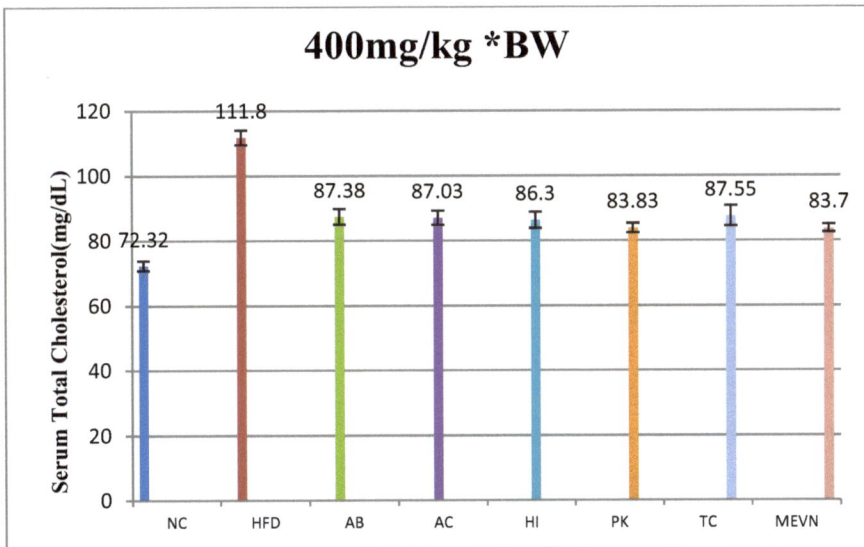

Fig. (4). Figure showing the effect of extract treatment on serum HDL-cholesterol in diet induced obese rats. NC, Normal control group; HFD, High fat diet group, AB, *A. bilimbi* extract treated group; AC, *A. calamus* extract treated group; HI, *H. integrifolia* extract treated group; PK, *P kurroa* extract treated group; TC, *T. chebula* extract treated group and MEVN, mevinolin treated positive control group. *BW: Body Weight. The values are mean ± s.d for ten rats.

Effect of Plant Extracts on LDL Cholesterol Levels

The pivotal role of LDL cholesterol in causing atherosclerosis and the complications caused by it has been unequivocally established. Lowering of LDL cholesterol also benefits in secondary and primary obesity prevention. Oral administration of these extracts brings down the serum LDL-c. The LDL-cholesterol of normal, HFD, extract and mevinolin treated groups are shown in Fig. (**5**). High dose (400 mg/kg BW) of *P. kurroa, H. integrifolia* and *T. chebula* shows high LDL-c reducing potential.

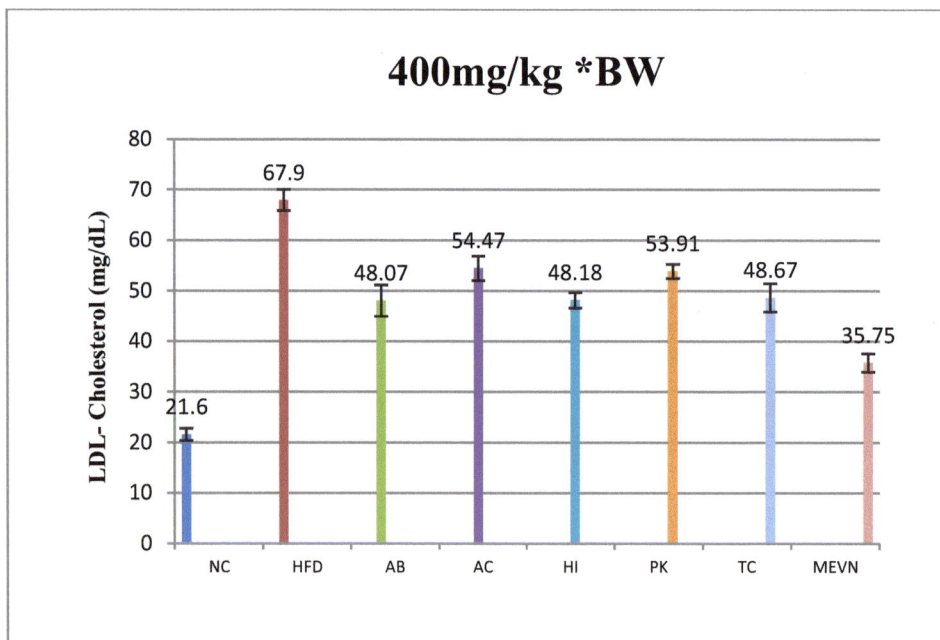

Fig. (5). Figure showing the effect of extract treatment on serum LDL-cholesterol in diet induced obese rats NC, Normal control group; HFD, High fat diet group, AB, *A. bilimbi* extract treated group; AC, *A. calamus* extract treated group; HI, *H. integrifolia* extract treated group; PK, *P kurroa* extract treated group; TC, *T. chebula* extract treated group and MEVN, mevinolin treated positive control group. *BW: Body Weight. The values are mean ± s.d for ten rats.

Effect of Plant Extracts on Apolipoproteins

Apolipoproteins play an important role in the formation, stabilization, and metabolism of lipoproteins. They are classified into six subcategories namely, apo A-1, apo A-2, apo B, apo C-2, apo C-3, and apo E. Apo A-I plays a prominent role in HDL-c metabolism as a primary acceptor of un-esterified cholesterol from the peripheral tissues. Apo A-I is a key marker of HDL-cholesterol levels and studies have shown that the level of apo A-I is more closely correlated with the reduced risk of atherosclerosis than other markers of HDL-cholesterol. This makes apo A-I, a very attractive biomarker candidate for implementation into clinical practice, taking into account its analytical advantages.

The level of apo A1 level in normal, HFD, extract and mevinolin treated groups after four weeks are shown in Fig. (**6**). From the graph, it is clear that high dose (400 mg/kg BW) of *T. chebula* extract significantly increases Apo A1. A parallel increase in HDL-c is also observed. On the other hand, *P. kurroa* treatment is not able to modify the Apo A1 levels in high fat diet rats. *A. calamus* and *A. bilimbi* extract is able to improve Apo A1 levels, but the activity is less compared to *T. chebula.*

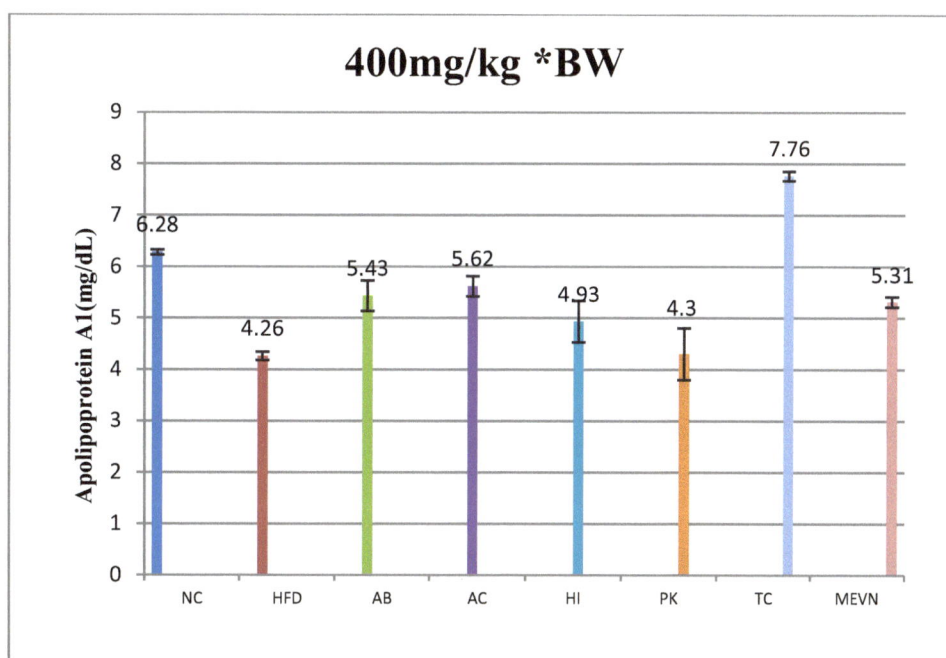

Fig. (6). Figure showing the effect of extract treatment on apo A1 in diet induced obese rats NC, Normal control group; HFD, High fat diet group, AB, *A. bilimbi* extract treated group; AC, *A. calamus* extract treated group; HI, *H. integrifolia* extract treated group; PK, *P kurroa* extract treated group; TC, *T. chebula* extract treated group and MEVN, mevinolin treated positive control group. *BW: Body Weight. The values are mean ± s.d for ten rats.

Although an increased concentration of LDL-c is the main risk factor for coronary heart disease, the constituents of LDL-C, mainly apolipoprotein B, may also play an important role in atherosclerosis. The serum Apo B concentration has decreased significantly after the use of extracts in diet induced obese rats. Apo B concentrations of normal, HFD, extract and mevinolin treated group are shown in Fig. (**7**).

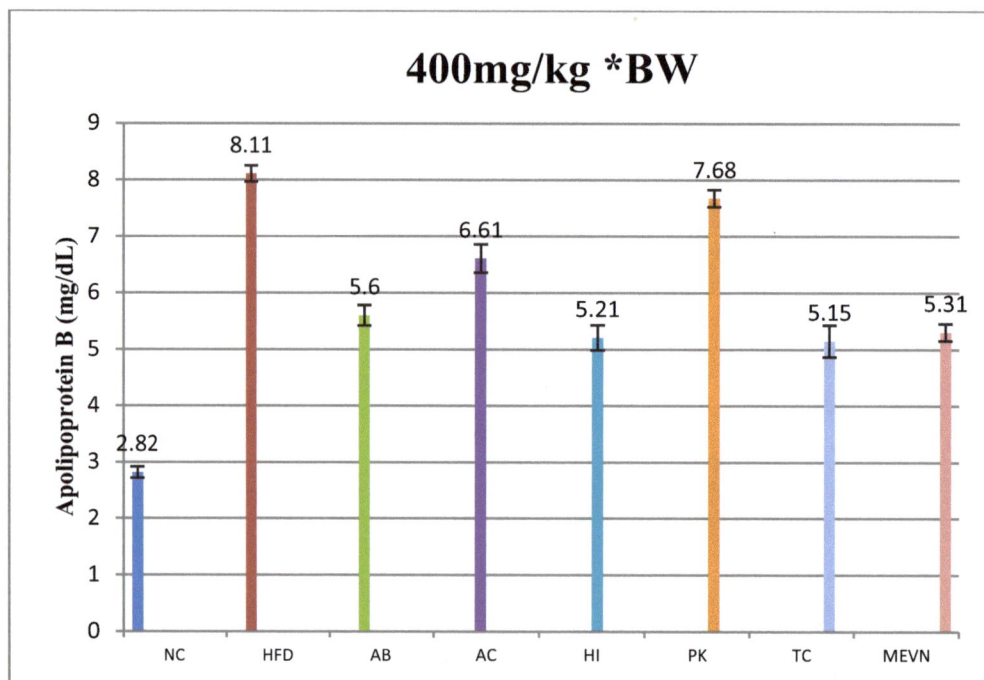

Fig. (7). Figure showing the effect of extract treatment on apo B in diet induced obese rats. NC, Normal control group; HFD, High fat diet group, AB, *A. bilimbi* extract treated group; AC, *A. calamus* extract treated group; HI, *H. integrifolia* extract treated group; PK, *P kurroa* extract treated group; TC, *T. chebula* extract treated group and MEVN, mevinolin treated positive control group. *BW: Body Weight. The values are mean ± s.d for ten rats.

All extracts except that of *P. kurroa* were able to significantly reduce Apo B levels after 4 week oral administration in a dose dependent manner and this decrease is parallel to that of serum LDL-c concentration. Current studies prove the fact that the reduction of LDL-c by *P. kurroa* was not due to the modification of Apo B levels.

Effect of Different Plant Extracts on Enzymes Involved in Cholesterol Pathway

HMG-CoA Reductase

The endoplasmic reticulum-bound enzyme, HMG-CoA reductase is the rate-limiting factor in endogenous cholesterol biosynthesis. Although this enzyme is expressed in all tissues, it is most abundant in the liver, which plays a critical role in regulation of plasma cholesterol level. Thus, a marked down-regulation of hepatic HMGR can contribute to hypocholesteremic effect. The present study addressed the effect of selected plant extracts in modulating HMGR activity. The

HMGR enzyme level of study groups is given in Fig. (**8**). Among the five extracts used, all showed HMGR inhibition activity. The high dose (400 mg/kg BW) of *H. integrifolia* extract showed remarkable HMGR inhibition potential that was found to be better than that of mevinolin (3 mg/kg BW). The study points to the use of *H.integrifolia* control cholesterol levels in blood.

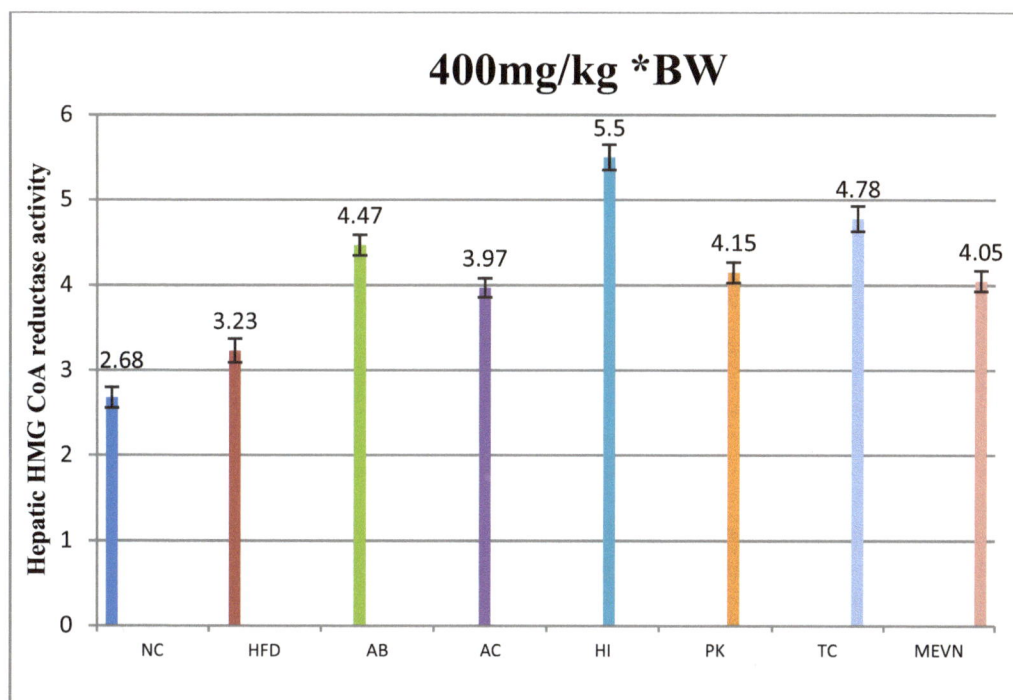

Fig. (8). Figure showing the effect of extract treatment on HMGR protein in diet induced obese rats NC, Normal control group; HFD, High fat diet group, AB, *A. bilimbi* extract treated group; AC, *A. calamus* extract treated group; HI, *H. integrifolia* extract treated group; PK, *P kurroa* extract treated group; TC, *T. chebula* extract treated group and MEVN, mevinolin treated positive control group. *BW: Body Weight. The values are mean ± s.d for ten rats.

Lecithin-Cholesterol Acyltransferase

LCAT plays an important role in HDL-mediated transport of surplus cholesterol from the peripheral cells for disposal in the liver, a phenomenon commonly referred to as reverse cholesterol transport. The extracts of *H. integrifolia*, *A. calamus* and *P. kurroa* were able to improve LCAT activity positively. *H integrifolia* treatment resulted in an increase in LCAT enzyme concentration by approximately 27.86%, compared to that of model control group (Fig. **9**).

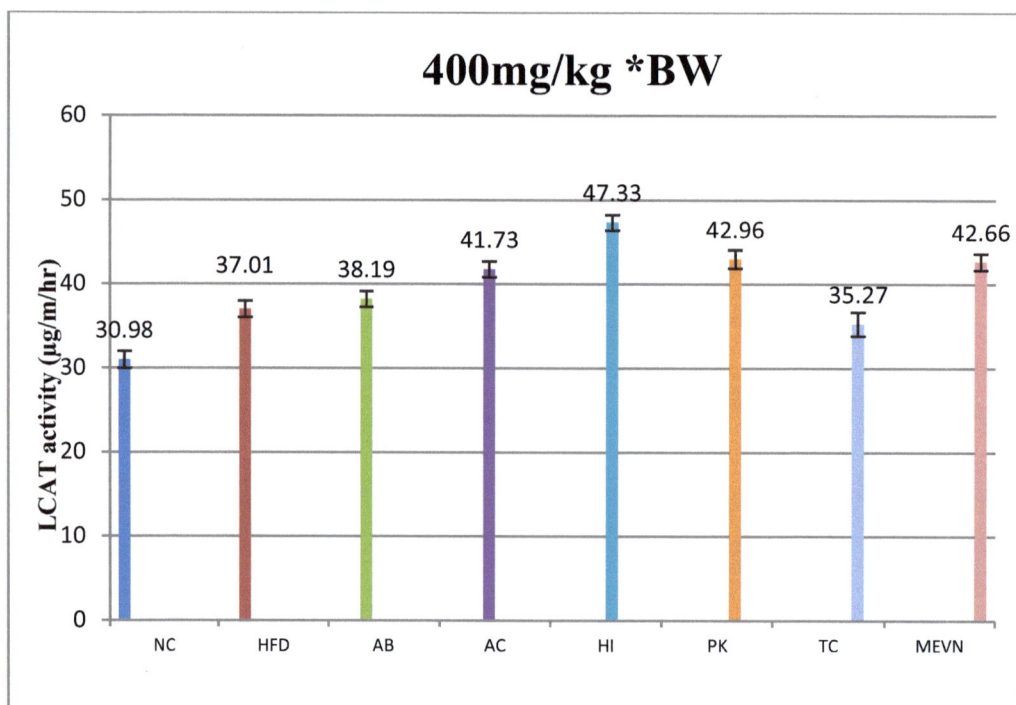

Fig. (9). Figure showing the effect of extract treatment on LCAT activity in diet induced obese rats.NC, Normal control group; HFD, High fat diet group, AB, *A. bilimbi* extract treated group; AC, *A. calamus* extract treated group; HI, *H. integrifolia* extract treated group; PK, *P kurroa* extract treated group; TC, *T. chebula* extract treated group and MEVN, mevinolin treated positive control group. *BW: Body Weight. The values are mean ± s.d for ten rats.

Lipoprotein Lipase

Triglycerides of dietary origin are transported through blood as large particles-called chylomicrons. There is good evidence that chylomicron triglycerides are rapidly cleared from the circulation through the action of the enzyme lipoprotein lipase. The function of this enzyme is to hydrolyze plasma triglycerides thereby facilitating the uptake of constituent fatty acids by extra hepatic tissues of the body.

Lipoprotein lipase acts on plasma triglycerides at the luminal surface of the endothelial cells that line the capillaries of extra hepatic tissues such as heart, lung and adipose tissue. The LPL assay results of different treatment groups are shown in Fig. (**10**). The results show that *A. bilimbi*, *H. integrifolia* and *P. kurroa* treatment significantly increase LPL level. *A. calamus* and *T. chebula* treatment does not show any impact on LPL activity thereby confirming that the hypolipidemic activity is not due to altering of LPL level.

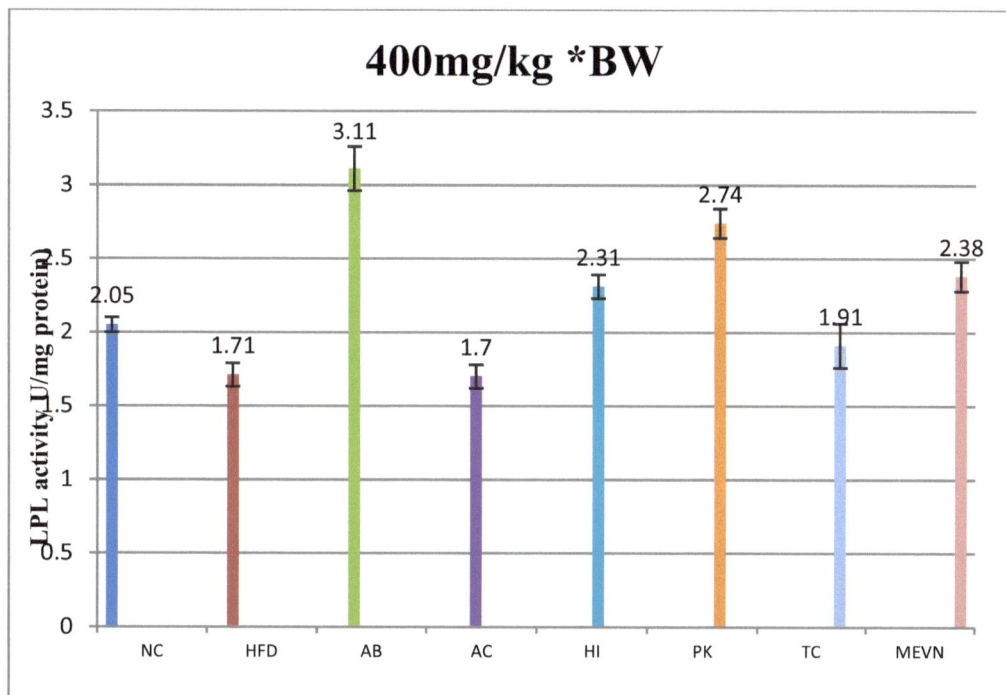

Fig. (10). Figure showing the effect of extract treatment on LPL activity in diet induced obese rats.NC, Normal control group; HFD, High fat diet group, AB, *A. bilimbi* extract treated group; AC, *A. calamus* extract treated group; HI, *H. integrifolia* extract treated group; PK, *P kurroa* extract treated group; TC, *T. chebula* extract treated group and MEVN, mevinolin treated positive control group. *BW: Body Weight. The values are mean ± s.d for ten rats.

Effect of Different Plant Extracts on Intestinal Fat Absorption

The role of dietary fat in the etiology of obesity is widely accepted. It is seen that the higher energy value of faeces observed in the *H. integrifolia, T. chebula* and *A. Bilimbi* extract treated groups resulted from a reduction in the apparent digestion of fat (Fig. **11** and **12**).

Effect of Different Plant Extracts on Inhibition of Adipogenesis and Adipogenic Factors

Adipose tissue is the biggest storage site for excess energy. Excessive growth of adipose tissue results in obesity which includes two growth mechanisms: hyperplastic (cell number increase) and hypertrophic (cell size increase).The ingestion of excessive energy causes obesity due to visceral fat accumulation, leading to the onset of symptoms of metabolic syndrome (MS), including insulin resistance, diabetes mellitus, lipid metabolism abnormalities, and hypertension.

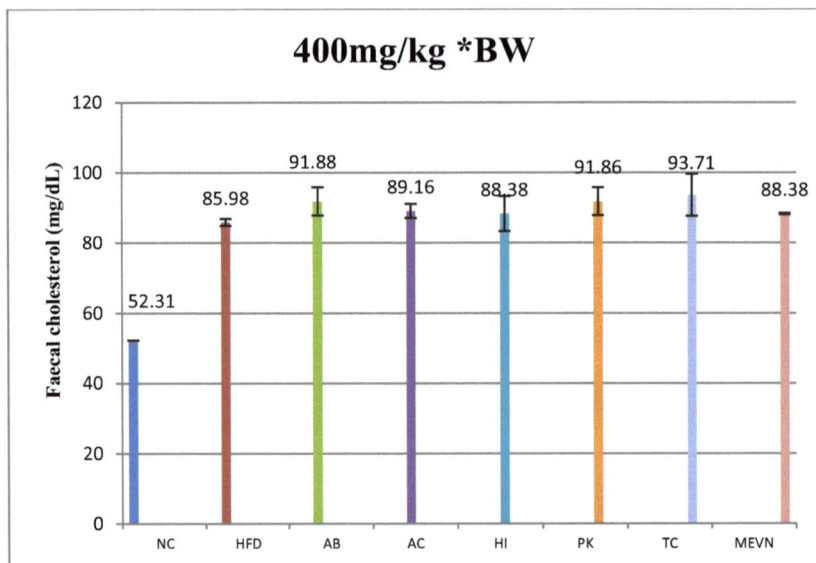

Fig. (11). Figure showing the effect of extract treatment on faecal cholesterol in diet induced obese rats. NC, Normal control group; HFD, High fat diet group, AB, *A. bilimbi* extract treated group; AC, *A. calamus* extract treated group; HI, *H. integrifolia* extract treated group; PK, *P kurroa* extract treated group; TC, *T. chebula* extract treated group and MEVN, mevinolin treated positive control group. *BW: Body Weight. The values are mean ± s.d for ten rats.

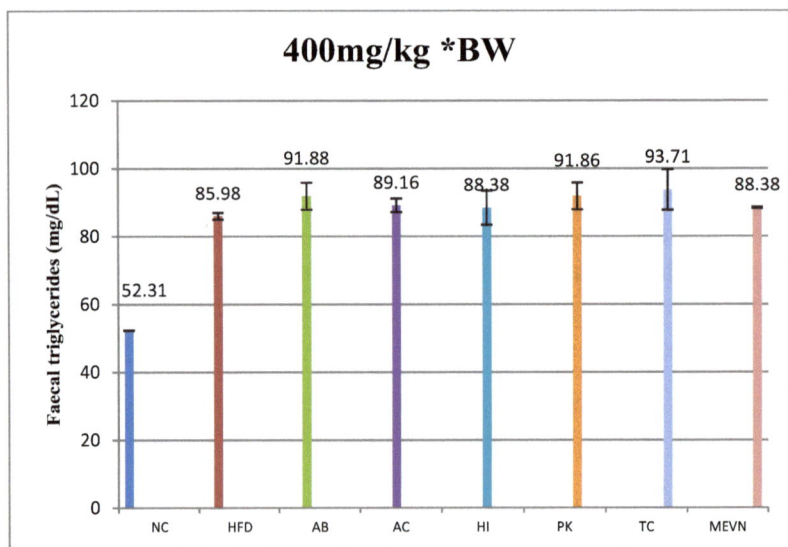

Fig. (12). Figure showing the effect of extract treatment on faecal triglycerides in diet induced obese rats. NC, Normal control group; HFD, High fat diet group, AB, *A. bilimbi* extract treated group; AC, *A. calamus* extract treated group; HI, *H. integrifolia* extract treated group; PK, *P kurroa* extract treated group; TC, *T. chebula* extract treated group and MEVN, mevinolin treated positive control group. *BW: Body Weight. The values are mean ± s.d for ten rats.

The distribution of body fat is an independent predictor of the adverse metabolic patterns of obesity, cardiovascular morbidity and mortality. More specifically, studies that have examined regional fat distribution have shown a close correlation between intra-abdominal fat deposition and indices of cardiovascular risk, including low HDL-c/total cholesterol ratio, hypertension, hypertrigly-ceridemia and hyperinsulinemia

The extracts of *P. kurroa* and *A. calamus* caused a notable decrease in visceral fat mass while the other extracts reduce visceral fat mass to lesser extents (Fig. **13**).

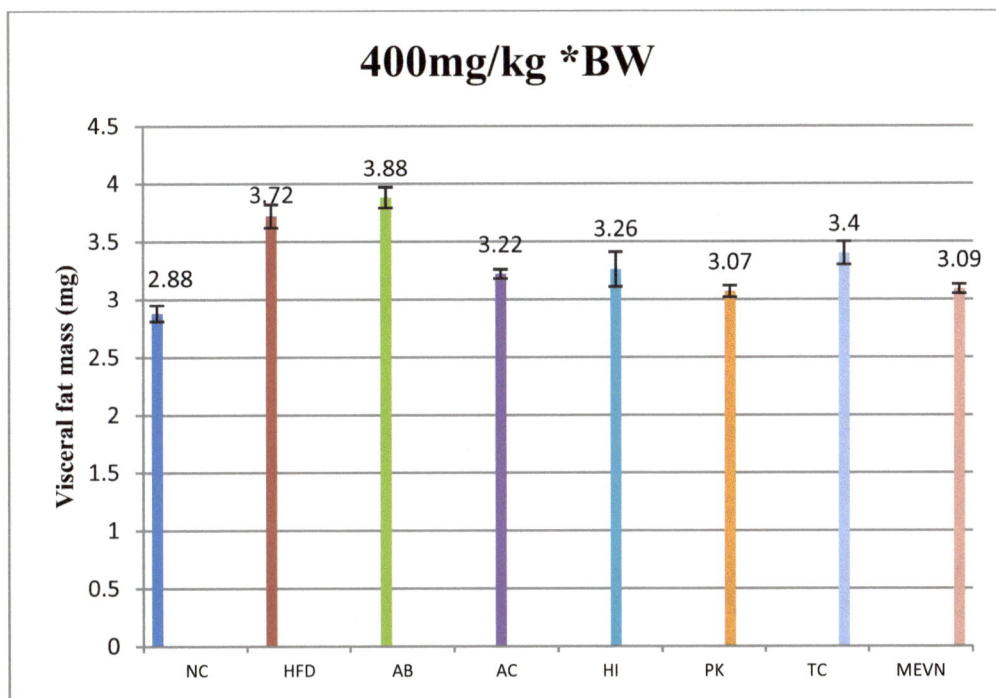

Fig. (13). Figure showing the effect of extract treatment on visceral fat mass in diet induced obese rats.NC, Normal control group; HFD, High fat diet group, AB, *A. bilimbi* extract treated group; AC, *A. calamus* extract treated group; HI, *H. integrifolia* extract treated group; PK, *P kurroa* extract treated group; TC, *T. chebula* extract treated group and MEVN, mevinolin treated positive control group. *BW: Body Weight. The values are mean ± s.d for ten rats.

The plant extracts from *H. integrifolia, A. bilimbi, T. chebula, A. calamus* and *P.kurroa* showed substantial reduction in the size of fat pads compared with high fat fed rats. In addition, the extract treated rats have significantly lower adipose depot weights than high fat fed rats (Fig. **14**).

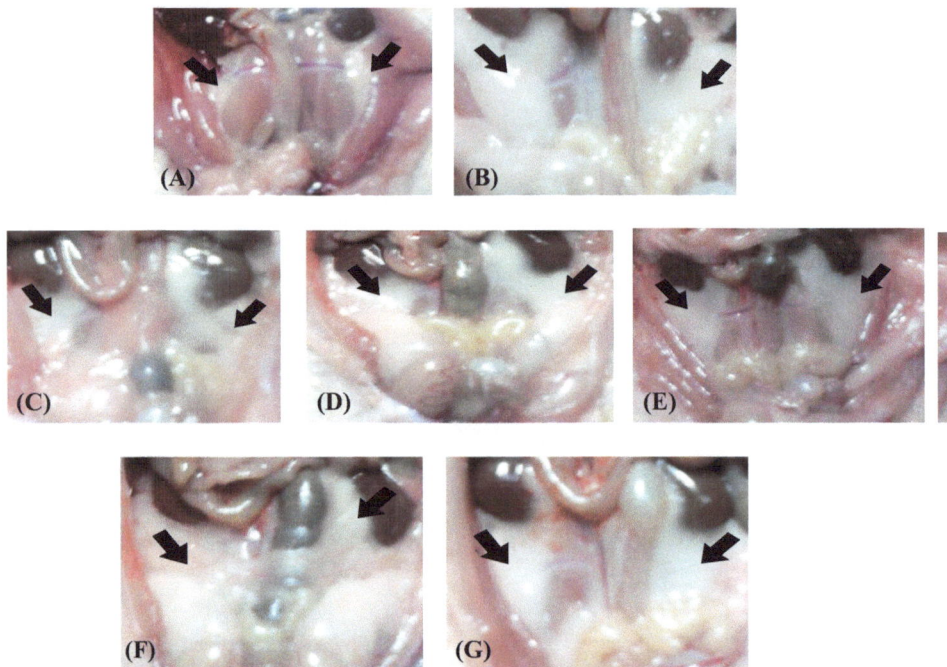

Fig. (14). Image showing the decreased adipocity in various plant extract treated group.The exposed ventral view of (A) Normal Control (B) High Fat Model (C) *H. integrifolia* (D) *A. bilimbi*(E) *T. chebula*(F) *A. calamus*(G)*P.kurroa.*The arrow represents the visceral fat pads (perirenal, periovaric, parametrial and perivescical).

CONCLUDING REMARKS

Treatment with methanol fraction of extracts from *A. calamus, H. integrifolia, P. kurroa, A. bilimbi* and *T. chebula* (at dosage of 200 and 400 mg/kg body weight), ameliorated the dyslipidemia and adipose cell lipid accumulation and reduced body weight gain accompanied by a significantly decreased visceral fat mass in HFD-fed rats. The treatment also positively modified enzyme activity involved in cholesterol pathway that enables a roll back to normal levels and ameliorates the ailments caused by high fat diet to a great extent. The present study provides a strong rationale for further evaluation of the potential therapeutic role of above mentioned plants in treating obesity. The central findings of this investigation is that the 4 week administration of extract reversed the excess adipose cell accumulation. The treatments also positively modified serum lipid profile, apolipoproteins and enzymes involved in cholesterol pathway, particularly HMGR and could correct hyperlipidemia and prevent weight gain in diet-induced obese rats. The result provides an impetus for future investigations to expand our understanding of the pharmacological consequences of HMGR inhibition by these natural products.

CONSENT FOR PUBLICATION

Not applicable.

CONFLICT OF INTEREST

The author (editor) declares no conflict of interest, financial or otherwise.

ACKNOWLEDGEMENTS

We are thankful for the funding provided by UGC as UGC-BSR fellowship and the infrastructural facilities provided by the School of Life Sciences, Kannur University and Inter University Centre for Biosciences, Kannur University.

REFERENCES

[1]   Seagle HM, Strain GW, Makris A, Reeves RS. Position of the American Dietetic Association: weight management. J Am Diet Assoc 2009; 109(2): 330-46.
[http://dx.doi.org/10.1016/j.jada.2008.11.041] [PMID: 19244669]

[2]   Decaria JE, Sharp C, Petrella RJ. Scoping review report: obesity in older adults. Int J Obes 2012; 36(9): 1141-50.
[http://dx.doi.org/10.1038/ijo.2012.29] [PMID: 22410960]

[3]   Kopelman PG. Obesity as a medical problem. Nature 2000; 404(6778): 635-43.
[PMID: 10766250]

[4]   Thompson WG, Cook DA, Clark MM, Bardia A, Levine JA. Treatment of obesity. Mayo Clin Proc 2007; 82(1): 93-101.
[http://dx.doi.org/10.1016/S0025-6196(11)60971-3] [PMID: 17285790]

[5]   Cooke D, Bloom S. The obesity pipeline: current strategies in the development of anti-obesity drugs. Nat Rev Drug Discov 2006; 5(11): 919-31.
[http://dx.doi.org/10.1038/nrd2136] [PMID: 17080028]

[6]   Kaplan LM, Klein S, Boden G, *et al.* Report of the American Gastroenterological Association (AGA) Institute Obesity Task Force. Gastroenterology 2007; 132(6): 2272-5.
[http://dx.doi.org/10.1053/j.gastro.2007.03.061] [PMID: 17498517]

[7]   Svetkey LP, Stevens VJ, Brantley PJ, *et al.* Comparison of strategies for sustaining weight loss: the weight loss maintenance randomized controlled trial. JAMA 2008; 299(10): 1139-48.
[http://dx.doi.org/10.1001/jama.299.10.1139] [PMID: 18334689]

[8]   Padma TV. Ayurveda. Nature 2005; 436(7050): 486-6.
[http://dx.doi.org/10.1038/436486a] [PMID: 16049472]

[9]   Sharma PV. CharakaSamhita. Varanasi, India: Chaukhamba Orientalia 1998; p. 4.

[10]   Valiathan MS. Ayurveda: Putting the House in Order. Curr Sci 2006; 90: 5-6. [Indian Academy of Sciences].

[11]   Bertisch SM, Wee CC, McCarthy EP. Use of complementary and alternative therapies by overweight and obese adults. Obesity (Silver Spring) 2008; 16(7): 1610-5.
[http://dx.doi.org/10.1038/oby.2008.239] [PMID: 18451783]

[12]   Valentino MA, Lin JE, Waldman SA. Central and peripheral molecular targets for antiobesity pharmacotherapy. Clin Pharmacol Ther 2010; 87(6): 652-62.
[http://dx.doi.org/10.1038/clpt.2010.57] [PMID: 20445536]

[13]　Sharma HM, Bodeker T, Gerard C. Alternative Medicine (medical system). 2008 ed. Encyclopedia Britannica 1997.

[14]　James WP. WHO recognition of the global obesity epidemic. Int J Obes 2008; 32 (Suppl. 7): S120-6.
[http://dx.doi.org/10.1038/ijo.2008.247] [PMID: 19136980]

[15]　Allison DB, Fontaine KR, Manson JE, Stevens J, VanItallie TB. Annual deaths attributable to obesity in the United States. JAMA 1999; 282(16): 1530-8.
[http://dx.doi.org/10.1001/jama.282.16.1530] [PMID: 10546692]

[16]　Wolf AM, Colditz GA. Current estimates of the economic cost of obesity in the United States. Obes Res 1998; 6(2): 97-106.
[http://dx.doi.org/10.1002/j.1550-8528.1998.tb00322.x] [PMID: 9545015]

[17]　Gallagher D, Heymsfield SB, Heo M, Jebb SA, Murgatroyd PR, Sakamoto Y. Healthy percentage body fat ranges: an approach for developing guidelines based on body mass index. Am J Clin Nutr 2000; 72(3): 694-701.
[PMID: 10966886]

[18]　Christopher G B, Andrew J W, Philippe F. The Genetics of Human Obesity 2005.

[19]　Jeffery RW, Baxter J, McGuire M, Linde J. Are fast food restaurants an environmental risk factor for obesity? Int J Behav Nutr Phys Act 2006; 3: 2-10.
[http://dx.doi.org/10.1186/1479-5868-3-2] [PMID: 16436207]

[20]　Grundy SM. Obesity, metabolic syndrome, and cardiovascular disease. J Clin Endocrinol Metab 2004; 89(6): 2595-600.
[http://dx.doi.org/10.1210/jc.2004-0372] [PMID: 15181029]

[21]　Guerre-Millo M. Adipose tissue hormones. J Endocrinol Invest 2002; 25(10): 855-61.
[http://dx.doi.org/10.1007/BF03344048] [PMID: 12508947]

[22]　Bujjirao G, Ratna Kumar PK. Anti-Obese Therapeutics from Medicinal Plants-A Review. Int J Bioassays 2013; 02(10): 1399-406.

[23]　Karasu SR. Of mind and matter: psychological dimensions in obesity. Am J Psychother 2012; 66(2): 111-28.
[PMID: 22876525]

[24]　Suzuki Keisuke, Jayasena Channa N, Bloom Stephen R. Obesity and Apetite control. Experimental Diabetes Research 2012; 2012: 1-19.

[25]　Hardeman W, Griffin S, Johnston M, Kinmonth AL, Wareham NJ. Interventions to prevent weight gain: a systematic review of psychological models and behaviour change methods. Int J Obes Relat Metab Disord 2000; 24(2): 131-43.
[http://dx.doi.org/10.1038/sj.ijo.0801100] [PMID: 10702762]

[26]　Abdollahi M, Afshar-Imani B. A review on obesity and weight loss measures. Middle East Pharmacy 2003; 11: 6-10.

[27]　Mahan LK, Escott-Stump S. Krause's food, nutrition, and diet therapy. WB Saunders: Philadelphia 2008; 12(11).

[28]　Hassler FA. Charakasamhita. Science 1893; 22(545): 17-8.
[http://dx.doi.org/10.1126/science.ns-22.545.17-a] [PMID: 17781231]

[29]　Bertisch SM, Wee CC, McCarthy EP. Use of complementary and alternative therapies by overweight and obese adults. Obesity (Silver Spring) 2008; 16(7): 1610-5.
[http://dx.doi.org/10.1038/oby.2008.239] [PMID: 18451783]

[30]　Woollett LA, Beitz DC, Hood RL, Aprahamian S. An enzymatic assay for activity of lipoprotein lipase. Anal Biochem 1984; 143(1): 25-9.
[http://dx.doi.org/10.1016/0003-2697(84)90552-9] [PMID: 6528997]

[31] Gooda Sahib N, Saari N, Ismail A, Khatib A, Mahomoodally F, Abdul Hamid A. Plants' metabolites as potential antiobesity agents. Sci World J 2012; 2012: 436039.
[http://dx.doi.org/10.1100/2012/436039] [PMID: 22666121]

[32] Avogaro P, Bon GB, Cazzolato G, Rorai E. Relationship between apolipoproteins and chemical components of lipoproteins in survivors of myocardial infarction. Atherosclerosis 1980; 37(1): 69-76.
[http://dx.doi.org/10.1016/0021-9150(80)90094-5] [PMID: 7426089]

[33] Kang SA, Shin HJ, Jang KH, *et al.* Effect of Garlic on serum lipids profiles and Leptin in rats fed high fat diet. Prev Nutr Food Sci 2006; 11: 48-53.
[http://dx.doi.org/10.3746/jfn.2006.11.1.048]

[34] Amin KA, Nagy MA. Effect of Carnitine and herbal mixture extract on obesity induced by high fat diet in rats. Diabetol Metab Syndr 2009; 1(1): 17.
[http://dx.doi.org/10.1186/1758-5996-1-17] [PMID: 19835614]

[35] Oben J, Kuate D, Agbor G, Momo C, Talla X. The use of a Cissus quadrangularis formulation in the management of weight loss and metabolic syndrome. Lipids Health Dis 2006; 5: 24.
[http://dx.doi.org/10.1186/1476-511X-5-24] [PMID: 16948861]

[36] Kannel WB, Castelli WP, Gordon T, McNamara PM. Serum cholesterol, lipoproteins, and the risk of coronary heart disease. The Framingham study. Ann Intern Med 1971; 74(1): 1-12.
[http://dx.doi.org/10.7326/0003-4819-74-1-1] [PMID: 5539274]

[37] Scharnagl H, Nauck M, Wieland H, März W. The Friedewald formula underestimates LDL cholesterol at low concentrations. Clin Chem Lab Med 2001; 39(5): 426-31.
[http://dx.doi.org/10.1515/CCLM.2001.068] [PMID: 11434393]

[38] Marcovina SM, Albers JJ, Henderson LO, Hannon WH. International Federation of Clinical Chemistry standardization project for measurements of apolipoproteins A-I and B. III. Comparability of apolipoprotein A-I values by use of international reference material. Clin Chem 1993; 39(5): 773-81.
[PMID: 8485867]

[39] Zheng JS, Yang J, Huang T, Hu XJ, Luo M, Li D. Effects of Chinese liquors on cardiovascular disease risk factors in healthy young humans. Sci World J 2012; 2012: 372143.
[http://dx.doi.org/10.1100/2012/372143] [PMID: 22919307]

[40] Judd JT, Baer DJ, Chen SC, *et al.* Plant sterol esters lower plasma lipids and most carotenoids in mildly hypercholesterolemic adults. Lipids 2002; 37(1): 33-42.
[http://dx.doi.org/10.1007/s11745-002-0861-y] [PMID: 11876261]

[41] Sung JH, Choi SJ, Lee SW, Park KH, Moon TW. Isoflavones found in Korean soybean paste as 3-hydroxy-3-methylglutaryl Coenzyme A reductase inhibitors. Biosci Biotechnol Biochem 2004; 68(5): 1051-8.
[http://dx.doi.org/10.1271/bbb.68.1051] [PMID: 15170109]

[42] Pyo YH, Seong KS. Hypolipidemic effects of Monascus-fermented soybean extracts in rats fed a high-fat and -cholesterol diet. J Agric Food Chem 2009; 57(18): 8617-22.
[http://dx.doi.org/10.1021/jf901878c] [PMID: 19697921]

[43] Shukla PK, Khanna VK, Ali MM, Maurya RR, Handa SS, Srimal RC. Protective effect of acorus calamus against acrylamide induced neurotoxicity. Phytother Res 2002; 16(3): 256-60.
[http://dx.doi.org/10.1002/ptr.854] [PMID: 12164272]

[44] Bishayee A, Chatterjee M. Hypolipidaemic and antiatherosclerotic effects of oral *Gymnemasylvestre* R. Br. Leaf extract in albino rats fed on a high fat diet. Phytother Res 1994; 8: 118-20.
[http://dx.doi.org/10.1002/ptr.2650080216]

[45] Bell FP, Hubert EV. Inhibition of LCAT in plasma from man and experimental animals by chlorpromazine. Lipids 1981; 16(11): 815-9.
[http://dx.doi.org/10.1007/BF02535035] [PMID: 7311740]

[46]   Weigle DS, Cummings DE, Newby PD, *et al.* Roles of leptin and ghrelin in the loss of body weight caused by a low fat, high carbohydrate diet. J Clin Endocrinol Metab 2003; 88(4): 1577-86.
[http://dx.doi.org/10.1210/jc.2002-021262] [PMID: 12679442]

[47]   Jun SC, Jung EY, Hong YH, *et al.* Anti-obesity effects of chitosan and psyllium husk with L-ascorbic acid in guinea pigs. Int J Vitam Nutr Res 2012; 82(2): 113-20.
[http://dx.doi.org/10.1024/0300-9831/a000100] [PMID: 23065836]

[48]   Kang YJ, Kim J, Kim D, Lee HS, Kwon O, Kim MK. Effect of dried garlic flesh and dried garlic juice on body fat and lipid metabolism in 9-month-old rats with diet-induced obesity. Food Sci Biotechnol 2010; 19: 589-94.
[http://dx.doi.org/10.1007/s10068-010-0083-1]

[49]   Yamamoto M, Shimura S, Itoh Y, Ohsaka T, Egawa M, Inoue S. Anti-obesity effects of lipase inhibitor CT-II, an extract from edible herbs, *Nomame Herba*, on rats fed a high-fat diet. Int J Obes Relat Metab Disord 2000; 24(6): 758-64.
[http://dx.doi.org/10.1038/sj.ijo.0801222] [PMID: 10878683]

[50]   Chantre P, Lairon D. Recent findings of green tea extract AR25 (Exolise) and its activity for the treatment of obesity. Phytomedicine 2002; 9(1): 3-8.
[http://dx.doi.org/10.1078/0944-7113-00078] [PMID: 11924761]

[51]   Gregoire FM, Smas CM, Sul HS. Understanding adipocyte differentiation. Physiol Rev 1998; 78(3): 783-809.
[PMID: 9674695]

[52]   Rayalam S, Della-Fera MA, Baile CA. Phytochemicals and regulation of the adipocyte life cycle. J Nutr Biochem 2008; 19(11): 717-26.
[http://dx.doi.org/10.1016/j.jnutbio.2007.12.007] [PMID: 18495457]

[53]   Murase T, Nagasawa A, Suzuki J, Hase T, Tokimitsu I. Beneficial effects of tea catechins on diet-induced obesity: stimulation of lipid catabolism in the liver. Int J Obes Relat Metab Disord 2002; 26(11): 1459-64.
[http://dx.doi.org/10.1038/sj.ijo.0802141] [PMID: 12439647]

[54]   Okuno M, Kajiwara K, Imai S, *et al.* Perilla oil prevents the excessive growth of visceral adipose tissue in rats by down-regulating adipocyte differentiation. J Nutr 1997; 127(9): 1752-7.
[PMID: 9278555]

[55]   Wang S, Noh SK, Koo SI. Epigallocatechin gallate and caffeine differentially inhibit the intestinal absorption of cholesterol and fat in ovariectomized rats. J Nutr 2006; 136(11): 2791-6.
[PMID: 17056802]

[56]   Xu G, Salen G, Shefer S, *et al.* Plant stanol fatty acid esters inhibit cholesterol absorption and hepatic hydroxymethyl glutaryl coenzyme A reductase activity to reduce plasma levels in rabbits. Metabolism 2001; 50(9): 1106-12.
[http://dx.doi.org/10.1053/meta.2001.25664] [PMID: 11555847]

[57]   Loftus TM, Jaworsky DE, Frehywot GL, *et al.* Reduced food intake and body weight in mice treated with fatty acid synthase inhibitors. Science 2000; 288(5475): 2379-81.
[http://dx.doi.org/10.1126/science.288.5475.2379] [PMID: 10875926]

[58]   Sharma S, Panzani RC, Gaur SN, Ariano R, Singh AB. Evaluation of cross-reactivity between *Holoptelea integrifolia* and *Parietaria judaica.* Int Arch Allergy Immunol 2005; 136(2): 103-12.
[http://dx.doi.org/10.1159/000083317] [PMID: 15650307]

[59]   Graham JG, Quinn ML, Fabricant DS, Farnsworth NR. Plants used against cancer - an extension of the work of Jonathan Hartwell. J Ethnopharmacol 2000; 73(3): 347-77.
[http://dx.doi.org/10.1016/S0378-8741(00)00341-X] [PMID: 11090989]

[60]   Sharma S, Lakshmi KS, Rajesh T. Evaluation of antidiarrhoeal potentials of ethanolic extracts of leaves of *Holopteleaintegrifolia* in mice model. Int J Pharm Tech Res 2009; 1: 832-6.

[61] Warrier PK, Nambir VP, Ramankutty C. Indian medicinal plants-a compendium of 500 species. Chennai: Orient Longman Pvt. Ltd 2004.

[62] Goh SH, Chuah CH, Mok JS, Soepadmo E. Malaysian Medicinal Plants for the Treatment of Cardiovascular Diseases. Malaysia: Pelanduk 1995; p. 63.

[63] Tan BK, Fu P, Chow PW, Hsu A. Effects of *A. bilimbi* on blood sugar and food intake in streptozotocininduced diabetic rats. Phytomedicine 1996; 3 (Suppl. 1): 271.
[PMID: 23195082]

[64] Rao NK, Nammi S. Antidiabetic and renoprotective effects of the chloroform extract of *Terminalia chebula* Retz. seeds in streptozotocin-induced diabetic rats. BMC Complement Altern Med 2006; 6: 17.
[http://dx.doi.org/10.1186/1472-6882-6-17] [PMID: 16677399]

[65] Parab RS, Mengi SA. Hypolipidemic activity of *Acorus calamus* L. in rats. Fitoterapia 2002; 73(6): 451-5.
[http://dx.doi.org/10.1016/S0367-326X(02)00174-0] [PMID: 12385866]

[66] Kim JK, So H, Youn MJ, *et al. Hibiscus sabdariffa* L. water extract inhibits the adipocyte differentiation through the PI3-K and MAPK pathway. J Ethnopharmacol 2007; 114(2): 260-7.
[http://dx.doi.org/10.1016/j.jep.2007.08.028] [PMID: 17904778]

[67] Pandit S, Mukherjee PK, Ponnusankar S, Venkatesh M, Srikanth N. Metabolism mediated interaction of α-asarone and *Acorus calamus* with CYP3A4 and CYP2D6. Fitoterapia 2011; 82(3): 369-74.
[http://dx.doi.org/10.1016/j.fitote.2010.11.009] [PMID: 21062640]

[68] Failla ML, Babu U, Seidel KE. Use of immunoresponsiveness to demonstrate that the dietary requirement for copper in young rats is greater with dietary fructose than dietary starch. J Nutr 1988; 118(4): 487-96.
[PMID: 3357064]

[69] Lien EL, Boyle FG, Wrenn JM, Perry RW, Thompson CA, Borzelleca JF. Comparison of AIN-76A and AIN-93G diets: a 13-week study in rats. Food Chem Toxicol 2001; 39(4): 385-92.
[http://dx.doi.org/10.1016/S0278-6915(00)00142-3] [PMID: 11295485]

[70] Xu C, Haiyan Z, Hua Z, Jianhong Z, Pin D. Effect of *Curcuma kwangsiensis* polysaccharides on blood lipid profiles and oxidative stress in high-fat rats. Int J Biol Macromol 2009; 44(2): 138-42.
[http://dx.doi.org/10.1016/j.ijbiomac.2008.11.005] [PMID: 19059430]

[71] Pahua-Ramos ME, Ortiz-Moreno A, Chamorro-Cevallos G, *et al.* Hypolipidemic effect of avocado (*Persea americana* Mill) seed in a hypercholesterolemic mouse model. Plant Foods Hum Nutr 2012; 67(1): 10-6.
[http://dx.doi.org/10.1007/s11130-012-0280-6] [PMID: 22383066]

SUBJECT INDEX

A

Abuse liability 42

Acetyl-CoA carboxylase (ACC) 125, 141, 158, 159, 160, 161, 163, 164, 165, 168, 169

Acorus calamus 197, 202

Activates BAT thermogenesis 154, 155

Active extract and 144, 145, 146, 147, 148, 149, 160, 161, 163, 164, 165, 166, 167, 168, 169

  compounds 160, 161, 163, 164, 165, 166, 167, 168, 169

  molecules 144, 145, 146, 147, 148, 149

Activity 150, 151, 173

  antiobesity 173

  transcriptional 150, 151

Acyl-CoA 157, 158, 159, 160, 163

  dehydrogenase 157, 158

  oxidase (ACO) 157, 159, 160, 163

Acyl-coenzyme 159, 161, 168

Adenophora triphylla 144, 159, 160, 163

Adenosine monophosphate (AMP) 125, 133, 156, 158

Adenylyl cyclase (AC) 155, 210, 211, 212, 213, 214, 215, 216, 217, 218

Adipocytes 7, 13, 64, 65, 76, 102, 122, 124, 125, 128, 133, 137, 138, 139, 141, 142, 144, 145, 146, 147, 151, 152, 153, 155, 157, 159, 160, 161, 162, 163, 164, 165, 166, 167, 168, 200, 204

Adipogenesis 13, 14, 62, 65, 67, 68, 70, 122, 137, 139, 140, 141, 142, 145, 148, 149, 150, 151, 152, 153, 168, 169, 172, 197, 202, 204, 216

  process of 139, 140, 142

  progression of 148, 168

  suppress 13, 142

Adipogenic transcription factors 146, 147, 166, 167

Adipokines 7, 25, 28, 29, 62, 74, 125, 142, 204

Adiponectin 7, 8, 22, 28, 29, 30, 122, 125, 132, 141, 142, 143, 144, 145, 146, 147, 148, 153, 160, 163, 165, 166, 167, 168, 169, 200

  and leptin 141, 142, 144, 146, 166

  circulating levels of 141, 142, 144

  expression of 142, 144

  levels 29, 144, 147, 167

  receptors 8, 143, 144

  secretion 142, 144, 147, 153, 160, 167

Adipose tissue 6, 7, 8, 12, 28, 29, 36, 57, 58, 59, 61, 63, 64, 66, 70, 78, 132, 133, 141, 142, 153, 155, 159, 160, 163, 204, 215, 216

  white 7, 8, 63, 153, 204

Aflatoxins 5

Agents 32, 34, 35, 43, 45, 133, 141, 201, 204

  insulin-sensitizing 34, 35

  natural antiobesity 204

Allium nigrum 159, 160, 163

Allosteric 122, 138, 139, 172

  PTP1B inhibitor 122, 172

  site 138, 139

Ameliorates 70, 160, 166, 219

Amorfrutin 150, 151

Amorpha fruticosa 150, 151

AMPK 157, 158, 159, 160, 161, 162, 163, 164, 165, 167, 168

  activation of 158, 159, 160, 162, 163, 164, 168

  increased activation of 157, 160, 165

  phosphorylation of 159, 161, 164, 167

Anemarrhena asphodeloides 130, 131

Antagonist, opioid receptor 42, 44

Antiobesity drugs 129, 136, 198, 202

  development of 129, 136

  innovative 198

  prescribed 202